Phenol-Croton Oil Peel

Carolina Marçon • Carlos Wambier

Phenol-Croton Oil Peel

A Comprehensive Guide to Principles and Practice

Springer

Carolina Marçon
Department of Dermatology
Santa Casa de São Paulo
São Paulo, São Paulo, Brazil

Carlos Wambier
Dr. Phillip Frost Department
of Dermatology and Cutaneous Surgery
University of Miami Miller
School of Medicine
Miami, Florida, USA

ISBN 978-3-032-25992-9 ISBN 978-3-032-25993-6 (eBook)
https://doi.org/10.1007/978-3-032-25993-6

The original submitted manuscript has been translated into English. The translation was done using artificial intelligence. A subsequent revision was performed by the author(s) to further refine the work and to ensure that the translation is appropriate concerning content and scientific correctness. It may, however, read stylistically different from a conventional translation.

This Springer imprint is published by the registered company Springer Nature Switzerland AG
The registered company address is: Gewerbestrasse 11, 6330 Cham, Switzerland

We dedicate this book to our families, friends, colleagues, and patients, whose trust and inspiration have guided our professional journeys. Their support has been the foundation upon which every page of this work has been built.

We also wish to honor, with deep admiration and gratitude, Dr Thomas J. Baker, Dr Howard Gordon, and Dr Gregory Hetter—pioneers who transformed the phenol–croton oil peel from an empirical practice into a true academic and scientific legacy. Their courage to challenge conventions, their relentless pursuit of excellence, and their commitment to sharing knowledge with the world have illuminated our path. This book exists because of the trail they blazed, and it is our hope that it continues the mission they began.

May this work contribute to the advancement of dermatology, to the safe and responsible use of chemical peels, and to the preservation of the scientific legacy of these pioneers.

Carolina Marçon & Carlos Wambier

Foreword

Phenol-croton oil peeling was inaugurated for physicians with its previous standard 65 years ago in 1961. When Dr. Gregory Hetter published and modified this standard 25 years ago in 2000, he brought forward new standards with reduced complications. His 2017 teaching and attendance at the International Peeling Society workshop in the USA 8 years ago sparked new revisions in the field of Dermatologic and Cosmetic Surgery. Dr. Carlos Wambier was present at that workshop. Since then, he and Dr. Carolina Marçon have honed and published new information to further focus the current techniques in deep chemical peeling. This new encyclopedic textbook is the most complete and extensively referenced textbook on the subject. Unlike the many atlas-type picture textbooks before it, the authors both explain in detail and illustrate the basic science and the clinical knowledge supporting one of the most dramatic and rewarding cosmetic procedures in the medical armaments against photoaging and scarring. The authors are to be congratulated for their successful effort to both sharpen the late Dr. Hetter's work and to combine it with their own published investigations. This book emphasizes safety and superb results, and when combined with inherent procedural cost-effectiveness, it outlines in detail how both segmental and full-face phenol-croton oil peeling can be tailored both for the physician's and the patient's needs.

Department of Dermatology of Emory University School of Medicine – Atlanta, GA

Harold J. Brody

Prologue

In the vast landscape of aesthetic dermatology, there exists a technique that stands apart, like a jewel polished over centuries: the Phenol–Croton Peel. Like an ancient art preserved in scrolls of knowledge and experience, its history is woven with threads of discovery and reinvention—a journey that traverses the annals of time and human culture.

Tracing its origins, one finds a path lost in the labyrinths of antiquity, where croton oil, ancestrally used for diverse medicinal purposes, revealed its rejuvenating power. The story unfolds as a captivating narrative, in which the sages of old recognized within its essence a transformative force.

Yet it was under the brilliant lights of Hollywood that the Phenol–Croton Peel found its stage, shimmering as a backstage secret for cinema stars. Its fame transcended the screen, reaching the hearts and minds of those who aspired to eternal youth, fueling fascination with its effectiveness and mystique.

And so, like a relic rescued from the ruins of time, the Phenol–Croton Peel reemerged in the modern era, revitalized by the skilled and innovative hands of Gregory Hetter. His refined formulations endowed the procedure with a new aura of safety and versatility, elevating it to a standard of excellence and trust.

Reflecting on its unparalleled results in rejuvenation and the treatment of acne scars, we are compelled to recognize that this technique transcends the boundaries of the conventional. More than a simple medical intervention, the Phenol–Croton Peel is an expression of art, where the physician becomes a painter, sculpting the contours of time upon the canvas of human skin.

In this pursuit of beauty and harmony, we encounter a profound truth, a philosophy interwoven into the very fabric of being: the Phenol–Croton Peel is more than an aesthetic procedure—it is a journey of self-discovery and transformation.

At the intersection of science and soul, we find the magic of restoring not only appearance, but also confidence and self-esteem. Here lies the true essence of this technique: its capacity to uplift not only the face, but also the spirit of those who seek it.

May this book be more than a record of knowledge—it is an invitation to explore the depths of this enchanted universe of the Phenol–Croton Peel. May each page be a journey of discovery and inspiration, a tribute to beauty that resides not only on the surface of the skin but also within the essence of the human soul.

May every word remind us that, at the heart of this procedure, lies not only science, but also art, passion, and compassion. For it is through the union of the technical and the human that we encounter the true magic of the Phenol Peel—a magic that transcends time and space, leaving behind a legacy of beauty and transformation.

São Paulo, Brasil & Miami, USA – 2026
Carolina Marçon & Carlos Wambier

Preface

The phenol–croton oil peel has always held a special place in dermatological surgery: feared for its potency, admired for its results, and often misunderstood outside small circles of experts. For decades, its practice remained limited to pioneers who transformed an empirical procedure into one of the most effective and enduring tools for skin rejuvenation. Yet, despite its impact, no complete textbook has ever been dedicated exclusively to this technique—until now.

This book was born from the conviction that the phenol–croton oil peel deserves a place in modern academic dermatology. Our goal was to gather the historical roots, the pharmacological science, the clinical indications, histological evidence, and the practical techniques into a single reference that can guide both seasoned practitioners and new generations of physicians. By uniting rigorous science with practical wisdom, we hope to dispel myths, establish safety standards, and reaffirm the value of this unique procedure.

The chapters are structured to lead the reader from the origins and evolution of the peel, through the chemistry and histology, to clinical applications, combinations with other treatments, patient selection, and management of complications. Each section is grounded in evidence, enriched with critical analysis, and written with the perspective of daily clinical practice.

We are deeply grateful to our mentors, colleagues, and patients, who have inspired and challenged us throughout this journey. Special thanks are extended to the pioneers, Dr Thomas J. Baker, Dr Howard Gordon, and Dr Gregory Hetter, whose courage and academic spirit paved the way for all of us. We also thank our families, whose support made this work possible.

It is our hope that this book not only provides knowledge but also fosters responsibility: to use the phenol–croton oil peel wisely, safely, and effectively, always with the patient's best interest in mind.

São Paulo, São Paulo, Brasil — Carolina Marçon
Miami, Florida, USA — Carlos Wambier

Acknowledgments

We are deeply grateful to the many individuals and institutions who made this book possible. Our sincere thanks go to our colleagues and peers in dermatology and dermatological surgery, whose discussions, questions, and shared experiences continually inspired us to look deeper into the science and practice of chemical peels.

We would also like to acknowledge the invaluable support of our patients, whose trust and willingness to embark on this therapeutic journey provided not only clinical insight but also the motivation to pursue excellence and safety in every aspect of our work.

The academic history of the phenol–croton oil peel was shaped by remarkable figures whose contributions transformed an empirical practice into evidence-based dermatology. Adolph Brown, Clyde Litton, Ed Truppman, Bernard Gross, and Phillip Stone pioneered early adaptations of formulas and clinical protocols. Samuel Stegman and Albert Kligman provided histological validation that established chemical peels, including phenol, on a firm scientific foundation. Zukowski and Stuzin broadened the clinical applications in facial rejuvenation, introducing technical refinement and surgical integration. Gregory Hetter redefined formulations and set modern safety standards, revolutionizing the understanding and practice of phenol–croton oil peels. More recently, Luitgard Weist, Harold Brody, Marina Landau, Oliver Kreiden, Richard Bensimon, Peter Rullan, J. Barton Sterling, Seaver Soon, and Carlos Wambier have advanced techniques, indications, and protocols, ensuring that the procedure continues to evolve within the highest standards of safety and efficacy. Each of these names represents a chapter in the collective history of phenol–croton oil peeling, and their legacy remains the foundation upon which this book is built.

Finally, our heartfelt gratitude goes to our families and close friends for their patience, encouragement, and unwavering support throughout the long process of research and writing. This work belongs as much to them as it does to us.

Contents

About the Authors

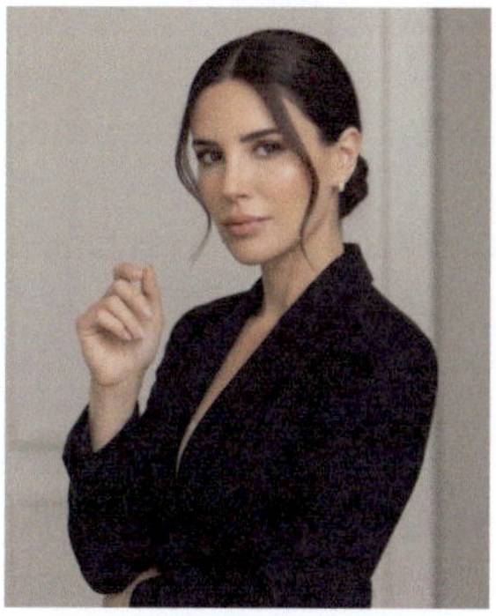

Carolina Marçon is a board-certified dermatologist and internationally recognized authority in aesthetic dermatology, skin aging, and chemical peels, with particular expertise in phenol–croton oil peels. She is the founder and medical director of Clinic CM in São Paulo, Brazil, where she integrates scientific rigor, clinical expertise, and a comprehensive approach to skin health in both medical and aesthetic dermatology.

She received her medical degree from the Pontifical Catholic University of São Paulo (PUC-SP) and subsequently completed her specialization in Internal Medicine and Dermatology at the prestigious Santa Casa de Misericordia de São Paulo (FCMSCSP), where she also earned her Master's and PhD degrees in Health Sciences. Early in her career, she served as Assistant Physician in the Emergency Department and Intensive Care Unit of Santa Casa de São Paulo, experiences that solidified her foundation in clinical medicine and patient safety.

Dr Marçon is a Specialist and Full Member of the Brazilian Society of Dermatology (SBD). She has held important leadership roles, including Coordinator of Communication for the SBD, Member of the Deliberative Council of SBD–São Paulo Regional, and Board Member of the Ibero-Latin American College of Dermatology (CILAD). She currently serves as a member of the Scientific Committee of the International Peeling Society (IPS).

In academia, she serves as Professor in the Department of Dermatology at Santa Casa de São Paulo and is the Coordinator of the Multidisciplinary Assistance Programme for People with Albinism (Pró-Albino/ISCMSP), a pioneering initiative that provides comprehensive care to patients with albinism, integrating dermatology, ophthalmology, genetics, and psychosocial support.

Dr Marçon is a frequent speaker at national and international congresses, where she lectures on advanced techniques in lasers, cosmiatry, and chemical peels, with special emphasis on phenol–croton oil peeling as one of the most powerful tools for skin rejuvenation. She has published extensively in dermatology, with contributions ranging from clinical dermatology to aesthetic procedures, consolidating her reputation as a voice of innovation, safety, and excellence.

Her professional journey combines over two decades of medical practice with academic and institutional leadership. Today, she is recognized as one of the foremost global experts in phenol–croton oil peels, advocating for their safe, evidence-based use, and inspiring a new generation of dermatologists to approach aesthetic medicine as both science and art.

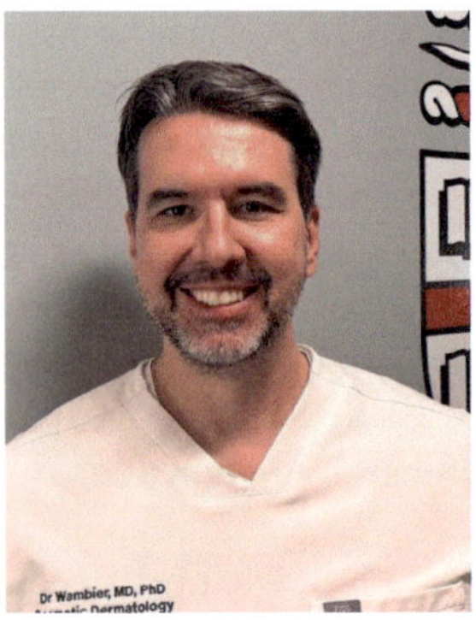

Carlos Wambier is a double board-certified dermatologist (Brazil & USA) who recently became faculty at the Dr. Phillip Frost Department of Dermatology and Cutaneous Surgery, University of Miami Miller School of Medicine, practicing in Coral Gables and West Palm Beach, Florida. Dr Wambier is also an Associate Professor of Dermatology, Clinician Educator at the Warren Alpert Medical School of Brown University. He was the Director of the Center for Lasers and Aesthetics at Brown Dermatology (2020–2026) and Medical Director of Dermatology Clinical Trials (2020–2025). He also has served as a dermatologist at the Rhode Island Burn Center, Rhode Island Hospital (2021–2026).

Dr Wambier has delivered over 100 lectures at national and international dermatology conferences and has published more than 150 peer-reviewed articles.

He received his Medical degree (2004), dermatology residency (2009), and Doctorate in Science in Dermatology (PhD, 2012) from the University of São Paulo, Brazil, and his Postdoctoral Fellowship (2018–2020) from Yale University School of Medicine, USA. He was the Vice-President of the International Peeling Society (2024–2026) and is currently the President of the International Peeling Society (2026–2028).

Dr Wambier has pioneered significant advances in dermatology, with a particular emphasis on phenol-croton oil peels. His research encompasses chemical and pharmaceutical studies, notably the emulsification of phenol-croton oil in water and the characterization of the activity of each ingredient in the formulation using porcine models. Dr Wambier's translational research has been instrumental in guiding randomized clinical trials, resulting in the publication of innovative clinical data.

His major contribution lies in the stabilization of phenol-croton oil emulsions, improving the safety and efficacy of these peels. This innovation has underpinned his mentorship of over 50 practical courses on deep peels, reigniting interest in phenol-croton oil peels, particularly Hetter's peels.

Through his scholarly publications, Dr Wambier has disseminated knowledge on various aspects of phenol-croton oil peels, including lip peeling for volume and eversion, and the nuances of repigmentation following deep peels. His extensive portfolio of peer-reviewed articles, CME reviews, commentaries, and book chapters reflects a deep commitment to advancing dermatological practice.

A highly sought-after speaker, Dr Wambier has shared his expertise through hundreds of lectures worldwide, making significant contributions to the global dermatology community. His work has not only advanced the science of phenol-croton oil peels but has also improved practical methodologies, impacting both clinical outcomes and patient care.

Dr Wambier is internationally recognized as an expert in procedural dermatology, with expertise in injectables (fillers, neurotoxins, and lipolysis), lasers, and drug-delivery procedures for both medical and cosmetic indications (such as scars and hair growth). He is acclaimed as a leader in chemical peels, with numerous publications on the subject, including the cover of the *Journal of the American Academy of Dermatology* in August 2019, which featured two CME articles on chemical peels for which he was the lead author. His innovations in techniques and research in chemical peels have sparked renewed interest in phenol-croton oil peels (also known as advanced or deep peels) within the dermatological academic community.

He developed expertise in hair growth, wound healing, inflammation, drug eruptions, photodynamic therapy, and leprosy during his research years at Ribeirão Preto Medical School, University of Sao Paulo. Subsequently, he focused on chemical peeling research as a tenure-track Associate Professor of Dermatology at the State University of Ponta Grossa (2013-18). Since 2018, Dr Wambier has been a principal investigator of clinical trials for novel JAK inhibitors in dermatology.

Dr Wambier has chaired major academic dermatology meetings worldwide, including the World Congress of Dermatology in Milan (2019), where he chaired the Basic Cosmetic Dermatology session, and the World Congress of Cosmetic Dermatology in Lima (2019), where he chaired the Pigmentary Lesions session. He has also chaired and lectured at AMWC (Monaco), IMCAS World Congress (Paris), IMCAS Americas, CILAD, RADLA, SINMELASMA, AAD, ASDS, SBCD and SBD meetings. He has served as an ad hoc consultant for funding agencies such as the WHO and the Araucaria Foundation.

Abbreviations and Acronyms

ACTH	Adrenocorticotropic hormone
ADSCs	Adipose-derived stem cells
AED	Automated external defibrillator
AGEs	Advanced glycation end-products
AH	Hyaluronic acid
AHA	Alpha hydroxy acid
AK	Actinic keratosis
ALT/GPT	Alanine aminotransferase
AMBU	Artificial manual breathing unit (manual resuscitator)
ANVISA	National Health Surveillance Agency
aPTT	Activated partial thromboplastin time
ARDS	Acute respiratory distress syndrome
AST/GOT	Aspartate aminotransferase
ATP	Adenosine triphosphate
BBL	Broadband light
BD	Bowen's disease
BDD	Body dysmorphic disorder
BHA	Beta hydroxy acid
BMI	Body mass index
BP	Blood pressure
BSA	Body surface area
CaHA	Calcium hydroxyapatite
CGU	Urinary gas chromatography
CME	Congress of Medical Education
CO	*Croton tiglium* oil
COL1	Type I collagen
COL3	Type III collagen
CO_2	Carbon dioxide (CO_2 laser, 10,600 nm)
COPD	Chronic obstructive pulmonary disease
CROSS	Chemical reconstruction of skin scars
CYP2E1	Cytochrome P450 2E1
DAG	Diacylglycerol
DAMPs	Damage-associated molecular patterns
DAXI	DaxibotulinumtoxinA (long-acting botulinum toxin)

DB	Bowen's disease
DEAE	Diethylaminoethyl (DEAE-cellulose resin)
DNA	Deoxyribonucleic acid
ECG	Electrocardiogram
ECM	Extracellular matrix
eGFR	Estimated glomerular filtration rate
ELISA	Enzyme-linked immunosorbent assay
EN	European Norm
EPD	Erosive pustular dermatosis
ESR	Erythrocyte sedimentation rate
Er:YAG	Erbium:YAG laser (2940 nm)
FDA	Food and Drug Administration
FFA	Frontal fibrosing alopecia
FWSS	Fitzpatrick Wrinkle Severity Score
GA	Glycolic acid
GAGs	Glycosaminoglycans
GAIS	Global Aesthetic Improvement Scale
GC-MS	Gas chromatography–mass sectrometry
GGT	Gamma-glutamyl transferase
HbA1c	Glycated hemoglobin A1c
H&E	Hematoxylin and eosin
HDL	High-density lipoprotein
HIFU	High-intensity focused ultrasound
HIV	Human immunodeficiency virus
HPI/PIH	Post-inflammatory hyperpigmentation
HPTLC	High-performance thin-layer chromatography
HR	Heart rate
ICAM-1	Intercellular adhesion molecule 1
IL	Interleukin (IL-1α, IL-6, IL-8, IL-10 etc.)
IL-1β	Interleukin 1 beta
INR	International Normalized Ratio
IPL/LIP	Intense pulsed light
IV/EV	Intravenous route
JAAD	Journal of the American Academy of Dermatology
JAMA	Journal of the American Medical Association
kDa	Kilodalton(s)
KIN	Keratinocytic intraepithelial neoplasia
LC-MS/MS	Liquid chromatography–tandem mass spectrometry
LD50	Lethal dose 50%
LDL	Low-density lipoprotein
MITF	Microphthalmia-associated transcription factor
mMASI	Modified Melasma Area and Severity IndexMMP Matrix metalloproteinase
MMP-1, MMP-3, MMP-8, MMP-9	Matrix metalloproteinase subtypes

MPO	Myeloperoxidase
MRF	Microneedling radiofrequency
MRM	Multiple reaction monitoring
MRSA	Methicillin-resistant *Staphylococcus aureus*
MTZ	Microscopic treatment zones
NB-UVB	Narrowband ultraviolet B
NBR	Brazilian Regulatory Standard
NETs	Neutrophil extracellular traps
NF-κB	Nuclear factor kappa B
NIOSH	National Institute for Occupational Safety and Health
NSAIDs	Non-steroidal anti-inflammatory drugs
NLRP3	NOD-like receptor family pyrin domain containing 3 (NLRP3 Inflammasome)
NMSC	Non-melanoma skin cancer
OCEBM	Oxford Centre for Evidence-Based Medicine
OSHA	Occupational Safety and Health Administration
OV	Organic vapors
PAVE	Peeling-assisted volume enhancing lift (volume-enhancing rhytidoplasty assisted by peeling)
PCL	Polycaprolactone
PCNA	Proliferating cell nuclear antigen
PCR	C-reactive protein
PDL	Pulsed dye laser
PDT	Photodynamic therapy
PFF2/N95/PFF3	Standards for particulate and vapor filtering masks
PKC	Protein kinase C
PLLA	Poly-L-lactic acid
PMA	Phorbol 12-myristate 13-acetate
PMMA	Polymethylmethacrylate
PO	Oral route
POSAS	Patient and Observer Scar Assessment Scale
PPE(s)	Personal protective equipment
PT	Prothrombin time
QS	Q-switched (high-power pulsed laser operating mode)
QTc	Corrected QT interval (preferably by Fridericia's formula)
RDC	Collegiate Board Resolution (ANVISA)
ROS	Reactive oxygen species
SDS-PAGE	Sodium dodecyl sulfate–polyacrylamide gel electrophoresis
SIRT-6/SIRT-7	Sirtuin-6/Sirtuin-7
SMAD	Family of signaling proteins (mentioned in the context of TGF-β/SMAD)
SMAS	Superficial musculoaponeurotic system
SpO_2	Peripheral oxygen saturation
TCA	Trichloroacetic acid
TCA/ATA	Trichloroacetic acid

TCLE	Informed consent form
TdP	Torsades de pointes (type of cardiac arrhythmia)
TGF-β	Transforming growth factor-beta
TGF-β1/TGF-β3	Transforming growth factor beta 1/3
TIMPs	Tissue inhibitors of metalloproteinases
TNF-α	Tumor necrosis factor-alpha
TPA	12-O-tetradecanoylphorbol-13-acetate
TSS	Toxic shock syndrome
TUNEL	Terminal deoxynucleotidyl transferase dUTP nick end labelling (technique for detecting apoptosis)
UEPG	State University of Ponta Grossa
UV/UVB	Ultraviolet/B
VEGF	Vascular endothelial growth factor

1 Phenol-Croton Oil Peel: Introduction, History and Contextualization in Modern Dermatology

1.1 Introduction

Deep chemical peeling with phenol combined with croton oil remains, to this day, one of the most effective procedures for severe facial rejuvenation. Although its early history is controversial and poorly documented, its efficacy has always been impressive, standing the test of time and the advent of modern technologies such as fractional lasers and collagen biostimulators (Fig. 1.1). This chapter aims to provide

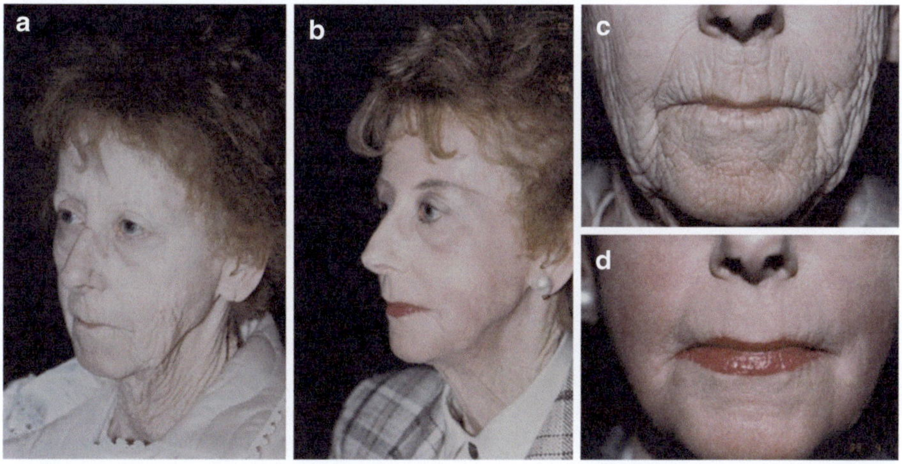

Fig. 1.1 Clinical outcome of deep phenol-croton oil peel. (**a–c**) The patient preoperatively, with marked photoaging and deep wrinkles. (**b–d**) Postoperatively, showing significant improvement in skin texture, smoothing of rhytids, and overall facial rejuvenation. (*Source: Adapted from Hetter GP. An examination of the phenol-croton oil peel: Part I. Dissecting the formula. Plast Reconstr Surg. 2000 Jan;105(1):227–39; discussion 249–51. doi:10.1097/00006534-200001000-00039. PMID: 10626996. Reproduced with permission from the publisher*)

C. Marçon, C. Wambier, *Phenol-Croton Oil Peel*,
https://doi.org/10.1007/978-3-032-25993-6_1

an in-depth overview of the origins of this technique, the chemical agents involved, and the key figures who, whether empirically or scientifically, paved the way for the consolidation of the phenol-croton oil peel in contemporary dermatological practice.

More than a chronological review, what follows is a detailed exploration of the historical trajectory of this formula—from the backrooms of unregulated beauty institutes in the 1920s to 1950s, to its formal incorporation into medicine by pioneering plastic surgeons. The journey from the empirical knowledge of lay "*peelers*" to academic legitimization is fundamental to understanding the potential, risks, and technical nuances of this procedure.

1.2 The Lay Origins of the Phenol-Croton Oil Peel

Phenol, or carbolic acid, is an organic compound derived from benzene, known for its caustic and antiseptic properties. Discovered in 1834 by Friedrich Ferdinand Runge through its isolation from coal tar, it gained clinical prominence in the nineteenth century when the British surgeon Joseph Lister introduced it in 1865 as a surgical antiseptic. Inspired by Louis Pasteur's discoveries on the germ theory of disease, Lister applied phenol to the cleaning of wounds and instruments, drastically reducing postoperative infection rates and transforming medical practice (Fig. 1.2).

Although initially adopted as an antiseptic and cauterizing agent, the use of phenol as a potent exfoliant for facial skin emerged in contexts parallel to official medicine, particularly in beauty salons, clandestine clinics, and informal aesthetic centers in Hollywood and Miami (Fig. 1.3). These lay "peelers," driven by empirical practices, sought skin rejuvenation through formulas passed on orally and kept as professional secrets, accessible only to close apprentices or family members. Knowledge circulated within restricted networks, but in some cases reached physicians through personal relationships or specific negotiations.

Among the most prominent names of this period is Jean DeDesley (Marie Elisabeth Larson), active in California from 1920, identified as the original source of formulas replicated by other lay practitioners. Antoinette LaGassé (Sarah Shaw) is said to have learned the technique and formula from DeDesley in 1926 and subsequently disseminated similar versions. Venner Kelsen, in the late 1940s, used a mixture that included Lysol (saponified cresol solution), vegetable oils, and phenol. Arthur Gradé (Arthur Gallo) was an assistant to DeDesley and later became a collaborator of Dr. Adolph Brown, playing an important role in the transition of the technique into the medical field. Maryanne Coopersmith, owner of the "Beau Rivage" in Fort Lauderdale, later passed the technique on to Clyde Litton, a physician who documented the transfer of this practice into medicine. Cora Galenti, convicted of practicing medicine illegally, used a formula reportedly containing 48% phenol, 50% water, and 2% impurities, and took refuge in Mexico (Tijuana), where she continued to perform peels.

Another notorious couple, Miriam and Francis Maschek, operated at the "House of Renaissance" in North Miami. Miriam revealed her formula to plastic surgeon Ed

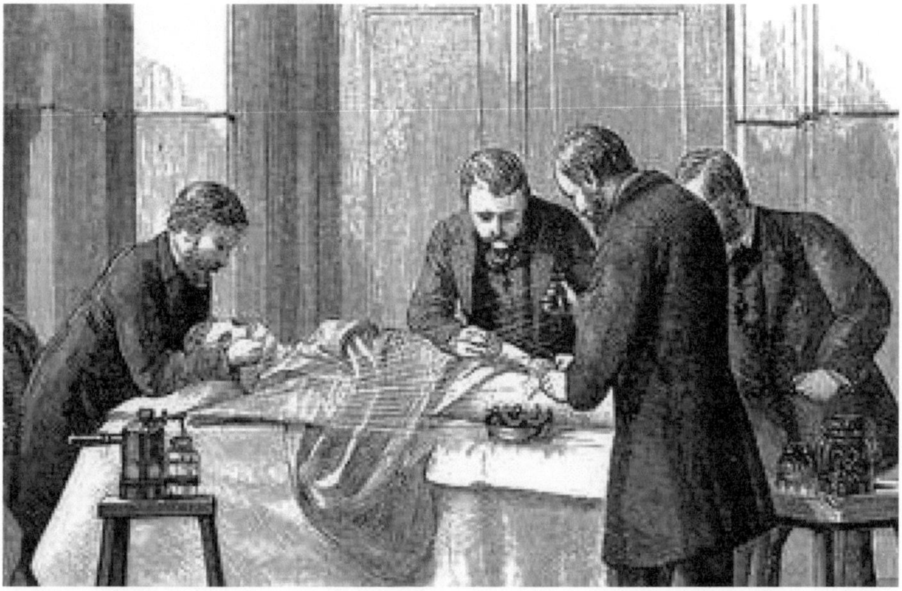

Fig. 1.2 Historical depiction of nineteenth-century surgery—phenol spray applied to the patient for antisepsis. Joseph Lister, inspired by Louis Pasteur's germ theory, introduced the use of phenol (carbolic acid) in 1865 as an antiseptic for cleaning wounds, instruments, and the surgical environment. This practice dramatically reduced postoperative infection rates—from around 50% to less than 15%—and established Lister as the "father of antiseptic surgery," marking a fundamental milestone in the transition to modern surgery. (*Source: Welcome Collection. Wikimedia Commons. CC-BY 4.0 license—Lister spray in use from Cheyne, Antiseptic Surgery*)

Truppman in exchange for a facelift, while Francis obtained it from Antoinette LaGassé. Jacqueline Stallone, mother of actor Sylvester Stallone, became an emblematic figure of this period after receiving the peeling formula from Francis Maschek, her husband, after Miriam's death. Stallone also claimed to have learned from Cora Galenti, with whom she worked in Tijuana. In the 1970s, Jackie and Francis opened the Derma-Lift Centre in Miami Beach, performing deep peels with medical backing from Dr. Bernard G. Gross. She even reported that Galenti had been assaulted by criminals in a failed attempt to obtain her secret formula, having provided false information to protect her method. Stallone continued performing procedures until the late 1980s, when B. G. Gross became involved in allegations related to the fatal outcome of a patient. This episode culminated in the closure of Derma-Lift's operations and led her to move to Las Vegas, where she continued to work in aesthetic centers, although there are no official records regarding the resolution of the case (Table 1.1).

Chemical analyses conducted by Gregory Hetter decades later revealed that, despite variations, these formulations shared core elements: phenol ranging from 45% to 62%, water from 28% to 52%, glycerin as an emulsifier and stabilizer, croton oil in estimated concentrations of 0.16–0.44%, and, in some cases, additives

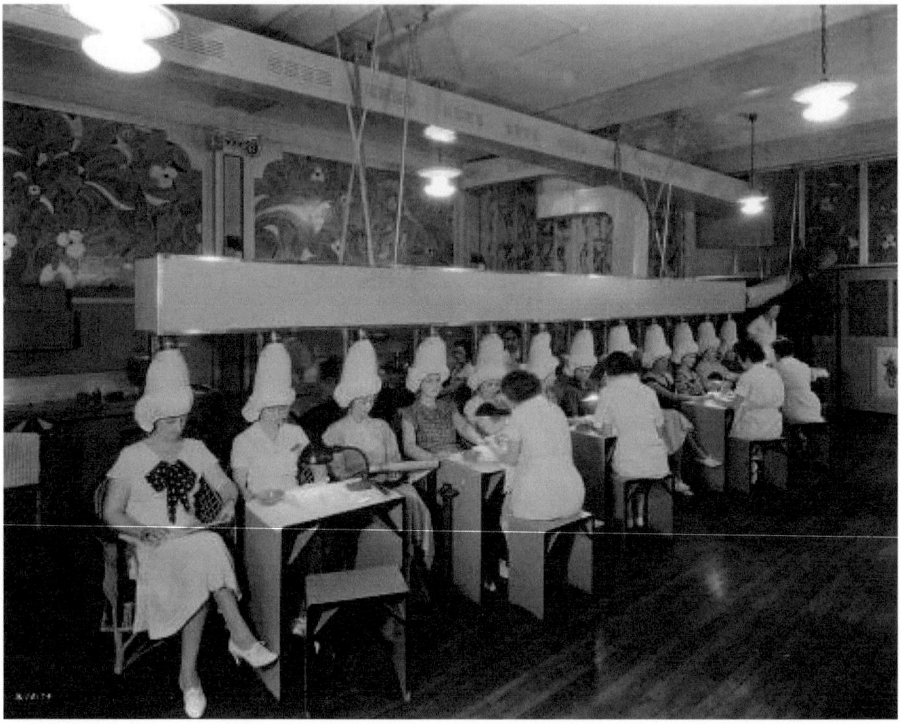

Fig. 1.3 Beauty salon setting (Miami, 1939), with simple furnishings, standardized service, and use of equipment—a typical scenario where, since the 1920s–30s, empirical skin rejuvenation practices circulated outside official medicine. Although phenol entered surgery as an antiseptic and cauterizing agent, its application as a deep peel spread in salons and informal clinics, carried out by lay *"peelers"* who preserved formulas and techniques in a secret and oral manner. (*Source: Fishbaugh, W. A. Women Getting their Hair Done at the Chez Marie Beauty Shop. Miami, 7 Aug. 1939. State Library and Archives of Florida;* via *World Digital Library/Library of Congress. "No known copyright restrictions." Available at: Library of Congress (ID: 2021669936)*)

such as Lysol, cresols, alcohol, and vegetable oils. Although now considered risky, these compositions produced striking clinical results, with intense blistering, thick crust formation, desquamation, and subsequent skin regeneration, resulting in notable improvement in texture, pigmentation, and deep wrinkles.

The application method followed a pattern that would later be systematized: use of cotton swabs or wooden sticks to apply the solution, occlusion with adhesive tape, removal of the dressing, application of powders such as thymol iodide, and then emollients or healing agents. The presence of croton oil, even in non-medical formulations, was constant. Extracted from the seeds of *Croton tiglium*, this oil is highly vesicant and inflammatory, as demonstrated by Joseph R. Spies and collaborators between 1935 and 1937. Soluble in organic solvents such as phenol, it enhanced the penetration and keratolytic action of the mixture. Despite its toxicity,

Table 1.1 Key figures of the lay phase of phenol-croton oil peels

Name	Activity/relevance
Madame DeDesley	Active in California from 1920; identified as the original source of formulas replicated by other lay practitioners
Antoinette LaGassé	Moved to California in 1926; disseminated similar versions of DeDesley's formula
Venner Kelsen	In the late 1940s, a mixture containing Lysol (saponified cresol), vegetable oils, and phenol used
Arthur Gradé	Trained by DeDesley; collaborator of Dr. Adolph Brown, participated in the transition of the technique into the medical field
Maryanne Coopersmith	Owner of *Beau Rivage* in Fort Lauderdale; passed the technique on to Clyde Litton, who documented its transfer into medicine
Cora Galenti	Practiced in Hollywood. Convicted of illegal medical practice, fled to Mexico
Miriam and Francis Maschek	Operated at the *House of Renaissance* in Miami; Miriam entrusted the formula to Ed Truppman in exchange for a facelift; Francis received a version from Antoinette LaGassé
Jacqueline Stallone	Received the formula from Francis Maschek and is said to have learned from Cora Galenti; opened the Derma-Lift Centre in Miami (1970s) with medical backing; involved in controversies, moved to Las Vegas

Summary of the main figures associated with the lay phase of phenol-croton oil peels, performed in beauty salons and informal clinics between the 1920s and 1970s. The information highlights the empirical circulation of formulas, the gradual transition to the medical field, and the risks associated with unregulated practice. (*Source: Table prepared by the author (Dr Carolina Marçon)*)

its clinical value was empirically recognized by these practitioners, becoming a key component in the evolution that would later lead to the development of the phenol-croton oil peel in academic medicine.

1.3 The Transition to Academic Medicine

The transition of the phenol-croton oil peel from lay aesthetics to academic medicine occurred between the late 1950s and early 1960s, with four central figures: Adolph Brown, Clyde Litton, Ed Truppman, and Thomas Baker.

Adolph Brown, an American plastic surgeon born in 1905, was the first physician to obtain and study in depth a formula containing croton oil from lay practitioners (Fig. 1.4). The son of Eastern European Jewish immigrants and inventive from a young age, he graduated in medicine in 1933 and, after an internship in Paris, distinguished himself as a plastic surgeon and university professor. In 1953, he settled in Beverly Hills, where he ran a prestigious aesthetic clinic alongside his wife Marthe Brown, a dermatologist. His contact with deep peels likely occurred through Arthur Gradé, and in 1959, he filed a patent that included phenol, vegetable oils, and emulsifying agents. The patent included different formulations, mentioning croton oil (in saponified form with cresol) in only one of them. The following year, he and his wife published two articles describing the histological effects of the peel in

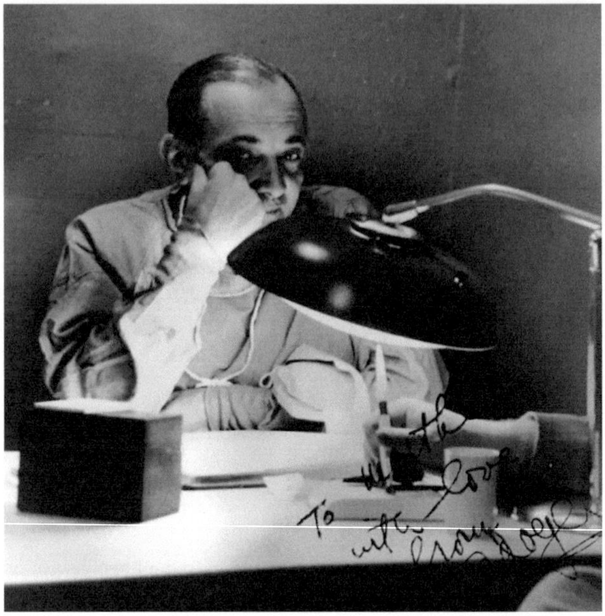

Fig. 1.4 Dr. Adolph Brown (1906–1963), a pioneer in the transition of empirical deep peel formulas to academic medicine, having learned them from Arthur Gradé. (*Source: Personal archive of the Brown family. Reproduced with permission from his daughter Dr Aimée Brown Price*)

humans and in rabbit ears. None of his published articles mentioned croton oil. One of these articles, rejected by the journal *Plastic and Reconstructive Surgery*, was published in the *British Journal of Plastic Surgery,* which limited its reach. Brown argued that more concentrated phenol solutions could, paradoxically, be safer by promoting rapid epidermal coagulation and reducing systemic absorption—a hypothesis that influenced generations but was later refuted. His pioneering contribution consisted of attempting to scientifically systematize the empirical knowledge of lay peelers, even if without fully disclosing the formula he used. He died prematurely in 1963, at the age of 57, leaving a legacy that remained overshadowed for decades.

Clyde Litton, M.D., in turn, was one of the first plastic surgeons to investigate the potential of phenol-croton oil facial peels, after direct contact with Maryanne Coopersmith during a visit to Fort Lauderdale in 1959, accompanied by colleagues Nick Georgiade and John Wilde. Fascinated by the remarkable rejuvenation of Coopersmith's skin—a woman who appeared decades younger—Litton sought to thoroughly understand the method she employed. Although she did not disclose the formula at that time, Litton later managed to reach an agreement with the Coopersmiths, who demonstrated the procedure on a patient of his choosing. The result was only moderately satisfactory, and the agreed fee was only partially paid. However, as part of the agreement, Litton received a written copy of the formula. Litton not only tested the technique but also conducted rigorous studies with pharmacists, pathologists, and toxicologists. He was among the first to understand that the vesicant effect observed was not caused by phenol alone, but rather by the presence of croton oil. Despite his pioneering work, he refrained from publicly disclosing the formula, due to ethical considerations and concerns about the trivialization of the practice.

According to Hetter's accounts, in 1960, Litton shared his findings with colleagues such as Tom Baker and John Drummond during a meeting of the Society of Plastic Surgery in Los Angeles. He presented clinical photographs and offered to send the formula, provided he was properly credited. Baker never requested the formula but would go on to publish his own variation of the technique the following year. Litton was also invited to publish his findings in the journal *Plastic and Reconstructive Surgery*, after learning that Brown's study had been rejected for personal reasons. Even so, he refused to give interviews to the press, maintaining a stance of integrity and discretion at a time when medical self-promotion was frowned upon.

Ed Truppman represented another important link in the transition from lay practice to medical documentation of the phenol-croton oil peel. In the late 1960s, he operated on Miriam Maschek—a central figure among the non-medical peelers of the time—performing a facelift when she was already around 70 years old. As a sign of trust, Maschek shared her original formula with Truppman, on the condition that he would not disclose it publicly before her death. After Miriam's passing in the mid-1970s, Truppman published the formula in 1979. Subsequently, Miriam's widower, Francis Maschek, began collaborating with Bernard G. Gross, a dermatologist who had already faced ethical controversies. In 1980, Gross and Francis Maschek published an article claiming that the formula had originally been obtained from a foreign woman in California, attributing its origin to the Frenchwoman Antoinette LaGassé—although this version sparked debate regarding its true provenance. Francis was also responsible for teaching Truppman the technique of applying the solution with large cotton swabs, which allowed for faster spreading of the solution—a technique that would later become characteristic of the approach adopted by other physicians.

Thomas Baker (Fig. 1.5) was introduced to the world of facial peels in 1960, after reading a report in the Chicago Tribune about Miriam Maschek. Intrigued by the results presented, he personally visited Maschek and other lay practitioners such as Maryanne Coopersmith and an operator from the "House of Beauty" in Miami. Although none of them revealed their formulas, Baker was able to closely observe the procedures, noting the use of phenol, croton oil, applicator sticks, occlusive tape, and thymol iodide. Based on these observations and influenced by articles such as those by Adolph Brown—which associated surfactant agents with increased skin penetration—Baker developed his own formula, incorporating Septisol (a detergent soap), which improved miscibility and enhanced the action of the mixture. In 1961, he presented his first cases to the *Plastic Surgery Research Council,* but was met with skepticism. Nevertheless, at the end of the same year, he published a preliminary report in the *Florida Medical Journal*, sharing his practice with colleagues in the region. In 1962, his article with the classic formula was finally published in *Plastic and Reconstructive Surgery*, formalizing his contribution. Interestingly, the new version of the formula contained twice as much croton oil as the previous one, although Baker himself could not recall the exact reason for the

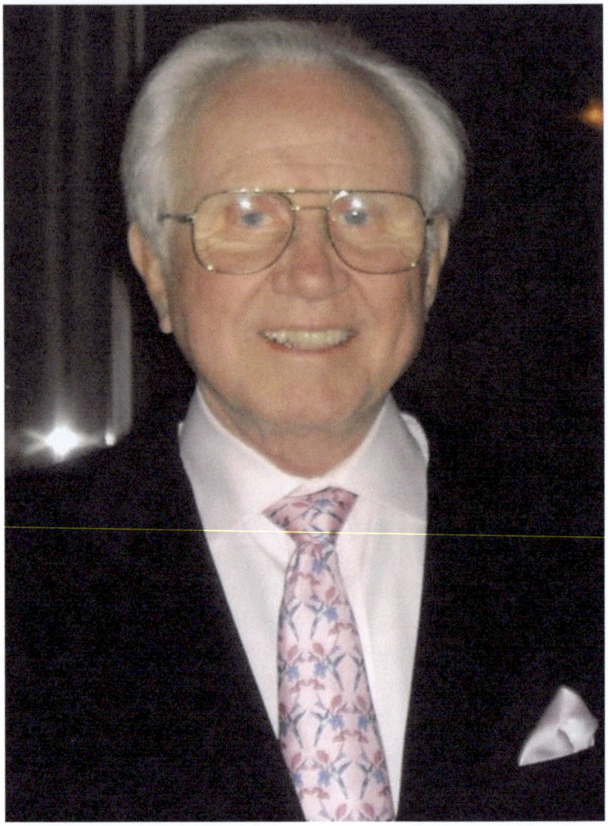

Fig. 1.5 Dr. Thomas J. Baker (1925–2020), a historical reference in the development of deep chemical peels and founder of the Baker Gordon Symposium. (*Source: Maspons Funeral Homes – Memorials. Available at:* https://memorials.masponsfuneral.com/thomas-baker/4474181/. *Reproduced with permission from the family – son Dr Tracy Baker*)

change. Due to its ease of preparation and the credibility of the journal, this formula became the gold standard for deep peels for more than three decades (Fig. 1.6).

The scientific consolidation of the phenol-croton oil peel was gradual. Originating in lay and marginal settings outside of medicine, it was later adopted by physicians who sought to understand, standardize, and disseminate the technique. The publication of Baker's formula in 1961 was a milestone, conferring legitimacy to the procedure, which quickly spread among plastic surgeons due to its superior efficacy compared to dermabrasion. Nevertheless, many concepts derived from empirical practice remained unproven for decades, such as Brown's assertion that higher concentrations of phenol would be less toxic. For a long time, the technique was supported more by case reports and clinical observations than by experimental studies.

Studies that challenged longstanding dogmas about the phenol-croton oil peel began to emerge in the 1970s, when a practice previously sustained by empirical observation started to be evaluated on an experimental basis. In 1970, Melvin Spira was the first to systematically test different concentrations of phenol and the presence of croton oil. Using human thigh skin, he found no significant differences in lesion depth between solutions containing 50% and 88% phenol but demonstrated

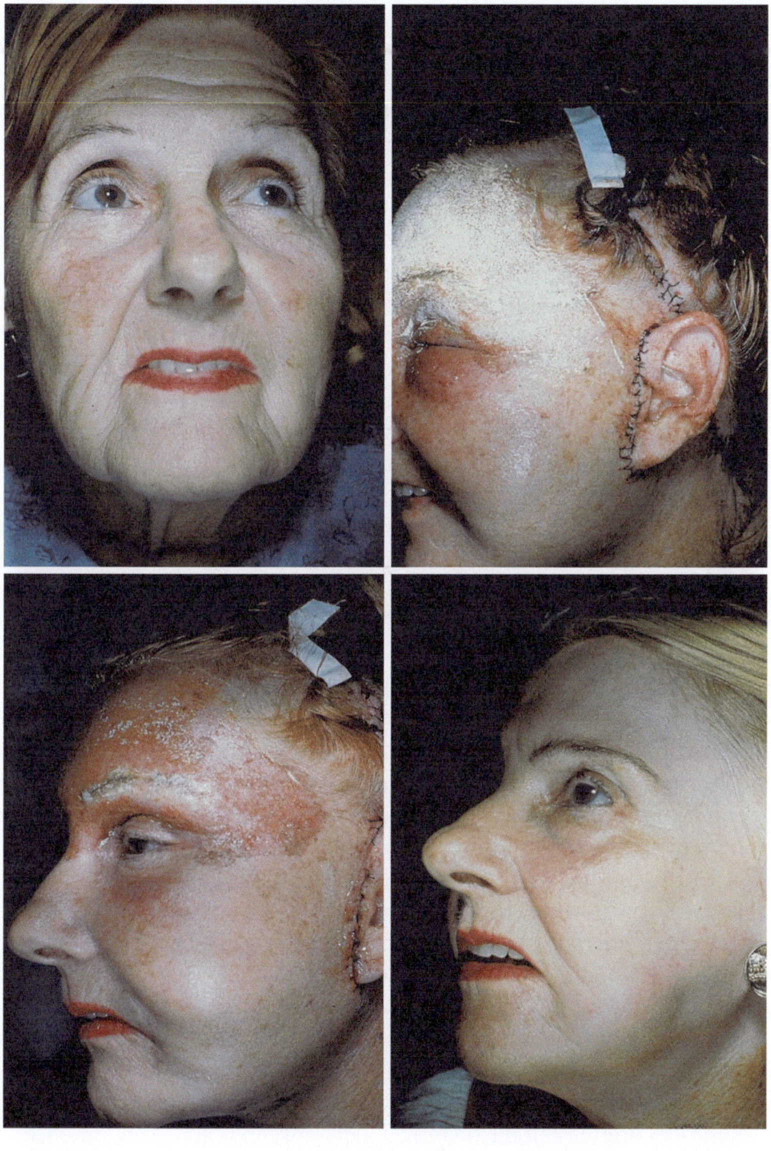

Fig. 1.6 First patient to undergo a phenol chemical peel in Dr. Thomas J. Baker's office, early 1960s. (Above, left) Preoperative. (Above, right) Immediate postoperative following classic rhytidectomy combined with phenol peel on the forehead, avoiding application to undermined skin. (Below, left) One week after the peel, with complete re-epithelialization, suggesting the safety of the technique. (Below, right) One year after rhytidectomy and subsequent phenol peel to the lower two-thirds of the face, demonstrating long-lasting results. (*Source: Baker TJ, Stuzin JM. Discussion: An Examination of the Phenol–Croton Oil Peel: Part IV. Face Peel Results with Different Concentrations of Phenol and Croton Oil. Plast Reconstr Surg. 2000 Mar;105(3):1084–1087. doi:10.1097/00006534-200003000-00044. Reproduced with permission from the publisher*)

that occlusion increased cutaneous penetration and that additives such as croton oil, at that time, lacked a clear scientific rationale—although there were already indications of its role in increasing the solution's aggressiveness.

In 1977, Behin and colleagues used an experimental model with minipigs to compare the phenol-croton oil peel to dermabrasion. Histological analysis revealed that chemical peeling promoted greater regeneration of dermal collagen, corroborating the clinical perception that its effects went beyond mere mechanical injury to the skin.

From 1980 onwards, Samuel Stegman, a dermatologist from San Francisco, published a series of experimental studies conducted in human volunteers and minipigs that dismantled several dogmas perpetuated since Brown. His findings demonstrated that occlusion enhanced the depth of dermal necrosis, that multiple passes increased the extent of the lesion, and that croton oil was decisive for the depth and histological pattern of the injury. Stegman showed that phenol alone, even at high concentrations, did not reproduce the effects observed with Baker's formula, and described necrosis involving the epidermis, papillary dermis, and part of the reticular dermis—a pattern characteristic of the association between phenol and croton oil.

In 1985, Kligman and colleagues reinforced these findings by demonstrating, in biopsies of patients who had undergone the procedure, the formation of a new dense band of collagen, persisting for long periods, suggesting prolonged dermal remodeling. Nevertheless, the authors acknowledged that the exact mechanisms, particularly the action of croton resin, remained poorly understood.

In the 1990s, further studies expanded this knowledge. Zukowski et al. showed that occlusion with ointments, such as bacitracin, produced effects comparable to those obtained with adhesive tape, questioning the necessity of traditional methods. Moy and colleagues confirmed that increasing the concentration of phenol intensified the depth of the lesion, but reaffirmed that the effect of the Baker-Gordon peel depended on the combination of ingredients and not on phenol alone.

Despite these contributions, the literature between 1962 and 1996 remained relatively scarce in experimental data. Most articles published during this period were based on the repetition of unreferenced concepts, such as the belief that lower concentrations of phenol would penetrate more deeply or that the addition of oils would act as a "buffer" in the formula—ideas that did not withstand scientific scrutiny. These six studies, however, were fundamental in initiating the scientific consolidation of the phenol-croton oil peel, paving the way for a safer, more effective, and technically standardized practice, although several aspects remain poorly understood, reflecting both its empirical origins and the historical gap between practice and science.

1.4 Contextualization in Modern Dermatology

The phenol-croton oil peel, once restricted to a closed circle of practitioners and kept as a secret behind the scenes of clinics and beauty salons, has gained legitimate standing among the deep ablative procedures of modern dermatology. Today, it stands out as one of the most effective techniques for the treatment of deep static rhytids, severe photodamage, acne scars, and cancerization field (Figs. 1.7 and 1.8).

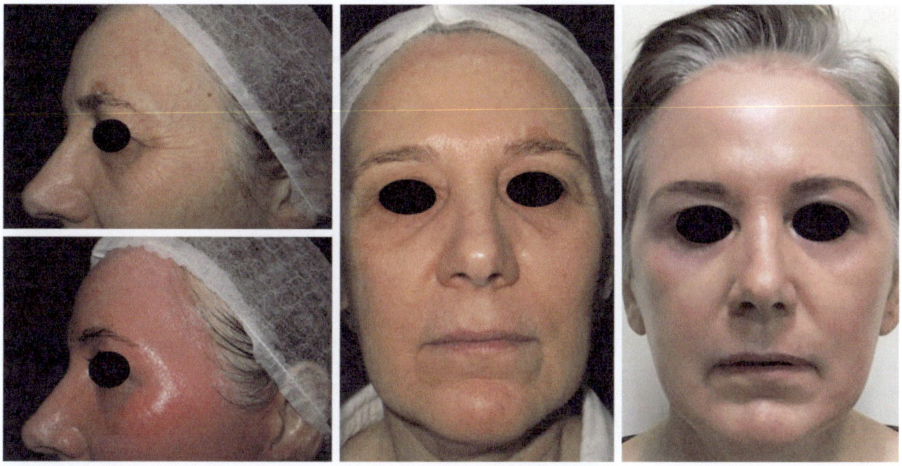

Fig. 1.7 Sixty-year-old patient treated with the Baker & Gordon formula. (Left) Profile views before and 1 month after the peel, showing initial erythema and the onset of improvement in rhytids. (Right) Frontal views before and 6 months after the procedure, demonstrating significant attenuation of wrinkles and overall improvement in skin texture. (*Source: Author's personal archive (Dr Carolina Marçon)*)

Fig. 1.8 Fifty-nine-year-old patient treated with peel segmenting the perioral area using Hetter's formula at 1.6%, with feathering for the cheeks. Pre-treatment and 3-month post-procedure photographs show significant improvement in perioral rhytids and skin texture. (*Source: Author's personal archive (Dr Carolina Marçon)*)

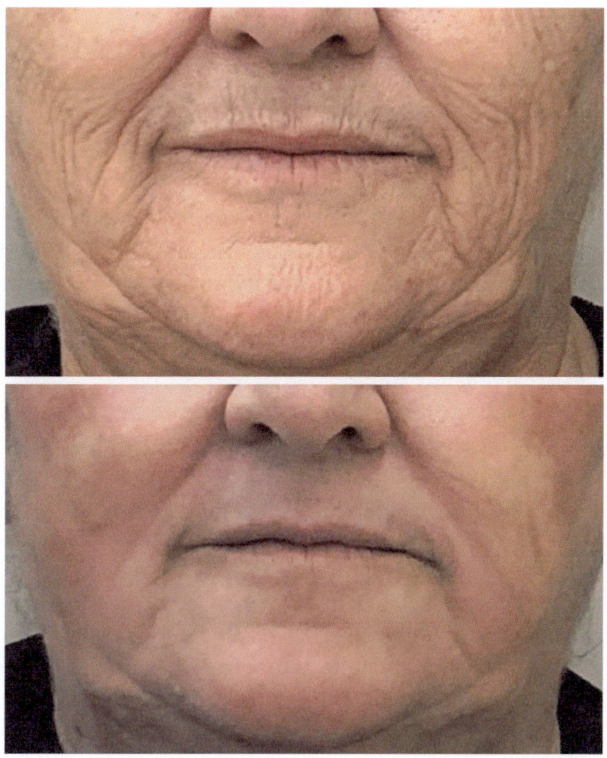

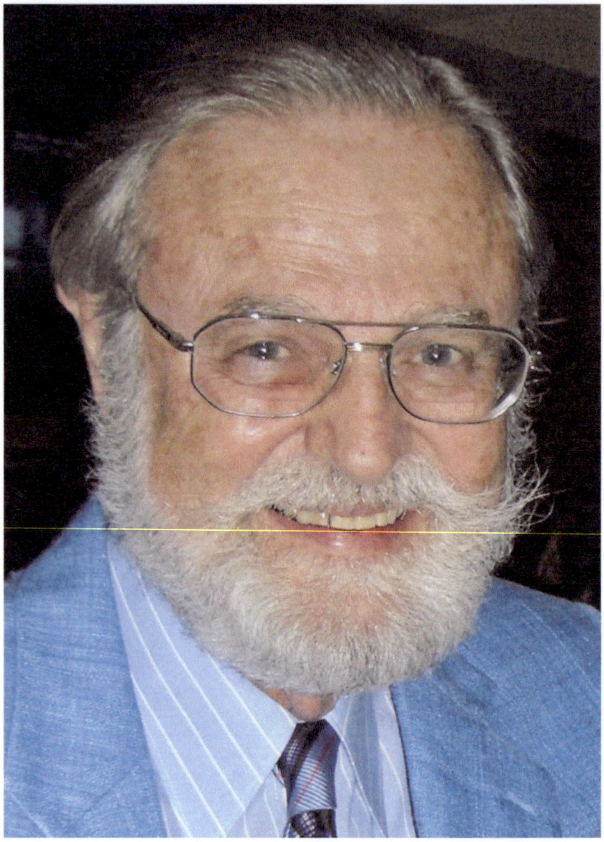

Fig. 1.9 Dr. Gregory Hetter (1936–2025), North American plastic surgeon, internationally recognized for his critical reassessment and fundamental contributions to the scientific understanding of the phenol-croton oil peel. His work redefined the approach to safety, efficacy, and refinement of formulations, influencing generations of specialists. (*Reproduced with permission from the family*)

This scientific and technical revival culminated in the studies and proposals of Hetter (Fig. 1.9) from the 2000s onwards (Fig. 1.10). Hetter demonstrated that the concentration of croton oil was the main determinant of the depth of dermal necrosis, proposing controlled dilutions (such as 0.4%, 0.8%, 1.6%, etc.) based on percentages rather than the number of drops—thus providing precision, reproducibility, and greater safety to the procedure (Fig. 1.11).

Furthermore, Hetter identified that different facial areas responded differently to the same peel, introducing the concept of individualization by anatomical zones, with adjustments in friction time, number of layers, and solution concentration. This standardization revolutionized the technique, allowing for greater predictability of results, better pain and recovery time management, reduced adverse effects—such as dyschromia and scarring—and the expansion of the technique to other indications, such as targeted treatment of perioral and periocular wrinkles, acne scars, extra-facial areas, etc. (Figs. 1.12 and 1.13).

Currently, the phenol-croton oil peel is among the most powerful interventions for deep dermal remodeling, with results often superior to those achieved by fractional lasers and various therapeutic combinations, provided it is performed by

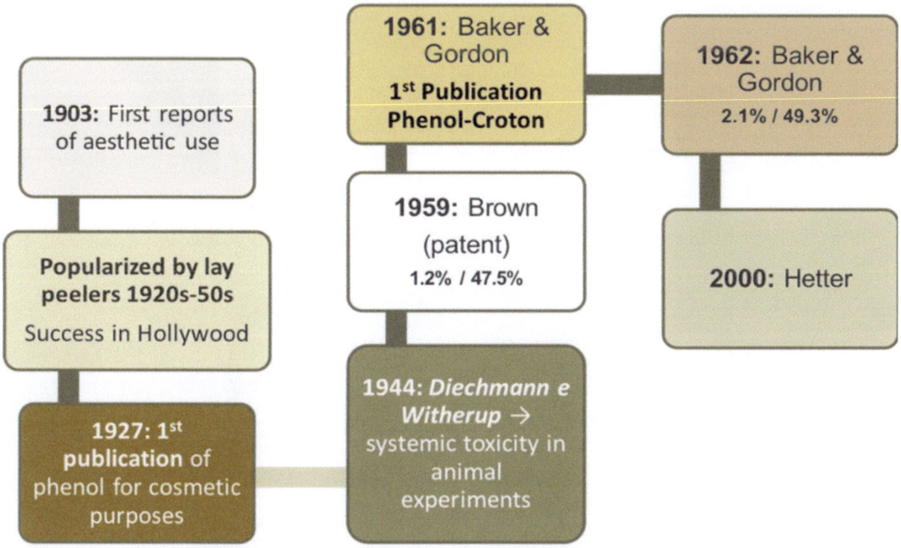

Fig. 1.10 Timeline of the evolution of the phenol-croton oil peel, from the first reports of phenol's aesthetic use in 1903, through its popularization among laypersons in the 1920s–1950s, the first publication for cosmetic purposes in 1927, and the description of systemic toxicity in 1944. Notable milestones include Brown's patent in 1959, the first publication by Baker and Gordon in 1961 with subsequent refinement in 1962, culminating in the modern standardizations proposed by Hetter in 2000. (*Source: Figure created by the author (Dr. Carolina Marçon)*)

qualified physicians with rigorous training, in a controlled environment, and with a full understanding of its pharmacokinetics and toxicology (Fig. 1.14).

However, its resurgence has also brought risks: the trivialization of the technique, the proliferation of formulations of unknown origin, and its performance by non-medical professionals have resulted in serious complications, including fatalities. Despite the remarkable results achieved with phenol, both in aesthetic treatments and other areas of dermatology, its use carries significant risks. The systemic toxicity of phenol can lead to severe complications, such as cardiac arrhythmias and renal failure. The recent ban on phenol in Brazil by ANVISA highlights this tension between efficacy and safety, and underscores the need for regulation, medical education, and technical accountability.

The phenol-croton oil peel thus represents the convergence of history, art, empiricism, chemistry, toxicology, and skin science. Its trajectory illustrates how marginal knowledge can be transformed into powerful therapeutic tools when integrated into medical practice, provided it is conducted with ethics, technical rigor, and scientific grounding. This book is born of that commitment: to preserve historical memory and knowledge, to strengthen evidence-based practice, and to prevent contemporary superficiality from trivializing a technique built upon decades of observation, risk, and refinement.

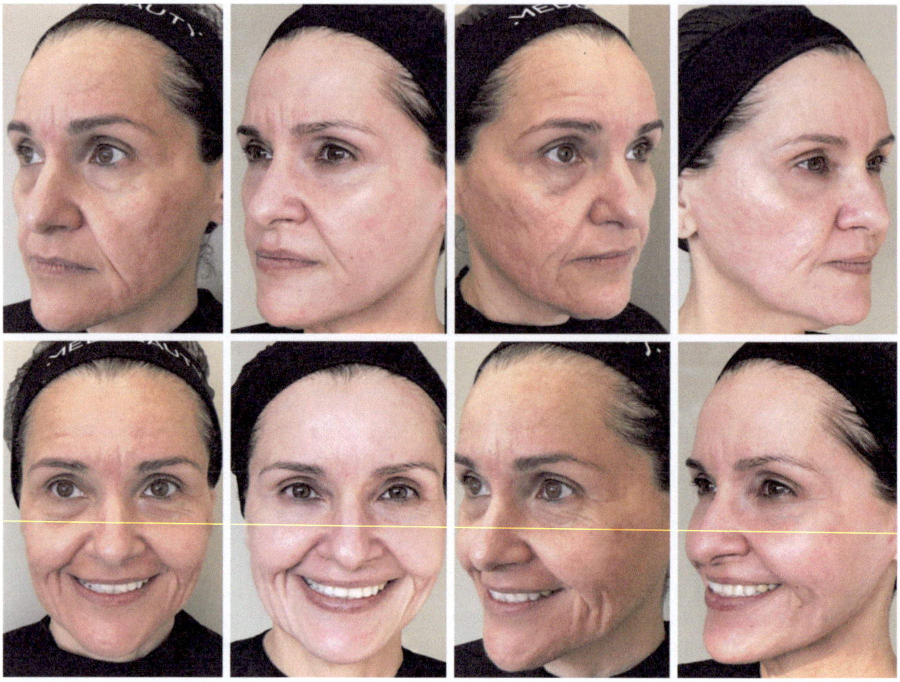

Fig. 1.11 Forty-nine-year-old patient with photoaging, melasma, and acne scars treated with phenol-croton oil peel using Hetter's formula at 1.2% on the entire face. Comparative photographs show results before and 1 year after the procedure, with marked improvement in skin texture, more even pigmentation, and attenuation of scarring. (*Source: Author's personal archive (Dr. Carolina Marçon)*)

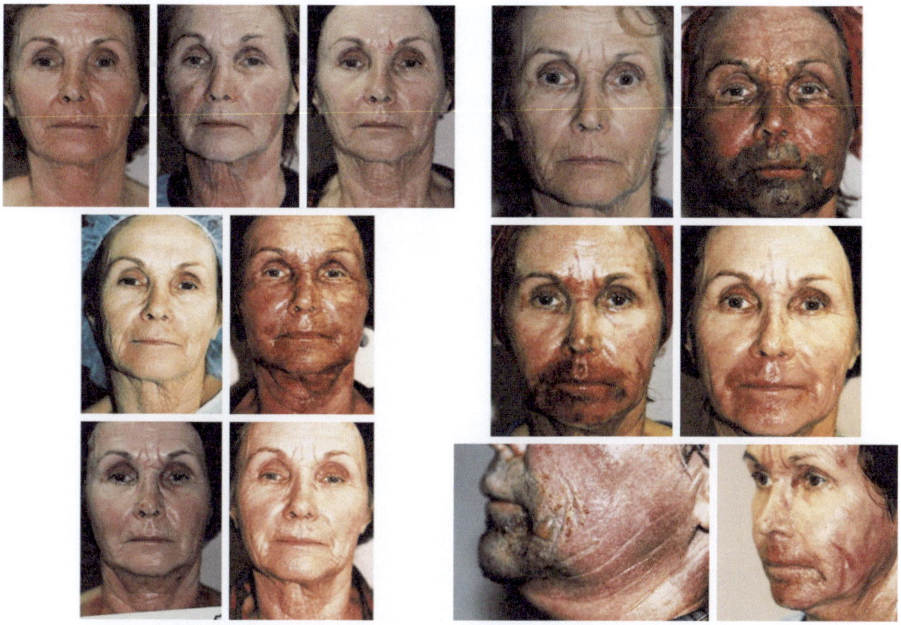

Fig. 1.12 Clinical evolution after serial peels with different concentrations of phenol alone and phenol combined with croton oil. While applications of 18% and 35% phenol without croton oil showed limited effect, with minimal and transient improvement of rhytids, the combination of croton oil with 50% phenol induced an intense cutaneous reaction, with crust formation, significant dermal injury, and more persistent clinical results, highlighting its decisive role in the depth and efficacy of the peel. (*Source: Hetter GP. An examination of the phenol-croton oil peel: Part I. Dissecting the formula. Plast Reconstr Surg. 2000 Jan;105(1):227–39; discussion 249–51. doi:10.1097/00006534-200001000-00039. PMID: 10626996. Reproduced with permission from the publisher*)

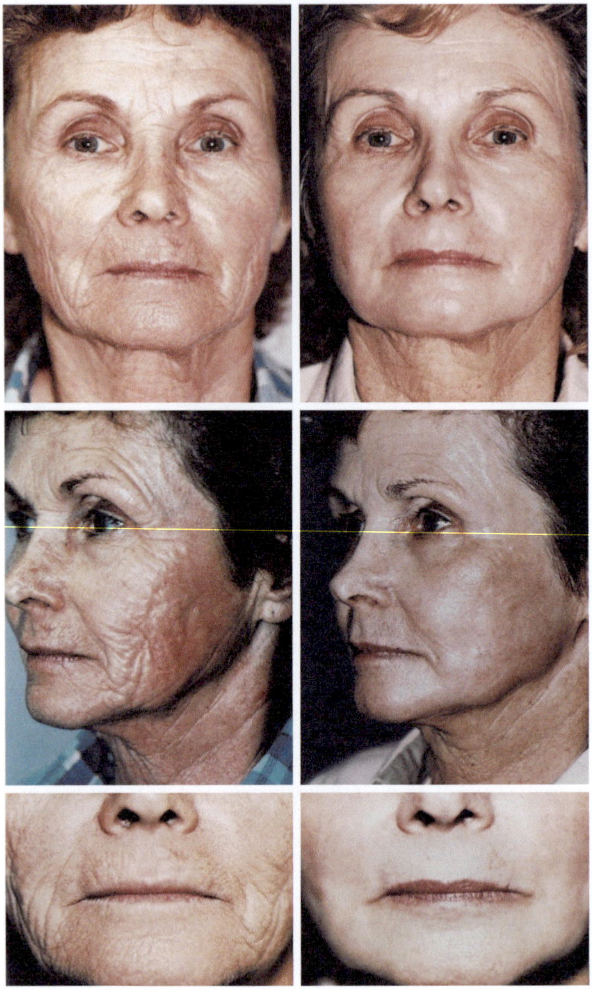

Fig. 1.13 Patient before the start of the peel series (Left) and 20 months after the fourth peel (Right). There is significant improvement in facial rhytids, near-complete obliteration of perioral and chin wrinkles, disappearance of preauricular redundancies, and a natural skin appearance without depigmentation or a glazed effect. (*Source: Hetter GP. An examination of the phenol-croton oil peel: Part I. Dissecting the formula. Plast Reconstr Surg. 2000 Jan;105(1):227–39; discussion 249–51. doi:10.1097/00006534-200001000-00039. PMID: 10626996. Reproduced with permission from the publisher*)

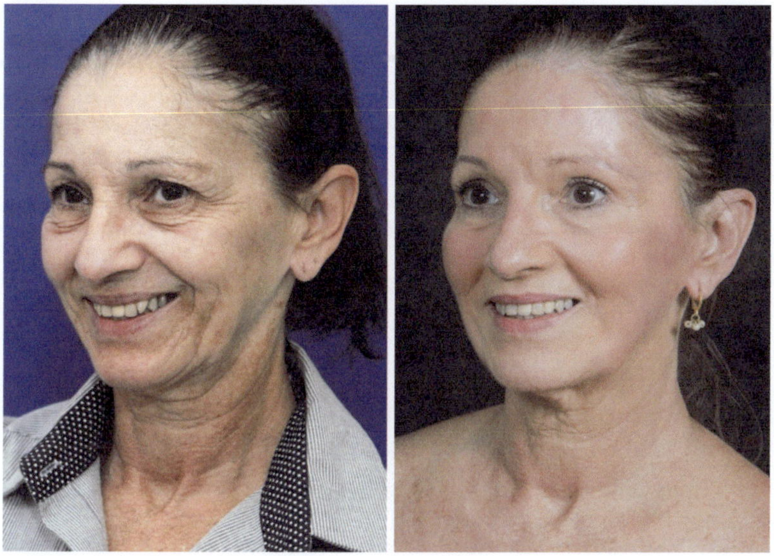

Fig. 1.14 Sixty-seven-year-old patient undergoing facial rejuvenation with Hetter peels. (Left) Preoperative (Glogau IV). (Right) 20 months postoperative (Glogau II), showing overall improvement in rhytids and skin texture. Different combinations of phenol and croton oil in graduated concentrations were used, with application to the periorbital, perioral, forehead, nose, and cheek areas. (*Source: Courtesy of Dr Tereza Cristina Celidonio, MD*)

Sources

1. Zukowski ML, Mossie RD, Roth SI, McKinney P. Pilot study analysis of the histological and bacteriological effects of occlusive dressings in chemosurgical peel using a minipig model. Aesthetic Plast Surg. 1993;17:53.
2. Moy LS, Peace S, Moy RL. Comparison of the effect of various chemical peeling agents in a minipig model. Dermatol Surg. 1996;22:429.
3. Hetter GP. An examination of the phenol-croton oil peel: Part I. Dissecting the formula. Plast Reconstr Surg. 2000;105(1):227–39; discussion 249–51.
4. Hetter GP. An examination of the phenol-croton oil peel: Part II. The lay peelers and their croton oil formulas. Plast Reconstr Surg. 2000;105(1):240–8; discussion 249–51.
5. Hetter GP. An examination of the phenol-croton oil peel: Part III. The plastic surgeons' role. Plast Reconstr Surg. 2000;105(2):752–63.
6. Wambier CG, Lee KC, Soon SL, et al. Advanced chemical peels: phenol-croton oil peel. J Am Acad Dermatol. 2019;81(2):327–36. https://doi.org/10.1016/j.jaad.2018.11.060.
7. Bensimon RH. Phenol-croton oil peels. In: Obagi S, editor. Procedures in cosmetic dermatology: chemical peels. 3rd ed. London: Elsevier; 2020. p. 81–99.
8. Frankel EB. Baker's phenol chemical peel. J Dermatol Surg Oncol. 1990;16(6):581–2. https://doi.org/10.1111/j.1524-4725.1990.tb02208.x. PMID: 2355140.

9. Shuster MM. The Baker phenol peel formula. Plast Reconstr Surg. 1998;102(1):268–9. PMID: 9655450.
10. Litton C. Chemical face lifting. Plast Reconstr Surg. 1962;29:371.
11. Baker TJ. The ablation of rhytids by chemical means: a preliminary report. J Fla Med Assoc. 1961;48:451.
12. Baker TJ. Chemical face peeling and rhytidectomy: a combined approach for facial rejuvenation. Plast Reconstr Surg. 1962;29:199.
13. Stone PA. The use of modified phenol for chemical face peeling. Clin Plast Surg. 1998;25:21.
14. Truppman ES, Ellenby JD. Major electrocardiographic changes during chemical face peeling. Plast Reconstr Surg. 1979;63(1):44–8.
15. Gross BG, Maschek F. Phenol chemosurgery for removal of deep facial wrinkles. Int J Dermatol. 1980;19:159.
16. Litton C, Szachowicz EH II, Trinidad GP. Present day status of the chemical face peel. Aesthetic Plast Surg. 1986;10(1):1–7.
17. Brown AM, Kaplan LM, Brown ME. Phenol-induced histological skin changes: hazards, technique, and uses. Br J Plast Surg. 1960;13:158–69.
18. The Dispensatory of the United States of America. 25th ed. Philadelphia: Lippincott; 1955.
19. McGrady PM Jr. The youth doctors. New York: Coward-McCann; 1968. p. 226.
20. Baker TJ, Gordon HL, Stuzin J. Surgical rejuvenation of the face. St. Louis: Mosby; 1996. p. 53.
21. Montgomery DW. Phenol J Cutan Dis Syphilol. 1917;35:157.
22. Barnes HO. Truth and fallacies of face peeling and face lifting. Med J Record. 1927;126:86.
23. Marmelzat WL. Bits of history, bits of mystery: a historical review of chemical rejuvenation of the face. In: Kotler R, editor. Chemical rejuvenation of the face. St. Louis: Mosby-Year Book; 1992.
24. Barnes HO. Aesthetic plastic surgery. Calif West Med. 1930;33:588.
25. Kron J. Lift. New York: Viking Press; 1998.
26. Boyd E. My experiences in wanting to be beautiful. Ladies Home J. 1908:179.
27. United States Patent 3,067,106 filed April 7, 1959. Issued December 4, 1962.
28. Spies JR. Croton resin: I. Toxicity studies using goldfish. J Am Chem Soc. 1935;57:180.
29. Spies JR. Croton resin: II. The toxic and vesicant action of certain of its derivatives. J Am Chem Soc. 1935;57:182.
30. Drake NL, Spies JR. Croton resin: III. The combined acids. J Am Chem Soc. 1935;57:184.
31. Spies JR. Croton resin: IV. The petroleum-ether-insoluble acids. J Am Chem Soc. 1937;59:62.
32. Eller JJ, Wolf S. Skin peeling and scarification. JAMA. 1941;116:934.
33. Urkov JC. Surface defects of the skin: treatment by controlled exfoliation. Ill Med J. 1946;89:75.
34. MacKee GM, Karp FL. Treatment of post-acne scars with phenol. Br J Dermatol. 1952;64:456.
35. Adelson S, Bonnett M, Brew G, et al. License to kill? People. 1982;26:20.
36. Spira M, Dahl C, Freeman R, et al. Chemosurgery: a histological study. Plast Reconstr Surg. 1970;45:247.
37. Behin F, Feuerstein S, Marovitz WF. Comparative histological study of mini pig skin after chemical peel and dermabrasion. Arch Otolaryngol. 1977;103:271.
38. Stegman SJ. A study of dermabrasion and chemical peels in an animal model. J Dermatol Surg Oncol. 1980;6:490.
39. Stegman SJ. A comparative histological study of the effects of three peeling agents and dermabrasion on normal and sun-damaged skin. Aesthetic Plast Surg. 1982;6:123.
40. Kligman AM, Baker TJ, Gordon HL. Long-term histological follow-up of phenol face peels. Plast Reconstr Surg. 1985;75:652.
41. Matarasso SL, Brody HJ. Deep chemical peeling. Semin Cutan Med Surg. 1996;15:155.
42. Stuzin JM. Phenol peeling and the history of phenol peeling. Clin Plast Surg. 1998;25:1.
43. Aronsohn RB. Facial chemosurgery. Eye Ear Nose Throat Mon. 1971;50:128.
44. Lister J. On the antiseptic principle in the practice of surgery. Br Med J. 1867;2:246–8.

45. Wambier CG, Lin E, da Costa Filho ARC, Beltrame FL, Döll-Boscardin PM, Celidonio TC, et al. Updates on level of evidence of clinical efficacy of facial phenol-croton oil peels and comments on history and mechanisms of action. Int J Dermatol. 2023;62:e383–6.
46. Rullan PP, Rullan JM. How we do it: carbolic acid (liquid phenol) 89% ring paint for boxcar and polymorphic acne scars. Dermatol Surg. 2024;50:785–7.
47. Brown AM, Kaplan L, Brown ME. Cutaneous alterations induced by phenol: a histologic bioassay. J Int Coll Surg. 1960;34(5):601–12.
48. Hetter GP. An examination of the phenol–croton oil peel: Part IV. Plast Reconstr Surg. 2000;105(3):1061–83; discussion 1084–7.

Physicochemical, Pharmacological and Molecular Aspects of Phenol and Croton Oil

2

2.1 Introduction

The phenol-croton oil peel is one of the most powerful and transformative procedures in aesthetic dermatology, with well-established clinical efficacy for the rejuvenation of photodamaged skin. The potency of this formulation is not solely due to the exfoliative action of phenol, but also to the profound pharmacological effects of *Croton tiglium* oil (CO). This chapter provides an in-depth exploration of the mechanisms of action, biochemical interactions, pharmacokinetics, toxicity, and stability of these two substances, with emphasis on the distinction between their cutaneous and systemic effects and the available experimental evidence.

2.2 Phenol

2.2.1 Chemical Structure and Physicochemical Properties

Phenol (C_6H_5OH), also known as carbolic acid, is a hydroxylated aromatic compound (Fig. 2.1), solid at room temperature, becoming liquid between 40 and 43 °C. It has a characteristic odor and is soluble in water, ethanol, and ether. In aqueous solution, it acts as a caustic and anesthetic agent.

2.2.2 Cutaneous Mechanism of Action

Phenol exerts a protein-denaturing effect, causing coagulative necrosis of the epidermis and the most superficial layers of the dermis, depending on its concentration and the number of passes. It acts initially by precipitating structural and cellular proteins, including keratin epidermal layer, which clinically manifests as rapid-onset, uniform blanching (Fig. 2.2). Its caustic effect results in deep dermal

C. Marçon, C. Wambier, *Phenol-Croton Oil Peel*,
https://doi.org/10.1007/978-3-032-25993-6_2

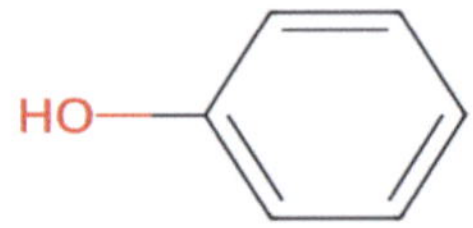

Fig. 2.1 Chemical structure of phenol (C_6H_5OH). Aromatic molecule consisting of a benzene ring bonded to a hydroxyl group. (*Source: Figure created by the author (Dr Carolina Marçon)*)

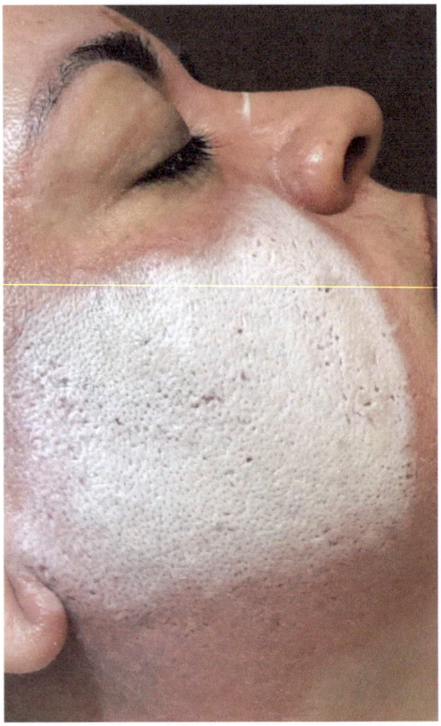

Fig. 2.2 Immediate clinical appearance following application of phenol peel, demonstrating the uniform blanching resulting from protein denaturation. Phenol induces coagulative necrosis of the epidermis and superficial dermis, while simultaneously triggering deep dermal remodeling with stimulation of collagen and elastin production. (*Source: Author's personal archive (Dr Carolina Marçon)*)

remodeling, stimulating the production of collagen and elastin. This mechanism is widely utilized in aesthetic procedures, such as facial rejuvenation, due to its ability to promote structural renewal of the skin with long-lasting results. Phenol also affects superficial dermal vessels, thereby limiting subsequent systemic absorption and creating a "pharmacological barrier" effect.

2.2.3 Clinical and Histological Effects of Different Phenol Concentrations

Phenol acts in a concentration- and volume-dependent manner, which directly influences the depth of necrosis, the duration of exfoliation, and the risk of systemic toxicity. At higher concentrations, phenol induces more rapid and deeper protein coagulation, blockade of nerve endings with a local anesthetic effect, and significant vasoconstriction, all of which contribute to reduced systemic absorption of substances applied concomitantly, such as croton oil.

Historically, the most commonly used formulations contain phenol at concentrations between 25% and 50%. The Baker-Gordon peel, for example, uses phenol at 88% in its stock solution, which is subsequently diluted with water, soap, and croton oil. Hetter's formula standardized final phenol concentrations between 27.5% and 35% (Table 2.1).

Comparative in vivo studies have shown that:

- Phenol at 35% without croton oil induces superficial necrosis, predominantly epidermal, with mild perivascular inflammation and no significant neocollagenesis—characterizing a medium-superficial peel.
- Phenol at 35% with 1.6% croton oil (as in Hetter's formula) induces thicker and more uniform necrosis, with a deep neutrophilic inflammatory band, vascular ectasia, and formation of a thick layer of type III neocollagen—demonstrating a much stronger and more regenerative effect.

Indiscriminate increases in phenol concentration do not necessarily intensify the clinical effect, as higher concentrations also increase superficial coagulation and the formation of an early protein barrier, which may paradoxically hinder the penetration of croton oil. Thus, there is an optimal balance between concentration and volume, so that the exfoliative action of phenol and the inflammatory response of the OC are complementary (Table 2.2).

In summary, phenol should not be regarded solely as a caustic agent; its role as a modulator of OC penetration and the resulting inflammation depends on its concentration, the volume applied, the vehicle, and the technique used. The choice of optimal concentration should balance safety, efficacy, and the desired tissue response.

2.2.4 Absorption and Toxicokinetics

Phenol absorption into the bloodstream following cutaneous application is rapid and intense, with 70% urinary recovery within 30 min and 85–95% within 24 h. Even small amounts can reach clinically relevant serum levels, making strict dose control and the use of segmented application techniques essential. The plasma

Table 2.1 Comparison between the Baker & Gordon Formula and Hetter's formulas

Component	Baker & Gordon 1961	Baker & Gordon 1962	Hetter 2000
Phenol (88%)	5 mL (47.5%)	3 mL (49.3%)	35%
Distilled water	4 mL	2 mL	q.s. to adjust
Septisol®	5 drops	8 drops	0.5 mL
Croton oil	3 drops (~1.2%)	3 drops (~2.1%)	0.4–1.6% (mild to extra strong)

The Baker & Gordon formula used fixed concentrations of phenol and croton oil, whereas Hetter standardized phenol dilutions at 35% and introduced graded variations of croton oil for greater predictability and safety. (*Source: Table prepared by the author (Dr Carolina Marçon)*)

Table 2.2 Comparison between Baker & Gordon (1962) and Hetter (2000)

Baker & Gordon (1962)	Hetter (2000)
Fixed concentrations of phenol and croton oil	Main ingredient: Croton oil
High risk of scarring	Variation in croton oil concentration → controls depth
Persistent hypopigmentation	Titration of intensity
	Reduction of phenol and croton oil → greater safety
	More subtle and natural results
	Segmentation
	Less pain and discomfort

The classic Baker & Gordon formulas used fixed concentrations and carried high risks, whereas Hetter introduced standardization and individualized adjustments, resulting in greater safety, natural appearance, and comfort during the procedure. (*Source: Table prepared by the author (Dr Carolina Marçon)*)

half-life is short, but potential toxicity depends on the concentration, rate of application, extent of the treated area, and the patient's hydration status and hepatorenal function.

Studies indicate that cutaneous absorption is less influenced by the concentration of the solution applied, depending largely on the area of skin exposed. In 1971, Piotrowski studied solutions containing phenol at concentrations of 5, 10, and 25 mg/m^3 and found that, regardless of concentration, the compound is rapidly absorbed both through the skin and the lungs.

2.2.5 Metabolism and Elimination

When applied to the skin, phenol is rapidly absorbed due to its lipophilic nature and low molecular weight, penetrating the stratum corneum and reaching the systemic circulation. Once absorbed, it undergoes hepatic detoxification, with approximately 75% metabolized mainly by glucuronidation, sulfonation, and oxidation via CYP2E1. Elimination occurs predominantly via the kidneys, with excretion in the urine mainly as glucuronides and sulfates. Approximately 25% of phenol undergoes further metabolism, being converted to carbon dioxide (CO_2) and water, while a small fraction may be excreted unchanged in the urine. In addition, in the first few minutes after absorption, some phenol may be eliminated via the lungs, which may be associated with the characteristic odor exhaled by patients. A smaller fraction of phenol is eliminated in the feces, resulting from biliary excretion of metabolites, although this route plays a secondary role in the compound's overall elimination. The half-life of phenol varies according to dose and route of exposure, but efficient renal elimination generally prevents accumulation in healthy individuals (Fig. 2.3). Therefore, adequate hydration and stimulation of diuresis are useful strategies to optimize its elimination. Furthermore, as respiratory, urinary, and biliary excretion occur relatively rapidly, it is essential to allow adequate intervals between

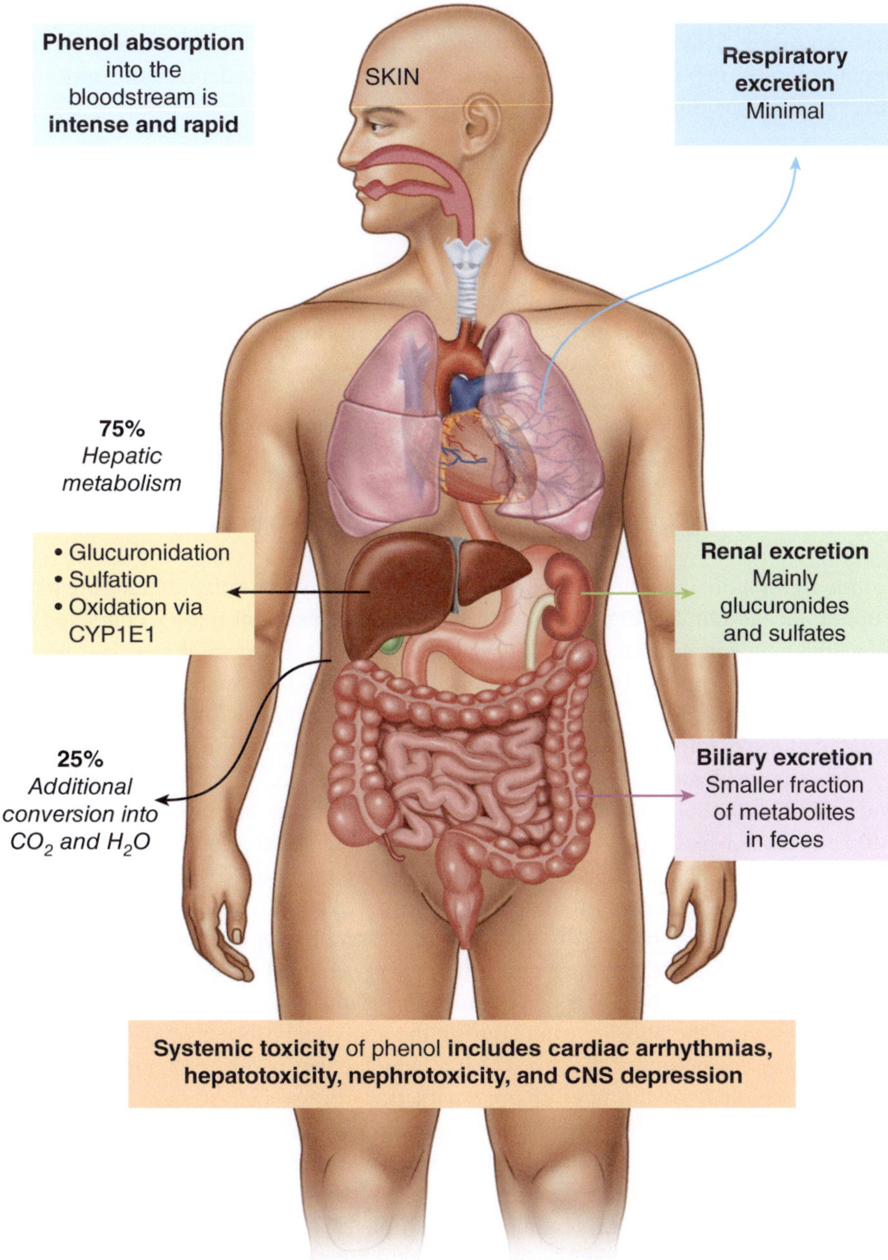

Fig. 2.3 Absorption, metabolism, and elimination of phenol. After cutaneous application, absorption is rapid and intense due to the lipophilicity and low molecular weight, with urinary recovery of 70% at 30 min and 85–95% at 24 h. Once in the circulation, small amounts already reach relevant serum levels, and the potential toxicity depends on the concentration, rate of administration, treated area, and renal and hepatic function. Metabolism occurs predominantly in the liver (≈75%) via glucuronidation, sulfonation, and oxidation through CYP2E1, while about 25% is converted into CO_2 and water. Elimination is mainly via the urine (as glucuronides and sulfates), with a small unchanged fraction, minimal initial respiratory elimination (characteristic odor), and secondary biliary excretion. (*Source: Figure prepared by the author (Dr Carolina Marçon)*)

successive applications to cosmetic units, ensuring complete elimination before further exposures. Systemic toxicity of phenol includes the risk of cardiac arrhythmias, hepatotoxicity, nephrotoxicity, and central nervous system depression, requiring strict precautions during the procedure.

2.2.6 Local Toxic Effects and Therapeutic Restrictions

Although highly effective, phenol alone is not capable of generating a sustained inflammatory effect or sufficient fibroblast stimulation for deep dermal remodeling. Its isolated use results in superficial, limited necrosis and offers less long-term benefit compared to its combination with croton oil.

2.3 Croton Oil (CO)

2.3.1 Chemical Composition and Molecular Structure

Croton tiglium oil, extracted from the seeds of the eponymous plant belonging to the Euphorbiaceae family (Fig. 2.4), constitutes a complex plant matrix characterized by a high concentration of biologically active diterpenes. Among these, the phorbol esters stand out, especially 12-O-tetradecanoylphorbol-13-acetate (TPA) and phorbol 12-myristate 13-acetate (PMA), compounds recognized for their potent pro-inflammatory, cytotoxic, and co-carcinogenic effects in experimental models.

These molecules share a central tetracyclic structure—the so-called tigliane core—and exhibit structural variations according to the acyl groups esterified at positions 12 and 13 of the phorbol skeleton. The intensity of the inflammatory response induced by these compounds depends directly on the nature and position of these groups, which confers functional specificity to the different forms of phorbol esters (Fig. 2.5).

Chromatographic analyses by liquid chromatography coupled with tandem mass spectrometry (LC-MS/MS) have confirmed the presence of these structures in commercial croton oil used in deep chemical peel formulations (Delasco®, USA). Fragmentation of the phorbol esters during the analytical process reveals characteristic patterns: formation of the m/z 311 ion, which corresponds to the basic phorbol skeleton after loss of the acyl chains (with transitions such as m/z 529 → 311, 501 → 311, and 473 → 311), and the subsequent m/z 311 → 293 transition, indicative of the loss of a water molecule, associated with the presence of free hydroxyl groups in the structure.

These spectrometric data, obtained by multiple reaction monitoring (MRM), not only validate the chemical composition of the oil but also support its potent biological activity, particularly its profound and sustained inflammatory effect, characteristic of phenol-croton oil peels. Confirmation of the presence of phorbol esters in this plant matrix is fundamental to understanding the histological mechanisms observed, such as neutrophil recruitment, NET formation, and the subsequent stimulated dermal regeneration.

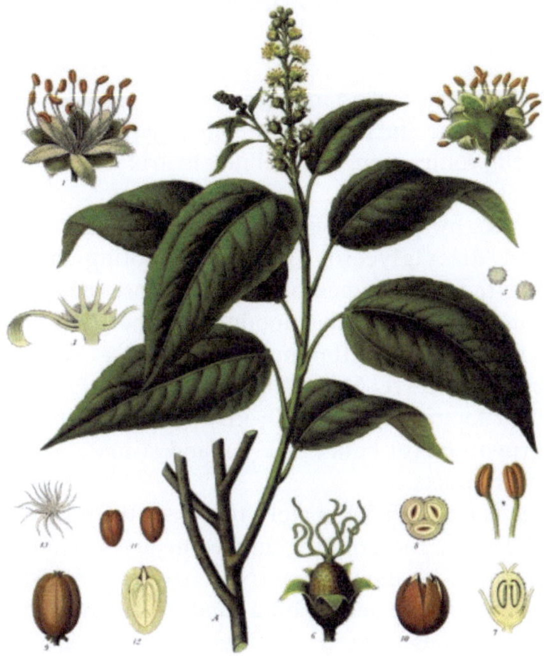

Fig. 2.4 Seeds of *Croton tiglium*, the botanical source of croton oil, a complex plant matrix rich in biologically active diterpenes, among which the phorbol esters (including 12-O-tetradecanoylphorbol-13-acetate, TPA, and phorbol 12-myristate-13-acetate, PMA) are prominent, compounds recognized for their pro-inflammatory, cytotoxic, and co-carcinogenic effects in experimental models. (*Source:* Köhler's *Medizinal-Pflanzen* (1897), *public domain*)

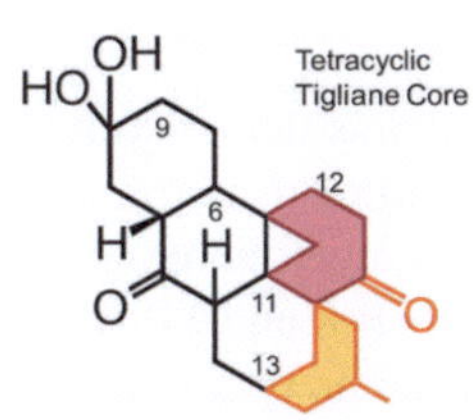

Fig. 2.5 Representative chemical structure of phorbol esters. All molecules share a common tetracyclic tigliane core, while structural variation occurs through esterification of different acyl groups at positions 12 and 13 of the phorbol skeleton. These modifications confer functional specificity, modulating the intensity of the inflammatory response and the potential to stimulate neocollagenesis. (*Source: Figure prepared by the author (Dr Carolina Marçon)*)

2.3.2 Cellular Mechanisms of Phorbol Esters and Their Regenerative Effects

The biological activity of phorbol esters begins with the activation of protein kinase C (PKC), a family of intracellular serine/threonine-dependent kinases involved in processes such as cell proliferation, extracellular matrix remodeling, inflammation, and tissue differentiation.

Activation of PKC by phorbol esters mimics signals physiological processes mediated by diacylglycerol (DAG), promoting the translocation of enzyme isoforms to the plasma membrane and, subsequently, the phosphorylation of intracellular substrates that modulate gene transcription. This process leads to the induction of inflammatory mediators such as interleukin-1 beta (IL-1β), interleukin-6 (IL-6), and tumor necrosis factor alpha (TNF-α), activation of nuclear factor kappa B (NF-κB) pathways, increased expression of transforming growth factor beta (TGF-β), and stimulation of collagen synthesis by dermal fibroblasts.

In addition to the classical inflammatory response, there is robust evidence for the induction of NETosis, a form of programmed neutrophil cell death resulting in the release of neutrophil extracellular traps (NETs), which are histologically visible as characteristic subcoagulative neutrophilic bands following application of croton oil. This mechanism, besides being an important component of innate immunity, contributes to the removal of damaged cutaneous structures such as solar elastosis, thereby promoting intense dermal renewal.

Recent studies have also revealed that phenol-croton oil peeling induces the expression of sirtuins, particularly SIRT-6 and SIRT-7, nuclear proteins associated with cellular longevity, DNA repair, epigenetic regulation, and the synthesis of type I and III collagen. The activation of these sirtuins appears to mediate, at least in part, the profound rejuvenating effects observed clinically, with reorganization of the extracellular matrix and improvement in the quality of photoaged skin (Table 2.3).

Additionally, experimental models demonstrate that topical application of 2.5% *Croton tiglium* oil leads to a significant increase in dermal inflammatory markers within the first few hours, such as myeloperoxidase (MPO) and matrix metalloproteinases (MMPs), particularly MMP-8 and MMP-9, involved in the controlled degradation of the extracellular matrix and tissue remodeling. The increased expression of these enzymes was confirmed by immunohistochemistry, ELISA, and proteomic analysis by mass spectrometry.

These findings confirm that croton oil acts as a potent inducer of targeted acute inflammation and intense tissue regeneration. Its synergistic action with phenol—which induces controlled necrosis and vasoconstriction—enhances these effects by creating a sterile microenvironment with limited systemic absorption and intense local stimulation, responsible for the clinical responses observed. This unique combination of pharmacological and histological effects distinguishes phenol-croton oil peels from any other deep chemical rejuvenation modalities available in contemporary dermatology (Figs. 2.6 and 2.7).

Table 2.3 Summary of croton (phorbol esters)

Aspect	Description
Biological activity of phorbol esters	Intense pro-inflammatory activity and stimulation of neocollagenesis via activation of protein kinase C, resulting in marked pro-inflammatory effects
Early medicinal applications	Historical reports date back to 1800
1918—Medical Use (France and Austria)	Treatment of gunpowder scars in First World War soldiers
Inflammatory mechanism	Inflammatory response resulting from the irritant activity of croton oil, sustained and intensified by secondary metabolites
Key metabolite	Phorbol 12-myristate 13-acetate (PMA) → induces subcoagulative neutrophilic band (NETosis)
Molecular effects	↑ cytokines → increased TGF-β → stimulation of collagen production
Phenol + croton oil	Increases penetration and acts synergistically with croton oil
Epigenetic effects	↑ expression of sirtuins SIRT-6 and SIRT-7
Collagen synthesis	↑ production of type III collagen

Main historical, pharmacological, and molecular aspects related to *Croton tiglium* oil and its phorbol esters. The table summarizes the earliest medicinal applications in the nineteenth century through to recently described molecular mechanisms, including activation of protein kinase C, induction of NETosis, stimulation of cytokine and TGF-β production, expression of sirtuins (SIRT-6 and SIRT-7), and synthesis of type III collagen, as well as the synergistic effect with phenol. (*Source: Table prepared by the author (Dr Carolina Marçon)*)

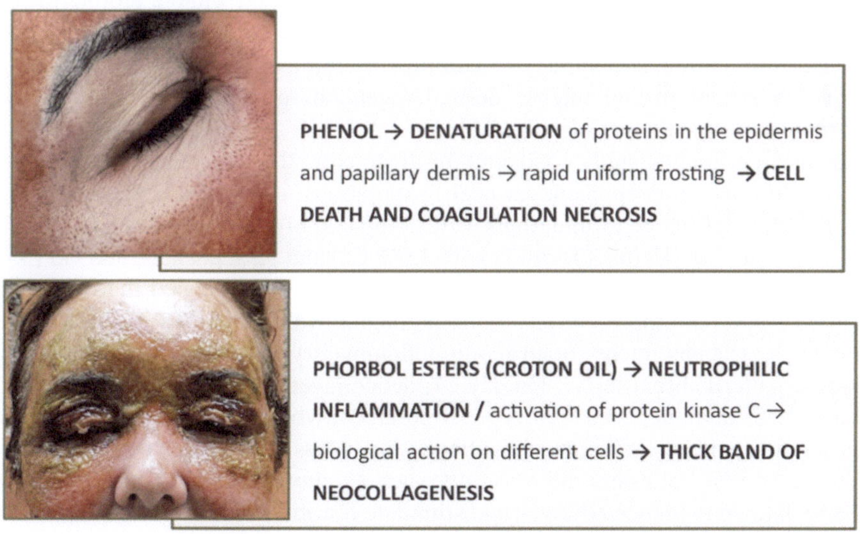

Fig. 2.6 Biological mechanisms of action of phenol and croton oil in deep chemical peeling. Phenol promotes protein denaturation in the epidermis and papillary dermis, resulting in uniform frosting and coagulative necrosis. The phorbol esters in croton oil trigger intense neutrophilic inflammation via protein kinase C activation, with amplified cellular action culminating in the formation of a thick band of neocollagenesis. (*Source: Author's personal archive/Figure created by the author (Dr Carolina Marçon)*)

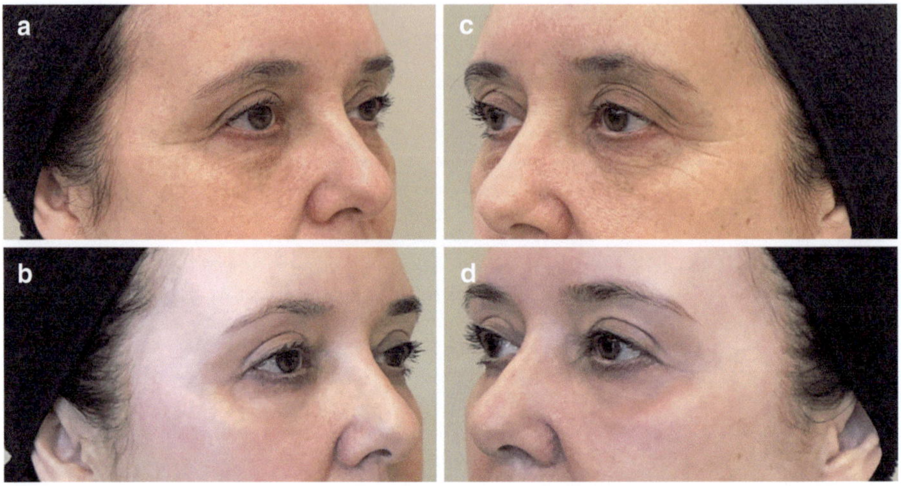

Fig. 2.7 Rejuvenation of the periocular region with 35% phenol/1.2% croton oil peel in a 58-year-old patient. Before and 6 months after: (**a**, **b**) (right hemiface); (**c**, **d**) (left hemiface). (*Source: Author's personal archive (Dr Carolina Marçon)*)

2.3.3 Experimental Evidence

Several comparative studies between formulations with and without croton oil confirm that phenol alone induces superficial and limited necrosis, without significant collagen stimulation. In contrast, the addition of croton oil induces deeper necrosis, dense inflammation, and intense dermal regeneration with greater neocollagen thickness and vascularization (Fig. 2.8).

In an experimental study conducted by Justo et al. the biological role of *Croton tiglium* oil (CO) in deep chemical peel formulations, especially Hetter's formula, was investigated. Three formulations were compared in a porcine animal model: G1 (5% Septisol), G2 (Hetter's formula with 1.6% CO and 35% phenol), and G3 (35% phenol with Septisol, without CO). Histological analysis revealed that group G2 showed deeper and more uniform dermal coagulative necrosis, as well as marked vascular ectasia and intense neutrophilic inflammatory infiltrate below the necrosis zone—a pattern absent in G3. On day 21, neocollagenesis in G2 was significantly greater, with thick deposition of type III collagen, whereas G3 showed superficial regeneration and insignificant neocollagenesis. Mass spectrometry identified the presence of phorbol esters in croton oil, such as phorbol 12-myristate 13-acetate (PMA), known to induce NETosis and stimulate fibroblasts. These data support that the profound regenerative effects observed in peels with CO are not due exclusively to phenol, but rather to the intense acute inflammatory response triggered by the bioactive compounds in CO, particularly the phorbol esters. The study also suggests that higher concentrations of phenol may paradoxically attenuate the effect of CO by promoting early coagulation of the vasculature, thereby limiting the local bioavailability of the oil (Figs. 2.9, 2.10, and 2.11).

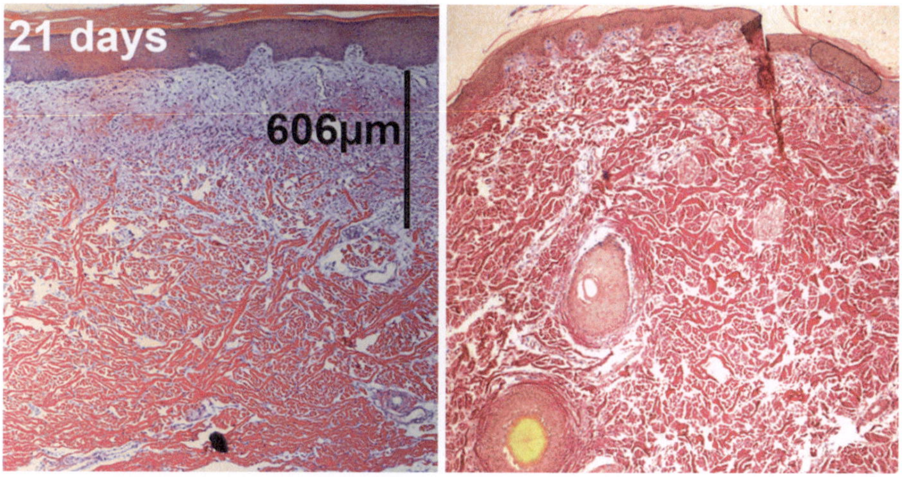

Fig. 2.8 On day 21 post-procedure, neocollagenesis (type III collagen, stained blue) was evident only in samples treated with 1.6% croton oil in 35% phenol. Isolated 35% phenol showed minimal neocollagenesis, consistent with the response of a superficial to medium-depth chemical peel. Herovici staining, 320× magnification. (*Source: Courtesy of Dr Flavio Beltrame, Dr Aline Justo & Dr Carlos Wambier*)

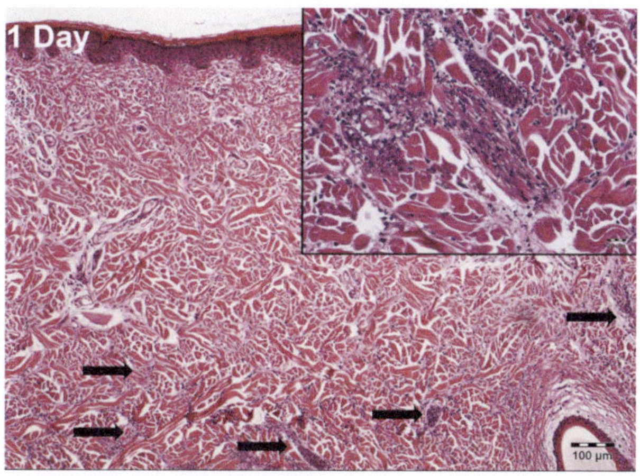

Fig. 2.9 First day post-procedure with 35% phenol peel: superficial and follicular coagulative necrosis, mild vascular ectasia, and sparse, mild perivascular mononuclear inflammatory infiltrate (white arrows). Hematoxylin–eosin, 100×; detail, 400×. (*Source: Courtesy of Dr Flavio Beltrame, Dr Aline Justo & Dr Carlos Wambier*)

2.3.4 Variability, Stability, and Quality Control

The composition of croton oil can vary substantially depending on its origin, extraction method, and storage duration, exhibiting high phytochemical variability between different batches and suppliers. Studies using liquid chromatography, mass spectrometry, and HPTLC (High-Performance Thin Layer Chromatography) have shown that many commercial products do not contain the same profile of phorbol esters—compounds directly responsible for the depth of action and inflammatory pattern of the peels—thus jeopardizing the safety and efficacy of the procedures.

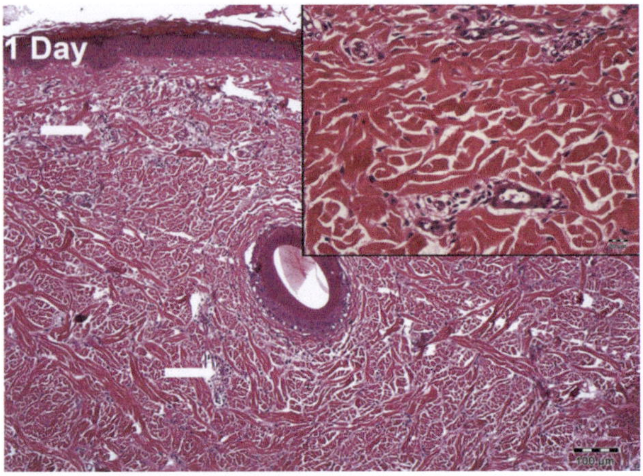

Fig. 2.10 First day post-procedure with 35% phenol peel: superficial and follicular coagulative necrosis, mild vascular ectasia, and sparse, mild perivascular mononuclear inflammatory infiltrate (white arrows). Hematoxylin–eosin, 100×; detail, 400×. (*Source: Courtesy of Dr Flavio Beltrame, Dr Aline Justo & Dr Carlos Wambier*)

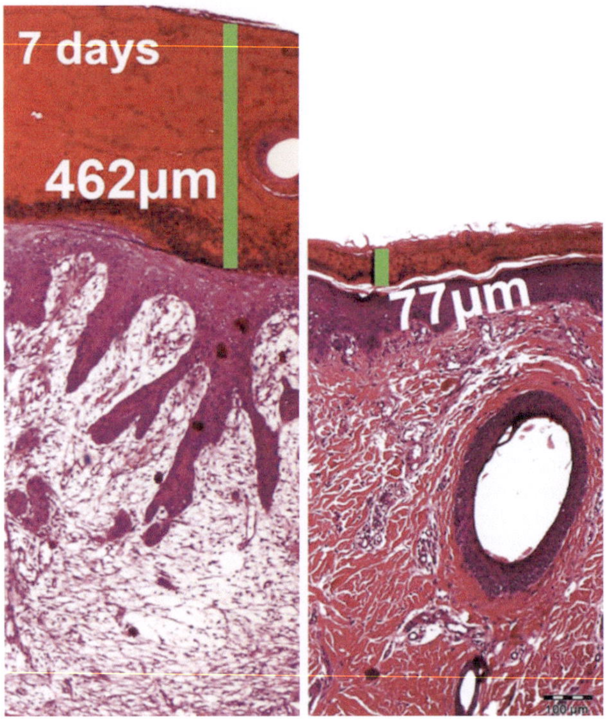

Fig. 2.11 Seventh day post-procedure with 35% phenol peel combined with 1.6% croton oil: complete re-epithelialization, intense neocollagenesis and neovascularization beneath a thick crust measuring 462 μm (long green bar, image on the left). Isolated 35% phenol peel: very superficial lesion, with a crust of 77 μm (short green bar, image on the right). The crust, stained deep red, highlights dehydrated structures. Hematoxylin–eosin, 100×. (*Source: Courtesy of Dr Flavio Beltrame, Dr Aline Justo & Dr Carlos Wambier*)

Furthermore, stability analyses have shown that the oil's composition changes over time during storage, resulting in the degradation of fatty acids and possible loss of the expected clinical effect. An experimental study evaluated the chemical integrity and biological efficacy of the stock solution of Hetter's formula (4% CO in 96% phenol (F—88%, w/v)) stored for 3 months. Histological assays were performed in an animal model, including assessment of epidermal thickness, fibroblast density, collagen production and organization, as well as physicochemical analyses by gas chromatography coupled with mass spectrometry (GC-MS).

The results revealed that, after 90 days of storage, there were significant changes in the lipid profile of CO, with degradation of fatty acids—especially unsaturated ones, which are susceptible to oxidation—and a marked reduction in phorbol ester levels (Fig. 2.12). These chemical changes were accompanied by less intense histological responses, with superficial inflammatory infiltrate, reduced cellular recruitment, less dense collagen fiber organization, and less structured type III collagen, when compared to the freshly prepared formulation.

These findings reinforce the need for strict control over the origin, purity, and storage of *Croton tiglium* oil used in dermatological procedures, as its instability may compromise the clinical efficacy of the formula. Therefore, the selection of reliable suppliers, with up-to-date analytical reports and rigorous purity control, is essential.

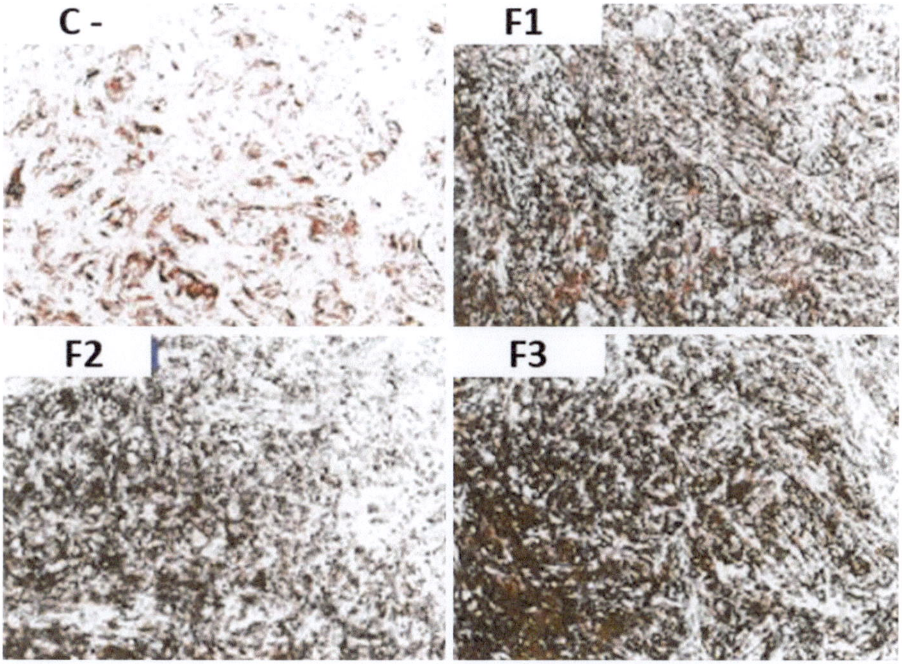

Fig. 2.12 Comparative histological analysis after 3 months of storage of *Croton tiglium* oil (CO), demonstrating, by gas chromatography coupled with mass spectrometry (GC/MS), a reduction in fatty acids resulting from the natural oxidation of oils during shelf life. (*Source: Adapted from Capote* et al. *(2023). Capote ACMO, Justo AS, Wambier CG, Beltrame FL. Evaluation of the shelf stability of Croton tiglium L. oil solution used in Hetter's formula for deep chemical peeling [poster presentation]. In: Congresso Científico da Universidade Estadual de Ponta Grossa – Banner Natal; 2023; Ponta Grossa, PR, Brasil. Reproduced with permission of the authors*)

2.4 Biochemical Interactions, Pharmacokinetics, and Safety

Phenol and croton oil interact synergistically. Phenol acts as a permeation enhancer, facilitating the penetration of phorbol esters, which in turn initiate and sustain the inflammatory process. This unique combination results in controlled necrosis, deep inflammation, and accelerated tissue regeneration (Figs. 2.13 and 2.14).

Systemic absorption of phorbol esters present in *Croton tiglium* oil appears to be limited in the context of chemical peeling, mainly due to the vasoconstrictive action of phenol, which reduces dermal perfusion and hinders systemic penetration of the applied compounds. However, even with low absorption, the local effects of phorbol esters are pronounced, including intense acute inflammation, NET formation, stimulation of cytokines such as TGF-β, and promotion of neocollagenesis. This potent local pharmacological action requires extreme care in the preparation of the formulation, particularly regarding the standardization of concentration, purity, stability, and source of the oil. Variations in these factors can significantly alter the clinical response and the safety profile of the procedure.

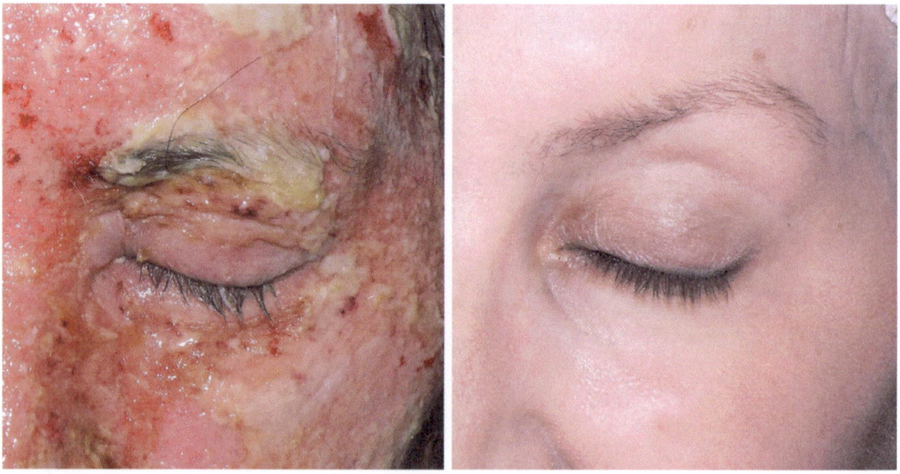

Fig. 2.13 Phenol and croton oil interact synergistically. Phenol acts as a coagulating agent and permeation enhancer, facilitating the penetration of phorbol esters, which trigger and sustain the inflammatory process. This combination results in controlled necrosis, deep inflammation, and accelerated tissue regeneration, providing significant clinical outcomes in skin rejuvenation. (*Source: Personal archive of Dr Carlos Wambier*)

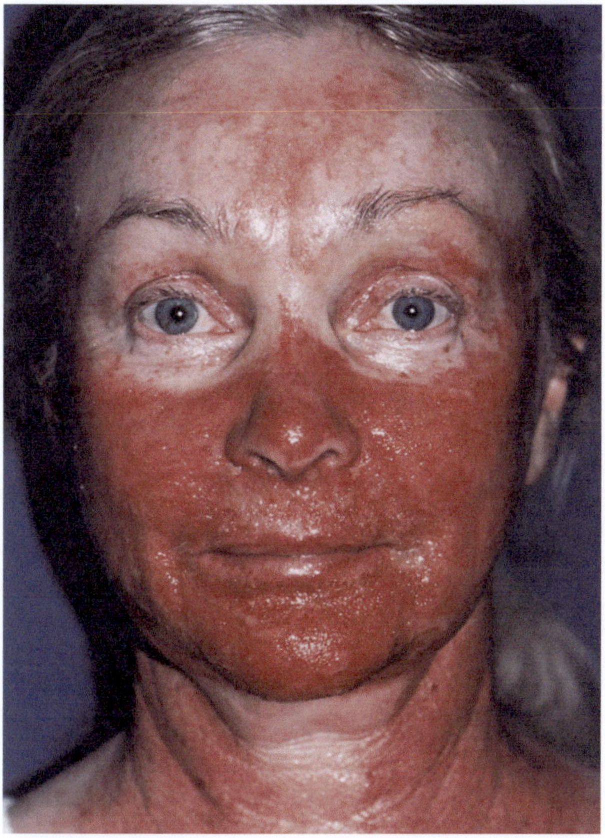

Fig. 2.14 Woman undergoing peeling with isolated 35% phenol on the forehead and 35% phenol combined with 0.4% croton oil on the nose and cheeks. No result is observed on the forehead, and significant dermal burn is seen in the areas treated with croton oil. (*Source: Adapted from Hetter GP. An examination of the phenol-croton oil peel: Part II. The lay peelers and their croton oil formulas. Plast Reconstr Surg. 2000 Jan;105(1):240–8; discussion 249–51. doi:10.1097/00006534-200001000-00040. Erratum in: Plast Reconstr Surg 2000 Mar;105(3):1083. PMID: 10626997. Reproduced with permission of the publisher*)

2.5 Final Considerations

The efficacy of the phenol-croton oil peel lies in the combined and synergistic action of two active principles with distinct yet complementary mechanisms of action. Phenol acts as a caustic agent, anesthetic, and vasoconstrictor, defining the depth of necrosis and controlling systemic absorption. Croton oil, in turn, is the true regenerative agent, responsible for the intense sterile inflammation and dermal remodeling.

Detailed knowledge of the chemistry, pharmacology, and stability of these substances is essential to ensure the safety, efficacy, and standardization of the procedure. The purity and provenance of croton oil, as well as strictness in formulation and application, are critical factors for clinical success and the prevention of adverse events.

Sources

1. Justo AS, Lemes BM, Nunes B, Antunes KA, Capote ACMO, Lipinski LC, Campagnoli EB, Emiliano J, Meurer EC, Ezemma O, Miot HA, Beltrame FL, Wambier CG. Characterization of the activity of *Croton tiglium* oil in Hetter's very heavy phenol-croton oil chemical peels. Dermatol Surg. 2021;47(7):944–6.
2. Kligman AM, Baker TJ, Gordon HL. Long-term histologic follow-up of phenol face peels. Plast Reconstr Surg. 1985;75:652–9.
3. Kadunc BV, Vanti AA. Evaluation of the systemic toxicity of phenol on facial peelings. Surg Cosmet Dermatol. 2009;1:10–4.
4. Downs JW, Wills BK. Phenol toxicity. In: StatPearls. Treasure Island, FL: StatPearls Publishing; 2023. https://www.ncbi.nlm.nih.gov/books/.
5. Agency for Toxic Substances and Disease Registry (US). Relevance to public health. In: Toxicological profile for phenol. Atlanta, GA: ATSDR; 2008. https://www.ncbi.nlm.nih.gov/books/NBK599443/.
6. Ruedemann R, Deichmann WB. Blood phenol level after topical application of phenol-containing preparations. JAMA J Am Med Assoc. 1953;152(6):506–9.
7. Hetter GP. An examination of the phenol-croton oil peel: Part I. Dissecting the formula. Plast Reconstr Surg. 2000;105(1):227–39; discussion 249–51.
8. Hetter GP. An examination of the phenol-croton oil peel: Part IV. Face peel results with different concentrations of phenol and croton oil. Plast Reconstr Surg. 2000;105(3):1061–83; discussion 1084–7.
9. Capote ACMO, Campos PM, Perera W, Strangman WK, Williamson RT, Beltrame FL. Authentication of commercial *Croton tiglium* L. oils used as raw material for peeling formulas. In: Abstracts of the ICSB & ISE 2025—joint meeting; 2025; p. [session PA-7].
10. Capote ACMO, Justo AS, Wambier CG, Beltrame FL. Effects of *Croton tiglium* oil as deep chemical peeling in skin rejuvenation [poster presentation]. In: XXII international congress of pharmaceuticals, cosmetics and natural products—CIFARP 2023; 2023 Oct; Ribeirão Preto, SP, Brazil. [abstract] [poster].
11. Capote ACMO, Justo AS, Wambier CG, Beltrame FL. Evaluation of the shelf stability of *Croton tiglium* L. oil solution used in Hetter's formula for deep chemical peeling [poster presentation]. In: Scientific congress of the State University of Ponta Grossa—Banner Natal; 2023; Ponta Grossa, PR, Brazil. [abstract] [poster].
12. Mao G, Douglas D, Prajapati M, Janardhanam Raghavendra Rao T, Zheng H, Zhao C, Billack B. Investigation of inflammatory mechanisms induced by croton oil in mouse ear. Curr Res Toxicol. 2024;7:100184.
13. Pagani A, Gaeta S, Savchenko AI, Williams CM, Appendino G. An improved preparation of phorbol from croton oil. Beilstein J Org Chem. 2017;13:1361–7.
14. Zhang XL, Khan AA, Wang L, Yu K, Li F, Wang MK. Four new phorbol diesters from *Croton tiglium* and their cytotoxic activities. Phytochem Lett. 2016;16:82–6.
15. Wang HB, Wang XY, Liu LP, Qin GW, Kang TG. Tigliane diterpenoids from the Euphorbiaceae and Thymelaeaceae families. Chem Rev. 2015;115:2975–3011.
16. Van Duuren BL, Langseth L, Sivak A, Orris L. The tumor-promoting principles of *Croton tiglium* L. II. A comparative study. Cancer Res. 1966;26(8):1729–33.
17. Spies JR. Croton resin: I. Toxicity studies using goldfish. J Am Chem Soc. 1935;57:180.
18. Spies JR. Croton resin: II. The toxic and vesicant action of certain of its derivatives. J Am Chem Soc. 1935;57:182.

19. Drake NL, Spies JR. Croton resin: III. The combined acids. J Am Chem Soc. 1935;57:184.
20. Spies JR. Croton resin: IV. The petroleum-ether-insoluble acids. J Am Chem Soc. 1937;59:62.
21. Zhang T, Liu Z, Sun X, Liu Z, Zhang L, Zhang Q, Peng W, Wu C. Botany, traditional uses, phytochemistry, pharmacological and toxicological effects of *Croton tiglium* Linn.: a comprehensive review. J Pharm Pharmacol. 2022;74(8):1061–84.
22. Neitzke IC, de Grande CD, Lin EM, Lee KC, Soon SL, Lunardelli Bittencourt AC, et al. Translational research on the role of formula stability in Hetter's phenol-croton oil peels: analysis of chemical studies and clinical outcomes from a randomized, double-blind, split-face controlled trial. J Am Acad Dermatol. 2021;84:854–6.
23. Cardoso FAMES, Moura RD, Pilar EFS, Moura ICG, Miot HA, da Costa A. Phenol-croton oil peel increases type-1 and type-3 collagen content by stimulating SIRT-6 and SIRT-7. Int J Dermatol. 2022;61:e71–4.
24. Butler PE, Gonzalez S, Randolph MA, Kim J, Kollias N, Yaremchuk MJ. Quantitative and qualitative effects of chemical peeling on photoaged skin: an experimental study. Plast Reconstr Surg. 2001;107:222–8.
25. Giese SY, McKinney P, Roth SI, Zukowski M. The effect of chemosurgical peels and dermabrasion on dermal elastic tissue. Plast Reconstr Surg. 1997;100:489–98.
26. Han SH, Kim HJ, Kim SY, Kim YC, Choi GS, Shin JH. Skin rejuvenating effects of chemical peeling: a study in photoaged hairless mice. Int J Dermatol. 2011;50:1075–82.
27. Wambier CG, Lin E, da Costa Filha ARC, Beltrame FL, Döll-Boscardin PM, Celidonio TC, et al. Updates on the level of evidence for the clinical efficacy of facial phenol-croton oil peels and comments on history and mechanisms of action. Int J Dermatol. 2023;62:e383–6.
28. Hetter GP. An examination of the phenol-croton oil peel: Part II. The lay peelers and their croton oil formulas. Plast Reconstr Surg. 2000;105(1):240–8; discussion 249–51.

3 Formulations: Components, Concentrations and Variations

Opening Remarks Rather than compiling a collection of formulas with minimal scientific rigor, this chapter will focus solely on the current standard (Hetter's formulas), which are part of a scientific continuum that began with the classic Baker-Gordon formula, now considered rarely used. By venturing into other premixed formulas or those with ingredients of questionable origin or utility, the physician assumes unnecessary risk.

Following studies in animal models, we identified the action of each active component.

Phenol is the coagulating agent that induces coagulative necrosis, permeating through the epidermis and follicles, coagulating even lymphatic vessels and capillaries. Due to its lipophilic nature, it also acts as a solvent for vegetable oils, enabling the delivery of croton oil even at phenol concentrations below the coagulative threshold. Below 8%, phenol does not coagulate cells during peeling unless injected and exhibits anesthetic and antiseptic properties. Previously used for oral hygiene and handwashing prior to the advent of surgical gloves, Joseph Lister introduced phenol (also known as carbolic acid) as a surgical antiseptic in 1865. At this concentration, phenol forms a solution in water. Only above 8% does phenol begin to precipitate at room temperature. The precipitate, when concentrated, is coagulative. For peels, concentrations above 20% are used, which always result in two phases. Above 80% at room temperature, phenol exists as a pure precipitated phase, referred to as liquid phenol. At low concentrations, it is a solution of phenol in water; at high concentrations, a solution of water in phenol. Between these two, dispersions of both components occur, resulting in a milky appearance that separates within minutes. As phenol is denser than water, the lower phase is always coagulative, while the upper phase has a phenolic odor and may act as an anesthetic, with a sensation similar to menthol.

Croton oil is crucial for inducing a pro-inflammatory response, with a band of neutrophil extracelular traps (NETosis) beneath the zone of coagulative necrosis. The combination of phenol and croton oil produces a deep level of injury while

C. Marçon, C. Wambier, *Phenol-Croton Oil Peel*,
https://doi.org/10.1007/978-3-032-25993-6_3

preserving follicular structures such as the bulb, where epithelial stem cells reside. NETosis is a characteristic form of neutrophilic inflammation discovered in 2004, observed following the action of Phorbol 12-myristate 13-acetate (PMA), a phorbol diester extracted from croton oil.

Through potent activation of PKC (Protein Kinase C), neutrophils release their DNA as a web that protects tissue from bacteria and other agents. Phorbol esters differentiate cells, induce apoptosis and necrosis of senescent cells, and stimulate cell proliferation.

Regarding the observed rejuvenation, neutrophils that undergo NETosis release elastase, an enzyme that digests solar elastosis. The roles of exosomes and cellular DNA in the extracellular matrix remain unclear. It appears that inflammation and cellular recruitment are triggered by the action of phorbol esters.

As Dr. Hetter often said, there were two shooting stars, phenol and croton oil, which crossed paths to create the platonic standard of facial rejuvenation. We do not know for certain who first combined these two ingredients.

There is reason to believe that the pioneers of the Vienna school of dermatology (von Hebra and possibly Unna) were involved in mixing the ingredients. Von Hebra had already published on both phenol and croton oil. During the First World War, much of Vienna's work was lost with the fall of the Austro-Hungarian Monarchy.

Some believe that French physicians were using these formulas during the First World War, a story recounted by individuals in the United States from the 1930s onwards who claimed French origins, such as Antoinette La Gasse, who claimed to be the daughter of a French physician from the First World War.

Formulations in 2026

The current standard is the **Hetter standardized formulas** (metric units), which comprise any formula containing the four primary ingredients in order of concentration: Distilled Water, Liquid Phenol (88–93%), Novisol emulsifying agent, and Croton Oil.

Dr. Gregory Hetter taught that what matters is understanding the % volume of each ingredient and mixing the formulas immediately before use.

Hetter Stock Solution (Fig. 3.1)

CAUTION: MAXIMUM STRENGTH (4% croton oil)—"Devil."

- 1 mL of croton oil mixed with 24 mL of phenol = Final Volume: 25 mL.
  This is a Stock Solution containing 1 drop of croton oil per mL of phenol.
- Or 0.5 mL of croton oil mixed with 12 mL of phenol = Final Volume: 12.5 mL.
- Or 0.25 mL of croton oil mixed with 6 mL of Phenol = Final Volume: 6.25 mL
  Shelf life: 3 months at room temperature, in an amber bottle, protected from light.

In in vitro experiments conducted at UEPG with the Pharmacognosy and Phytotherapy group led by Prof. Dr. Flávio Beltrame, we observed oxidation of fatty acids in croton oil after just 3 months; therefore, we consider this an appropriate shelf life.

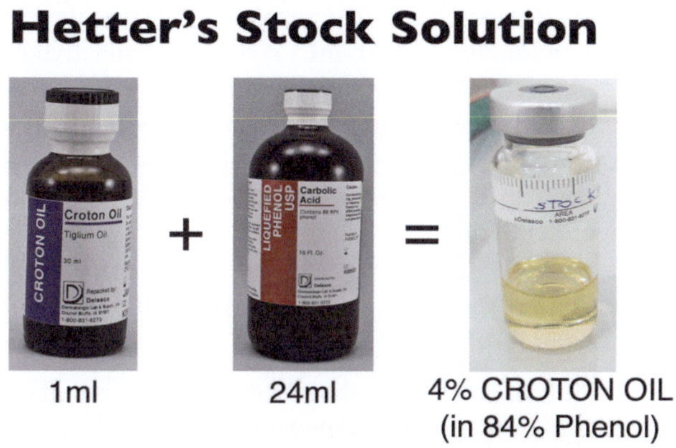

Fig. 3.1 Ingredients of the stock solution. *Source: Author's personal archive (Dr Carlos Wambier)*

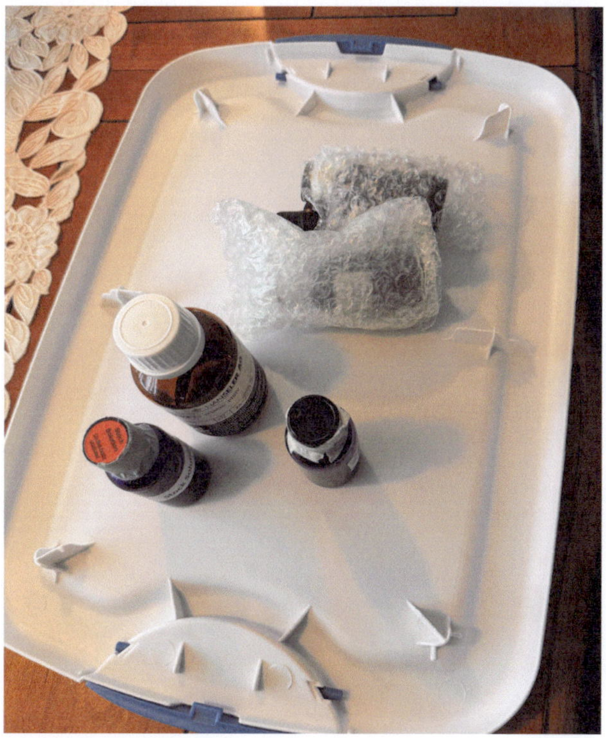

Fig. 3.2 Dr. Hetter's "Stock Solution." (labeled in the blue bottle). Material donated for research on the shelf life of the formulas, during my last visit to his home in Sarasota, on 10 March 2025. Dr. Hetter passed away at the age of 88 on 22 June 2025. This stock solution relic is preserved at Amanda Manipulações Farmacêuticas, Paraná, Brazil. *Source: Author's personal archive (Dr Carlos Wambier)*

We are currently conducting a chemical profile analysis of stock solutions mixed over 25 years ago, such as the stock prepared by Dr. Hetter while he was still active (Fig. 3.2), before his retirement in Sarasota. If the active substances in croton oil (phorbol esters) are preserved, we will conduct a comparative in vivo experiment.

When we dilute the stock with phenol, we vary the final formula, and it is crucial to understand that the variable component determines the potency, defined by the concentration of croton oil. Here, we will prepare a 10 mL formulas, where 40%

(4 mL) is the variable active part, as it contains the two active ingredients, phenol and croton oil, and 60% (6 mL) is the fixed, inactive part, used to increase the volume and safety of the formula, and to reduce the coagulation time of phenol for a more gradual depth, in the wet technique, which is the method used by Dr. Hetter and Dr. Wambier. We begin by diluting the Stock Solution to prepare 10 mL of Formulas with 35% Phenol, emulsified with 5% Novisol (Fig. 3.3). See Table 3.1 for ingredient volumes.

Variable component: (stock + dilution with liquid phenol—*see the list below*) = **4 mL**

- 1 mL of stock diluted in 3 mL of phenol results in 0.4% croton oil—Light
- 2 mL of stock diluted in 2 mL of phenol results in 0.8% croton oil—Medium
- 3 mL of stock diluted in 1 mL of phenol results in 1.2% croton oil—Heavy
- 4 mL of stock results in 1.6% croton oil—Very Heavy

Fixed component: Add 0.5 mL of Novisol (mix) and then add 5.5 mL of distilled water (mix) = **6 mL.**
Total = 10 mL.

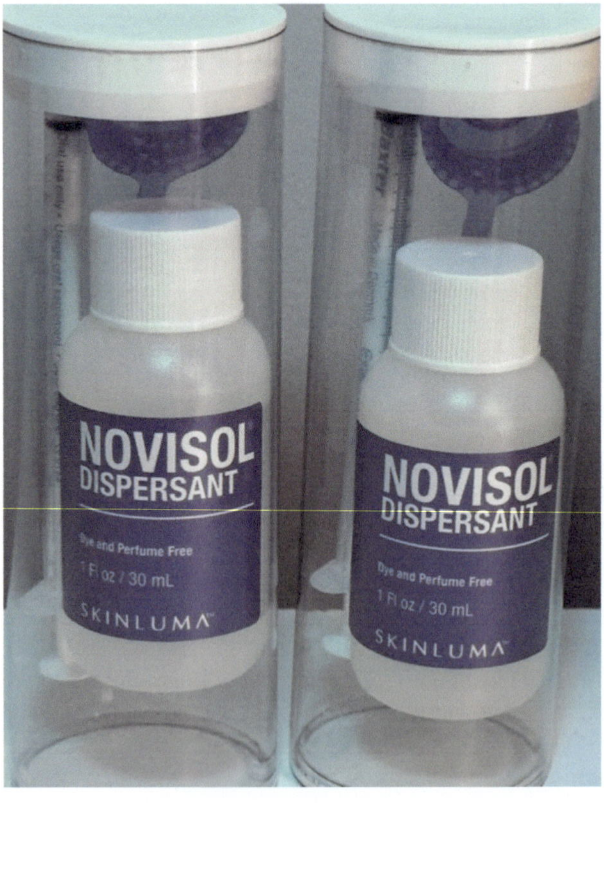

Fig. 3.3 Novisol. Available since 2018 from Young Pharmaceuticals, Inc./SkinLuma LLC in Connecticut, United States, and since 2019 compounded in Brazil by Amanda Manipulações Farmacêuticas, in Paraná, Brazil. *Source: Author's personal archive (Dr Carlos Wambier)*

Table 3.1 Standardized Hetter formulas containing 35% phenol in 10 mL

	Very heavy	Heavy	Medium	Light	Very light
Croton oil concentration	1.6%	1.2%	0.8%	0.4%	0.1%
Stock solution*	4 mL	3 mL	2 mL	1 mL	0.25 mL
Liquid phenol	0 mL	1 mL	2 mL	3 mL	3.75 mL
Distilled water	5.5 mL	5.5 mL	5.5 mL	5.5 mL	5.5 mL
Novisol	0.5 mL	0.5 mL	0.5 mL	0.5 mL	0.5 mL

*Hetter stock solution: 1 mL of *croton* oil mixed with 24 mL of liquid phenol containing at least 89% phenol in water. Final concentration: 4% croton *oil* in phenol. Each mL of stock contains 0.04 mL of croton oil, resulting in increments of 0.4% in formulas with a total volume of 10 mL. *Source: Table prepared by the author (Dr Carlos Wambier)*

NOVISOL® Emulsion Dosing

% Croton oil	**0.2**	**0.4**	**0.8**	**1.0**	**1.2**	**1.6**	**%**
% Novisol	**3.0**	**3.0**	**5.0**	**7.0**	**7.0**	**7.0**	**%**
mL Novisol per 10 mL	**0.3**	**0.3**	**0.5**	**0.7**	**0.7**	**0.7**	**mL**

Fig. 3.4 Floating dose (more precise) for emulsifying phenol and croton oil with water. In this way, the emulsion becomes more stable. The amount of distilled water to be added, together with the amount of Novisol, remains fixed at 60%, i.e., 6 mL when the final volume is 10 mL. *Source: Figure prepared by the author (Dr Carlos Wambier)*

Optional: to improve stability, the surfactant concentration can be varied as follows (Fig. 3.4):

Dr. Hetter also described all 35% formulas with 48.5% phenol for those who prefer a smaller volume and faster coagulation (such as those using only a semi-dry wooden swab). To prepare formulas close to 50% phenol, use a total of 5.5 mL of phenol and croton oil and 4.0 mL of distilled water, 0.5 mL of Novisol (for a total volume of 10 mL).

Figures 3.5 and 3.6 show the appearance of the formula during emulsification.

Hetter's 1996 formulas (obsolete, coined by Dr. Hetter as "Heretic" Formulas, as they were the first to challenge the higher phenol and croton oil concentrations of the classic Baker-Gordon formula).

Using the Delasco dropper (fine tip) to titrate croton oil:

- 1 drop = 0.04 mL (~25 drops = 1 mL).
- 4 mL of phenol + (1 to 3 drops of croton oil). Results in 0.35%, 0.7%, and 1.1% croton oil in 33% phenol.
- Problem: Each drop is different.
- FYI: I added the 4th drop at the JAAD CME with Dr. Hetter's authorization (not previously described), to make a "very heavy" formula similar to 1.6%.

Contrary to my practice, Dr. Hetter did not use the 1.6% concentration. It is my favorite formula, despite its slower penetration and frosting compared to 1.2% or

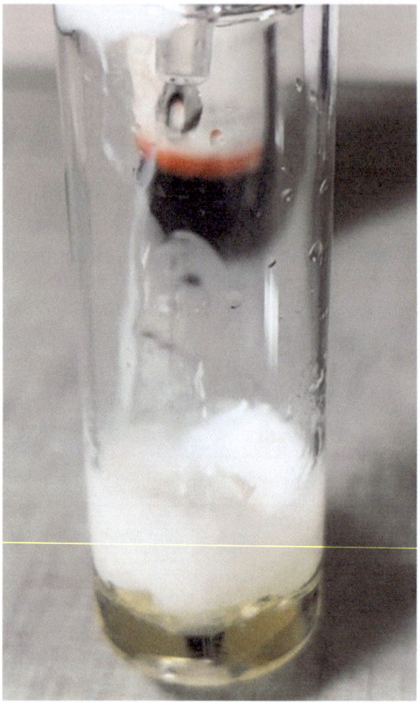

Fig. 3.5 Formula with 1.6% croton oil being mixed; detail of when Novisol is added before shaking; a creamy appearance is observed. *Source: Author's personal archive (Dr Carlos Wambier)*

0.8%. At the endpoint, 1.6% provides more inflammation and more interesting results than simply increasing the phenol concentration or switching to the Baker-Gordon formula.

Using Hetter's Methods to Prepare the Old Baker-Gordon Formula

Interestingly, the Hetter formula with 35% phenol and 1.6% croton oil and the Baker-Gordon formula contain the same concentration of croton oil in phenol (not considering the inactive phase). The only difference is the amount of water. Hetter contains 35% phenol and Baker 50% phenol. Due to the lower water volume, the concentration of phenol in Baker's formula increases to 2.1%.

To prepare Baker's formula using Hetter's standardized method, add 3 mL of stock solution with 0.25 mL of Novisol, mix until homogeneous, add 2 mL of distilled water, and mix.

In the Heretic method: 3 mL of liquid phenol, 3 drops of croton oil, mix, 0.25 mL of Novisol, mix, 2 mL of distilled water, and mix.

On the evolution of the emulsifying agent.

The first surfactant to be included in phenol-croton oil formulas was Lysol, which at the time contained cresol, akin to using bathroom disinfectant in a chemical peel formula today. This was used by Brown and others ("saponified phenol"). Lysol changed its composition over the decades. Baker introduced the antibacterial soap he used for pre-surgical handwashing, called Septisol, which at the time contained traces of alcohols and a toxic agent, Hexachlorophene, later banned by the

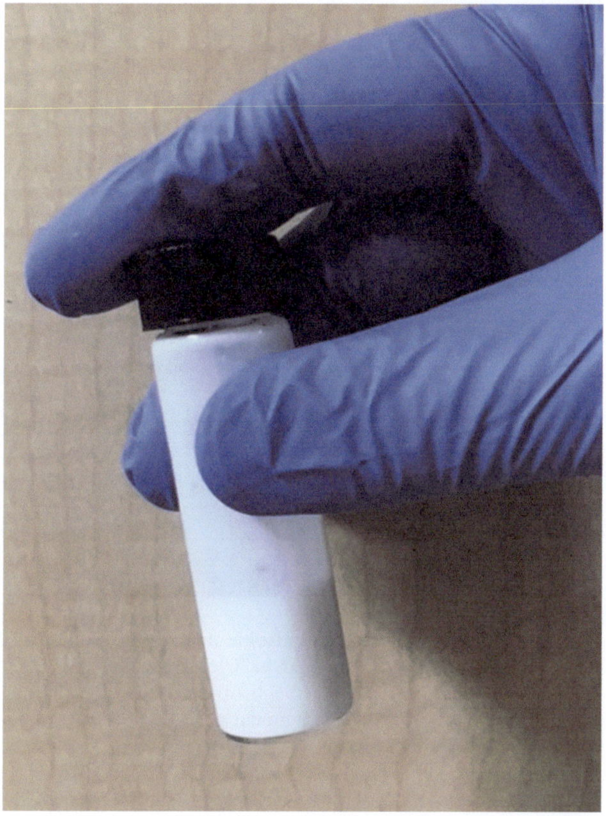

Fig. 3.6 Formula after the addition of distilled water and agitation (here containing 1.6% croton oil and 35% phenol). Uniform milky appearance. "The milk of rejuvenation." *Source: Author's personal archive (Dr Carlos Wambier)*

FDA. Septisol was reformulated to include Triclosan, which, after several decades, was also banned by the FDA for being an endocrine disruptor. Septisol was then withdrawn from the market. (Fig. 3.7) At that time, I observed in vitro and in vivo experiments that Septisol was not suitable for emulsifying phenol. It produced an extremely unstable formula with rapid separation, in less than 1 minute, compromising the safety of the procedure—a fact unknown until 2016. In 2017–18, many experiments were conducted until we arrived at Novisol, patented in 2022, the first emulsifying agent developed specifically for phenol-croton oil emulsions. (Figs. 3.8 and 3.9).

Any other formula currently known to the author (Stone, Fintzi, etc.) fails due to containing inactive ingredients that interact directly with phenol, such as alcohols like glycerol or edible fatty acids, which dilute the croton oil (akin to diluting gold with a cheaper metal). I will not mention any of these formulas as they do not meet the scientific rigor nor have histopathological analysis. Given the potential for oxidation of active ingredients in croton oil (Fig. 3.10), it is recommended that formulas be prepared immediately prior to application, versus using premixed formulas with no study of phorbol esters decay during shelf life (commercial products).

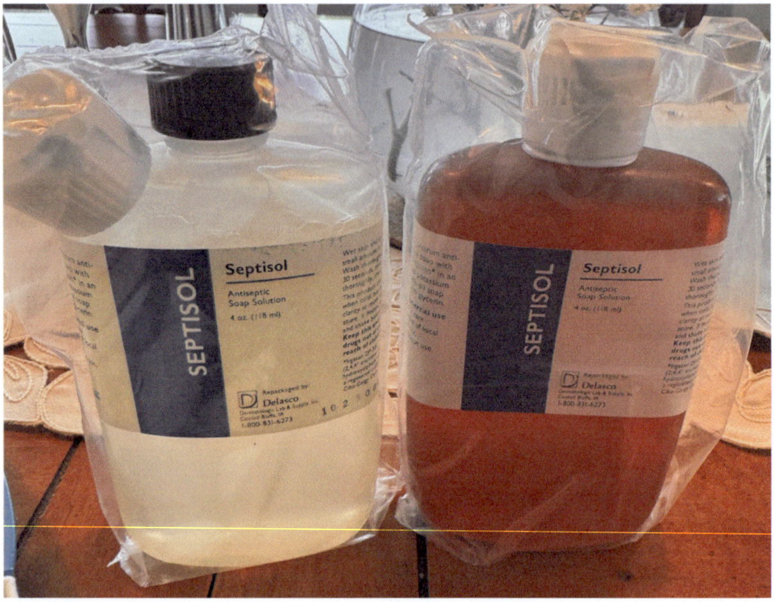

Fig. 3.7 From a distant past. Septisol in its multiple colors and formulations. Left: Septisol containing triclosan, banned by the FDA in 2016. Right: Original Septisol, containing Hexachlorophene, banned by the FDA in 1972. This Septisol was used for pre-surgical handwashing and was adopted, with little scientific basis, for chemical peels, probably to replace some other alchemical agent (such as bathroom disinfectants or glycerin) used by lay practitioners in Florida before physicians adopted the procedure. Novisol replaced Septisol in the formulas in 2018. Photograph of historical material from the collection of Dr. Gregory Hetter. *Source: Personal archive of the author (Dr Carlos Wambier)*

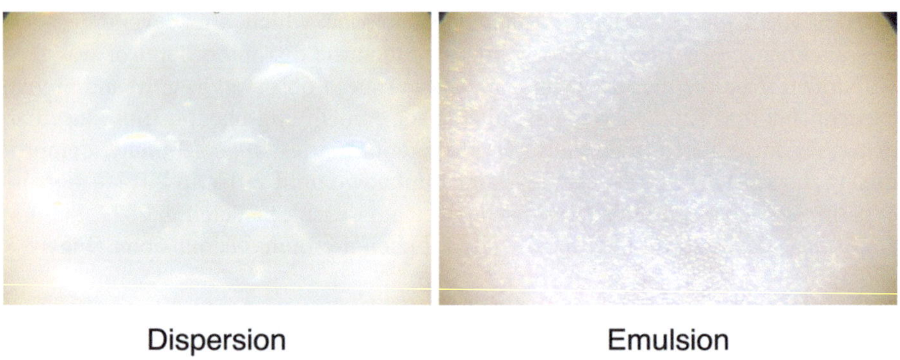

Fig. 3.8 Left: Unstable dispersion of phenol-croton oil droplets coalescing with Septisol and an emulsion of microdroplets maintaining the formula well mixed and relatively stable. *Source: Personal archive of the author (Dr Carlos Wambier)*

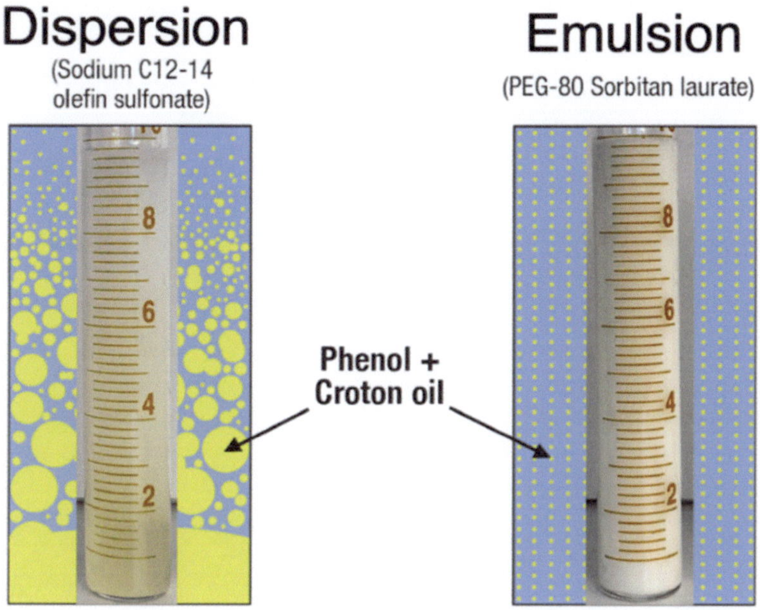

Fig. 3.9 Very heavy Hetter formulas mixed with 5% Septisol (left) and 5% Novisol (right). Demonstrating the instability present in formulas with Septisol, with evident separation within 1 minute. *Source: Personal archive of the author (Dr Carlos Wambier)*

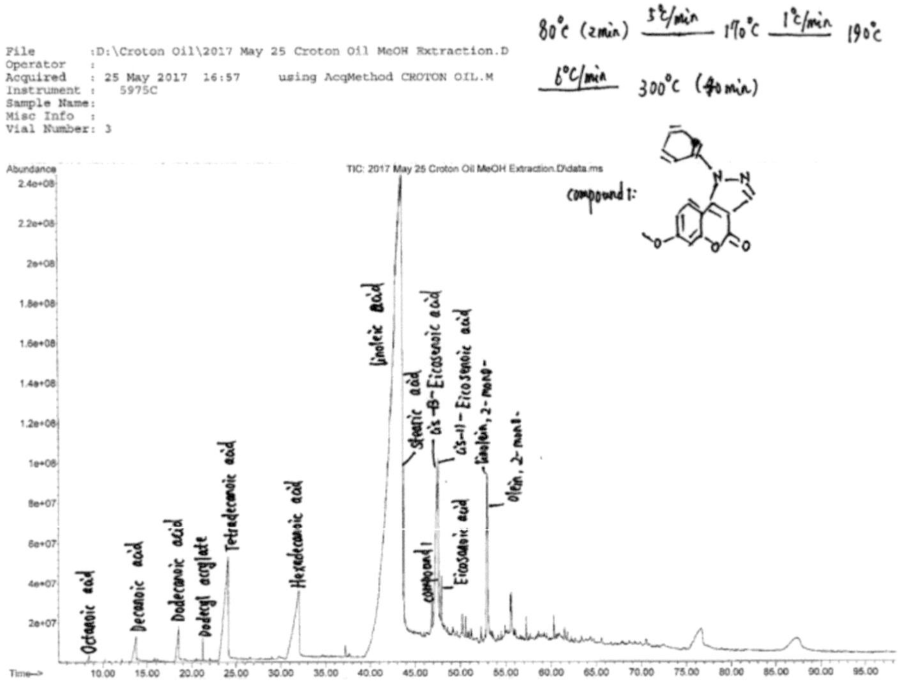

Fig. 3.10 Chemical analysis of the components of croton oil by gas chromatography with methanol extraction. Croton oil is a complex matrix of metabolites present in the seeds of *Croton tiglium*. The major peaks are fatty acids. Compounds such as phorbol esters are found in the smaller peaks. *Source: Personal archive of the author (Dr Carlos Wambier)*

Sources

1. Justo A d S, Lemes BM, Nunes B, et al. Depth of injury of Hetter's phenol-croton oil chemical peel formula using 2 different emulsifying agents. J Am Acad Dermatol. 2020;82(6):1544–6. https://doi.org/10.1016/j.jaad.2020.02.064.
2. Justo AS, Lemes BM, Nunes B, et al. Characterization of the activity of *Croton tiglium* oil in Hetter's very heavy phenol-croton oil chemical peels. Dermatol Surg. 2021; https://doi.org/10.1097/DSS.0000000000002990.
3. Brinkmann V, Reichard U, Goosmann C, et al. Neutrophil extracellular traps kill bacteria. Science. 1979;303(5663):1532–5. https://doi.org/10.1126/science.1092385.
4. Yang H, Biermann MH, Brauner JM, Liu Y, Zhao Y, Herrmann M. New insights into neutrophil extracellular traps: mechanisms of formation and role in inflammation. Front Immunol. 2016;7(AUG):1–8. https://doi.org/10.3389/fimmu.2016.00302.
5. Polliack A. 12-0-Tetradecanoyl Phorbol-13-Acetate (TPA) and its effect on Leukaemic cells, in-vitro—a review. Leuk Lymphoma. 1990;3(3):173–82. https://doi.org/10.3109/10428199009050993.
6. Evans. Naturally occurring phorbol esters. CRC Press; 2018. https://doi.org/10.1201/9781351074940.
7. Goel G, Makkar HPS, Francis G, Becker K. Phorbol esters: structure, biological activity, and toxicity in animals. Int J Toxicol. 26(4):279–88. https://doi.org/10.1080/10915810701464641.

8. Zhang XL, Khan AA, Wang L, Yu K, Li F, Wang MK. Four new phorbol diesters from *Croton tiglium* and their cytotoxic activities. Phytochem Lett. 2016;16:82–6. https://doi.org/10.1016/j.phytol.2016.03.008.
9. Totterman TH, Nilsson K, Sundstrom C. Phorbol ester-induced differentiation of chronic lymphocytic leukaemia cells. Nature. 1980;288(5787):176–8.
10. Majumder PK, Pandey P, Sun X, et al. Mitochondrial translocation of protein kinase C delta in phorbol ester-induced cytochrome c release and apoptosis. J Biol Chem. 2000;275(29):21793–6. https://doi.org/10.1074/jbc.C000048200.
11. Takei H, Araki A, Watanabe H, Ichinose A, Sendo F. Rapid killing of human neutrophils by the potent activator phorbol 12-myristate 13-acetate (PMA) accompanied by changes different from typical apoptosis or necrosis. J Leukoc Biol. 1996;59(2):229–40. https://doi.org/10.1002/jlb.59.2.229.
12. Justo AS, Lemes BM, Nunes B, et al., *Croton tiglium* oil is responsible for the intense inflammation and deep neocollagenesis in Hetter's phenol-croton oil chemical peel. Mendeley Data
13. Capote ACMO, Campos PM, Costa CC, et al. Liquid crystals as a vehicle for *Croton tiglium* L. oil in deep chemical peel formulations. Brazil. Arch. Biol. Technol. 2023;66(spe) https://doi.org/10.1590/1678-4324-ssbfar-2023230034.
14. Paiva ML, Justo AS, Lemes BM, et al. Skin of color repigmentation after phenol-croton oil chemical peel. J Am Acad Dermatol. 2023;89(5):1068–70. https://doi.org/10.1016/j.jaad.2023.06.053.
15. Neitzke IC, de Grande CD, Lin EM, et al. Translational research on the role of formula stability in Hetter's phenol-croton oil peels: Analysis of chemical studies and clinical outcomes from a randomized, double-blinded, split-face controlled trial. J Am Acad Dermatol. 2021;84(3):854–6. https://doi.org/10.1016/j.jaad.2020.10.024.
16. Wambier CG. Segmental phenol-croton oil peels for brow lifting, eyelid tightening, and lip eversion. In: Obagi S, editor. Procedures in cosmetic dermatology series: chemical peels. 3rd ed. Elsevier LTD; 2020. p. 173–82.
17. Bensimon RH. Phenol-croton oil peels. In: Obagi S, editor. Procedures in cosmetic dermatology series: chemical peels. 3rd ed. Elsevier LTD; 2020. p. 81–99.
18. Wambier C, Brown Dermatology Phenol-croton oil Peeling - Standard Operating Procedure v1.1. International Peeling Society. https://www.peelingsociety.com/fileadmin/user_upload/pdf/press/2024/Brown_SOP_Phenol-croton_oil_2023.pdf. Preprint posted online May 7, 2023
19. Wambier CG, Lin E, da Costa Filho ARC, et al. Updates on level of evidence of clinical efficacy of facial phenol-croton oil peels and comments on history and mechanisms of action. Int J Dermatol. 2023;62(7) https://doi.org/10.1111/ijd.16485.
20. Hetter GP. An examination of the phenol-croton oil peel: part IV. Face peel results with different concentrations of phenol and croton oil. Plast Reconstr Surg. 2000;105(3):1061–83.; discussion 1084-7. https://doi.org/10.1097/00006534-200003000-0003.

Systemic Toxicity of Phenol and Croton Oil

4

4.1 Introduction

The phenol-croton oil peel, despite its superior clinical effects in skin rejuvenation, is an intervention involving substances with significant potential for systemic toxicity. Although its application is topical, phenol has a high capacity for transcutaneous absorption, potentially reaching the systemic circulation at dangerous concentrations. *Croton tiglium* oil, even when used in minimal doses, contains extremely potent bioactive compounds such as phorbol esters, with intense and unpredictable pharmacological effects, which also warrant caution.

This chapter aims to discuss in depth the systemic risks of these substances, drawing on a broad base of clinical, toxicological, and experimental evidence. The analysis will be divided into two main sections: the first dedicated to the systemic toxicity of phenol and the second to the toxicity of *Croton tiglium* oil, whose actions are often underestimated. The routes of absorption, target organs, molecular mechanisms involved in adverse effects, the most relevant clinical reports, as well as preventive measures and recommended safety protocols will be addressed.

Given the increasing use of these substances by non-medical professionals and the irregular marketing of ready-made formulations, it is even more urgent to systematize technical and scientific knowledge regarding their risks. The aim of this chapter is to contribute to the conscious, safe, and qualified use of the phenol-croton oil peel, emphasizing that the aesthetic results obtained must never be dissociated from medical responsibility and a thorough understanding of their possible systemic implications.

C. Marçon, C. Wambier, *Phenol-Croton Oil Peel*,
https://doi.org/10.1007/978-3-032-25993-6_4

4.2 Systemic Toxicity of Phenol

4.2.1 Overview of Systemic Toxicity

Reports in the literature regarding phenol toxicity have been documented since the nineteenth century. Numerous publications have highlighted the fatal potential of phenol formulations, whether due to accidental or therapeutic exposures, via cutaneous, intravenous, oral, or inhalational routes. From the 1940s to the present day, publications have addressed the two opposing characteristics of the substance: the excellent effects of cutaneous applications and the serious risks resulting from systemic absorption and toxicity.

Early reports in animal models, such as those by Deichmann et al., point to the severe toxic effects of phenol when absorbed in large quantities, ranging from cardiac alterations to multiple organ failure. Historical accounts such as those by Lucas and Lane described cases of coma following dermal absorption of phenol. In 1922, Turtle and Dolan reported a fatal case in which a bottle containing phenol broke in a young man's pocket during his train journey home. Another case published by Miller in 1942 described an 18-year-old man with mycosis, whose housekeeper applied a mixture of phenol and camphor to his shoulders and trunk, resulting in death within 15 min. In 2016, Giri et al. published a report of four cases of acute phenol poisoning in children in India.

These cases highlighted the multiple routes of absorption of the substance, as well as its complications in multiple organs. The severity of intoxication was more closely correlated with cutaneous exposure than with oral ingestion. The authors concluded that cutaneous exposure can rapidly progress to multiple organ failure, and that severity appeared to vary according to the degree of skin exposure and the time interval to intervention (Fig. 4.1).

Cases of dermal exposure to phenol resulting in lethargy and coma, nausea and vomiting, hypotension, cardiac arrhythmias, seizures, intravascular hemolysis, pulmonary edema, tracheal and bronchial inflammation, acidosis, methemoglobinemia, renal dysfunction, and coma have been reported. The reason why certain organs are preferentially affected over others in different patients remains unclear (Fig. 4.2).

4.2.2 Systemic Risks

4.2.2.1 Central Nervous System

Neurological toxicity from phenol ranges from mild symptoms, such as lethargy, to seizures and coma. Phenol can exert a central narcotic effect, affecting both medullary and higher centers, resulting in rapid loss of consciousness and profound collapse.

Griffiths reported a fatal case involving a 23-year-old man who died within minutes of accidental dermal exposure to phenol, highlighting the risk of severe neurological toxicity. A 1900 publication by Abrahams described the case of a 7-day-old

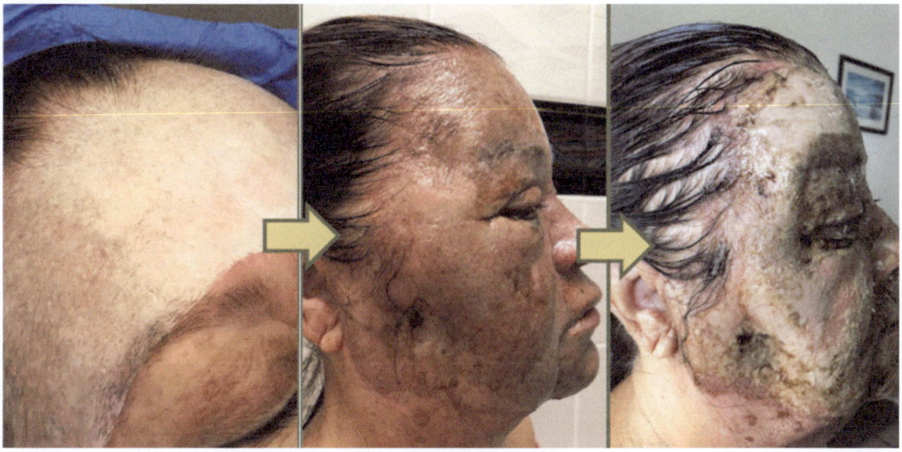

Fig. 4.1 Intense cutaneous inflammation following phenol-croton oil peel. The inflammatory response observed in the skin illustrates the potential for systemic absorption of phenol and its capacity to trigger inflammation in multiple organs, correlating visible skin damage with internal toxic effects. *Source: Author's personal collection (Dr Carolina Marçon)*

infant who was touched in the right inguinal region by a nurse with phenol on her fingers. The child died 10 hours later, developing seizures and coma.

4.2.2.2 Cardiac System

Phenol can exert direct toxicity on the myocardium, causing cardiac arrhythmias, and on blood vessels, causing hypotension. Studies in rats have shown reduced myocardial contraction and electrical activity following systemic exposure to the compound. The most frequent symptoms of phenol-induced cardiotoxicity are: tachycardia, bradycardia, bigeminy, and premature contractions, which may progress to ventricular tachycardia and atrial fibrillation.

Sex, age, previous cardiac history, and blood phenol levels have not been accurate predictors of susceptibility to cardiac arrhythmia during phenol peeling. Several authors agree that absorption and cardiac toxicity are primarily influenced by the extent of skin exposed over a given period—rather than the concentration of the phenol solution—and recommend safety measures such as cardiac monitoring, slow and spaced applications, and forced diuresis. However, some studies have shown that cardiac changes were observed even with slow applications.

A study by Truppman and Ellenby investigated factors associated with the development of cardiac arrhythmias during facial phenol peels, focusing on variables such as procedure duration, size of the treated area, and formulation used. The study demonstrated that peels performed in less than 30 min, with 50% or more of the facial area treated, were highly correlated with the onset of arrhythmias. The use of saponified versus non-saponified formulations did not significantly influence the incidence of arrhythmic events, suggesting that the response is more dependent on the rate of phenol absorption than on individual characteristics or formulation.

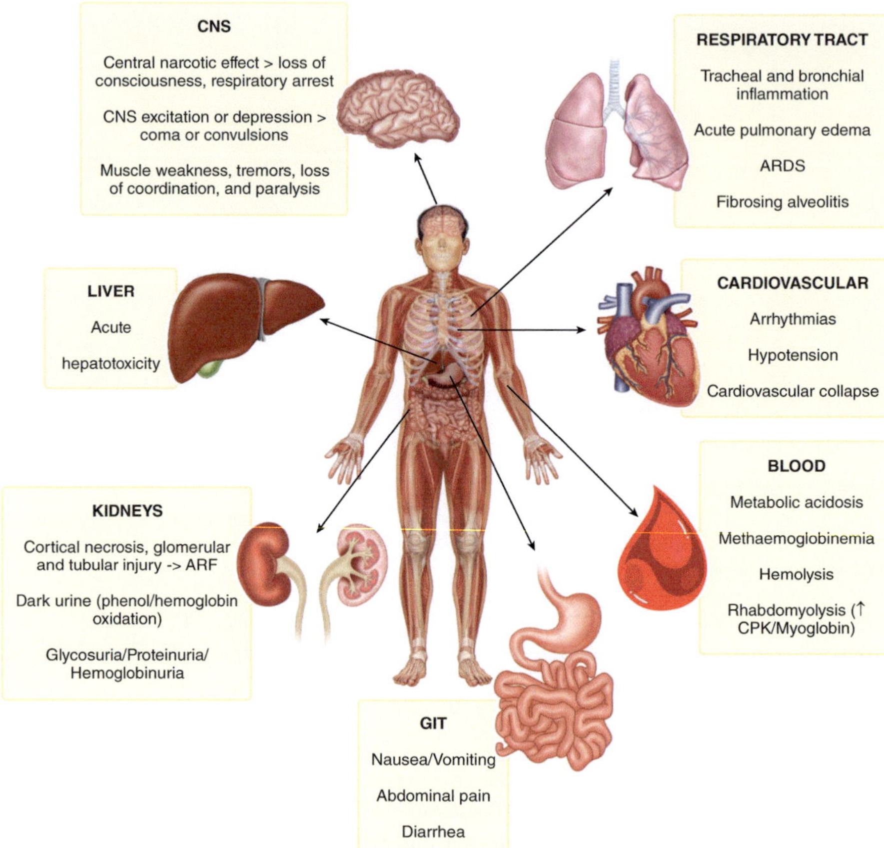

Fig. 4.2 Systemic toxicity of phenol in different organs. In the CNS**,** it may cause loss of consciousness, seizures, paralysis, and respiratory arrest. In the respiratory tract, it induces tracheobronchial inflammation, acute pulmonary edema, and ARDS. In the cardiovascular system**,** it leads to arrhythmias, hypotension, and circulatory collapse. The liver exhibits acute hepatotoxicity, while the **kidneys** undergo cortical necrosis, acute renal failure, and urinary changes. In the **GIT**, nausea, vomiting, abdominal pain, and diarrhea may occur. In the blood, metabolic acidosis, methemoglobinemia, hemolysis, and rhabdomyolysis are observed. *Source: Figure prepared by the author (Dr Carolina Marçon)*

Gross reported that 30% of 54 patients treated rapidly with phenol peels developed some form of cardiac arrhythmia. Gross also noted that there were no predictable results regarding serum phenol levels and the occurrence of cardiac arrhythmia. However, there appeared to be suggestive evidence that segmental facial peeling, at intervals allowing for metabolism and excretion of absorbed phenol, would reduce the risk.

Beeson evaluated 43 consecutive patients who underwent deep peels with phenolic formulations. Ten developed cardiac arrhythmias, including premature ventricular contractions, bigeminy, paroxysmal atrial tachycardia, and ventricular tachycardia, highlighting the need for monitoring to identify and manage these potentially serious complications.

A retrospective study evaluated 181 patients who underwent phenol peeling. Patients were monitored using multiparametric methods throughout the procedure, received potent analgesics, conscious sedation, and intravenous hydration, and the room was adequately ventilated. Cardiac arrhythmia was recorded in 6.6% of patients, being more prevalent in those with diabetes mellitus, hypertension, and depression.

Kadunc and Vanti investigated the systemic toxicity of phenol in facial peels, analyzing 60 women monitored by Holter and Urinary Gas Chromatography (UGC), as well as assessments of renal and hepatic function. The study revealed rapid elimination of phenol, with a half-life of 6–8 h, and no significant changes in renal or hepatic function after 30 days. However, four patients developed sustained ventricular tachycardia, highlighting the risk of cardiac complications. The authors concluded that, although phenol is effective, its use requires strict precautions and continuous monitoring to ensure patient safety.

A recent study by Rullan et al. (2024) assessed the safety of facial phenol peels in 196 patients who underwent multiparametric monitoring during the procedure. Of the participants, 10 (5%) experienced benign and transient arrhythmias: four had premature atrial contractions, two had premature ventricular contractions (one of whom also developed supraventricular tachycardia), and one presented with sinus tachycardia. One patient with initial sinus bradycardia experienced a temporary reduction in oxygen saturation, and three patients developed hypertension during the procedure. The results underscore the importance of intraoperative monitoring to mitigate cardiac and systemic risks associated with phenol use.

Li et al. reported a fatal case of phenol toxicity in a 21-year-old man following an attempt to remove a tattoo using an idiosyncratic method of subcutaneous injection of a "tattoo removal solution" containing phenol at an unknown concentration. The session lasted 3 h, after which he suffered sudden collapse and died within minutes. There were no signs of underlying organ disease that could have contributed to the death. Toxicology revealed the presence of phenol in cardiac blood and liver tissue. Internal examination showed congestion and pulmonary edema. Death was attributed to acute cardiotoxicity induced by phenol.

During the Second World War, phenol was systematically employed by physicians and nurses of the Schutzstaffel (Nazi Protection Corps, a paramilitary organization affiliated with the Nazi Party) as a method of mass murder. In Auschwitz, experiments with intravenous and intracardiac phenol injections were conducted with the aim of finding a rapid and "efficient" means of execution. Intracardiac injections proved particularly lethal and were routinely administered in rooms designated for this purpose (known as Behandlungszimmer, especially in Block 20 of the main camp). This practice was also widely used in Birkenau, where thousands of prisoners were killed by this technique. Chief nurse Josef Klehr, a member of the Schutzstaffel, became notorious for administering lethal phenol injections, often selecting his victims arbitrarily, sometimes merely out of personal dislike. Similarly, physician Friedrich Entress, also of the Schutzstaffel, implemented and systematized the use of intracardiac phenol injections in Auschwitz and Mauthausen, executing up to one hundred prisoners per day, and using the method to conceal the deaths of individuals subjected to failed medical experiments. This practice demonstrates not only the lethal toxicity of phenol but also its instrumentalization in crimes against humanity, revealing one of the darkest uses of this substance in the history of medicine (Fig. 4.3).

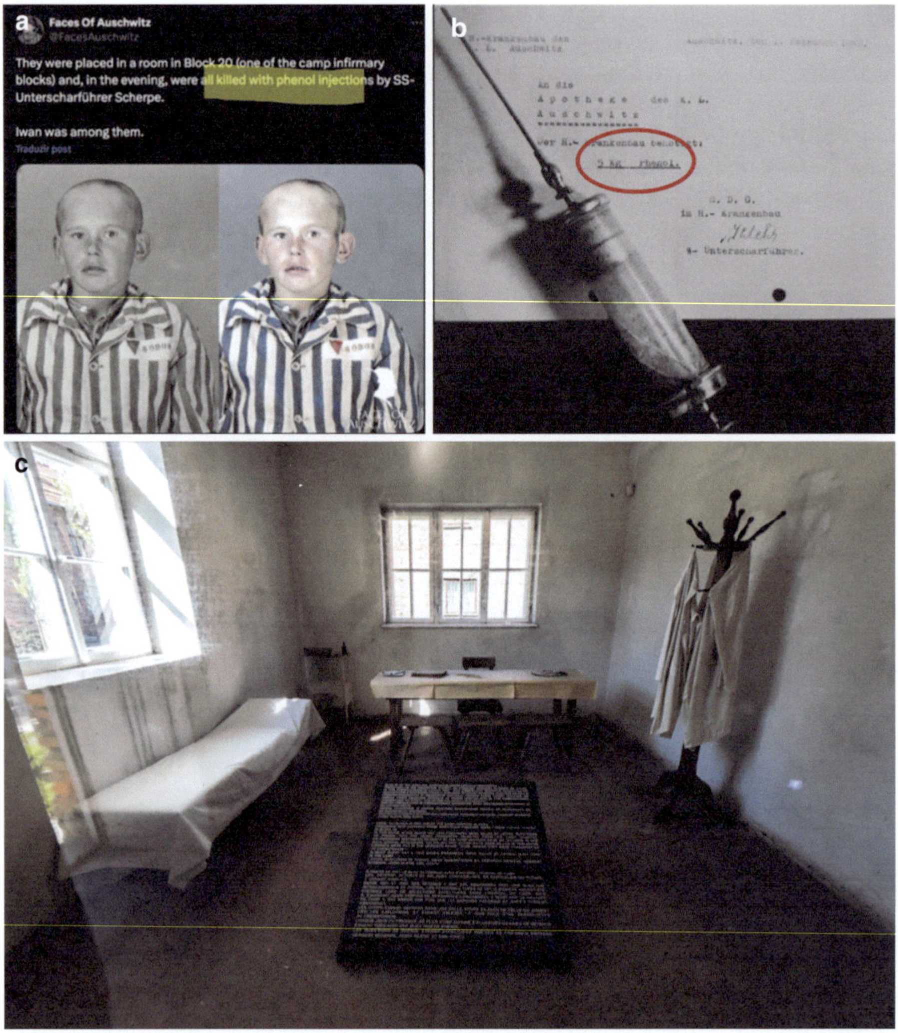

Fig. 4.3 Use of phenol as a method of extermination in Auschwitz during the Second World War. (**a**) Portrait of a child prisoner, victim of a lethal phenol injection in Block 20, administered by members of the Schutzstaffel (*Faces of Auschwitz Project*). (**b**) Syringe used for lethal injections, placed on a document requisitioning phenol for the camp (*Auschwitz-Birkenau Memorial Museum*). (**c**) Room in Block 20, known as the *Behandlungszimmer*, where intracardiac phenol injections were administered to selected prisoners (*Auschwitz-Birkenau Memorial Museum*). *Reproduction authorized by permission*

4.2.2.3 Renal System

The mechanism by which phenol induces renal injury is not clearly understood. Damage to renal tubular epithelial cells by phenol intermediate free radicals, the inability of epithelial cells to generate sufficient reduced glutathione to clear these intermediates, glomerular injury due to excretion of unconjugated phenol, renal ischemia, cast formation due to hemoglobin precipitation, extensive rhabdomyolysis and/or hemoglobinuria due to intravascular hemolysis have all been proposed as possible mechanisms. Seak et al., Foxall et al., and Cohen et al. have documented cases of renal failure in individuals with dermal exposure to phenol.

4.2.2.4 Respiratory System

Inhalation of phenol vapors can cause damage to both the upper and lower airways. In more severe cases, inhalation of high concentrations may lead to glottic edema and acute pulmonary edema, both serious and potentially fatal conditions. These effects are attributed to the corrosive nature of phenol, which damages the epithelial tissue of the airways and can induce a marked inflammatory response.

Laryngeal edema is an extremely rare but potentially serious complication following deep chemical peels with phenol. Klein and Little (1983) reported three cases among 245 patients treated between 1965 and 1975, all female smokers, who developed laryngeal stridor, hoarseness, and tachypnoea within 24 h of the procedure. Symptoms resolved with heated vapor inhalation therapy, without the need for tracheostomy, orotracheal intubation, or permanent sequelae. The authors associated this phenomenon with hypersensitivity in larynges chronically irritated by tobacco. Since the introduction of a prophylactic protocol with diuretics and oral antihistamines, the authors have not observed new episodes in their case series. Early recognition of this condition and appropriate respiratory support are essential to prevent severe outcomes.

Although pulmonary toxicity due to inhalation is more frequently discussed, cutaneous absorption of high concentrations can also lead to respiratory compromise. The systemic distribution of phenol and its inflammatory action on target tissues, such as the lungs, are the main factors responsible for these complications. Reports have documented cases of dermal and oral exposure to phenol associated with acute pulmonary edema and tracheobronchial inflammation. Studies by Fu et al. and Gupta et al. described cases of fibrosing alveolitis and acute respiratory distress syndrome (ARDS) following phenol exposure (Fig. 4.4), highlighting the severity of pulmonary involvement, particularly in the absence of adequate ventilatory support.

A recent fatal case in Brazil, published by Marçon et al. in the Journal of the American Academy of Dermatology (2024), highlighted the extreme risks of improper use of phenol peels by non-medical individuals. A previously healthy 27-year-old man underwent a procedure involving topical anesthetics, microneedling, and subsequent application of an unidentified chemical formula containing phenol, performed by a social media influencer without medical training. The patient developed tremors, profuse sweating, and loss of consciousness in the treatment room, progressing to cardiorespiratory arrest and death. The clinic lacked even basic life support resources. Post-mortem examination revealed extensive chemical necrosis of the face (Fig. 4.5),

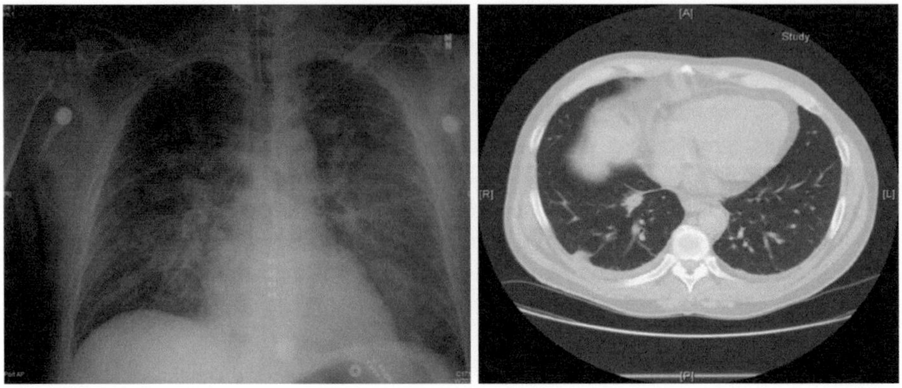

Fig. 4.4 Pulmonary changes following acute injectable phenol intoxication. Chest radiograph (left) performed 30 h after accidental administration of 10 ml of 89% phenol, showing bilateral alveolar opacities. Non-contrast chest computed tomography (right), on the 15th day of hospitalization, demonstrating multiple bilateral nodules in the upper and lower lobes, associated with a small right pleural effusion and a 1 cm peritracheal lymph node, consistent with an inflammatory process secondary to phenolic toxicity. *Source: Reproduced with permission from*: Gupta S, Guha A, Chandra D, Gupta AK, Finkel KW, Guntupalli JS. *Acute phenol poisoning: A life-threatening hazard of chronic pain relief.* Clin Toxicol (Phila). 2008;46 (3):250–253

pulmonary congestion and edema with alveolar hemorrhage, as well as erosions and inflammatory infiltrate in the laryngeal and tracheal mucosa, confirming systemic phenol toxicity. Toxicological analysis identified phenol as the sole substance involved. This case not only underscores the need for strict safety protocols and segmented application with pauses, but also warns of the risks of exacerbated systemic absorption due to inappropriate techniques such as prior microneedling. The fatality led to the prohibition of phenol in Brazil, emphasizing the urgency of regulation and medical education regarding the responsible use of this potent substance, whose benefits can only be achieved under specialist supervision.

Phenol-induced pulmonary toxicity can be particularly severe when associated with oral ingestion, as demonstrated in the case of a 28-year-old male patient who attempted suicide with 5% household phenol (phenyl). The clinical course rapidly progressed with dysphagia, dysarthria, hypotension, tachypnoea, and miosis, culminating in death 5 h after admission. Autopsy revealed extensive corrosion of the oropharyngeal and gastrointestinal mucosa, coagulative necrosis of internal organs, cerebral and renal edema, and acute pulmonary edema with diffuse congestion, corroborating phenol's capacity to trigger systemic corrosive inflammation and multiorgan failure. These findings reinforce that, in addition to cutaneous absorption, the oral route can precipitate fulminant pulmonary compromise, with a lethal outcome within hours.

4.2.2.5 Hepatic System

Phenol can induce acute hepatotoxicity due to the accumulation of toxic metabolites in the liver, which generate oxidative stress and mitochondrial dysfunction, leading to cellular necrosis. Manifestations such as elevated liver enzymes, jaundice, and, in

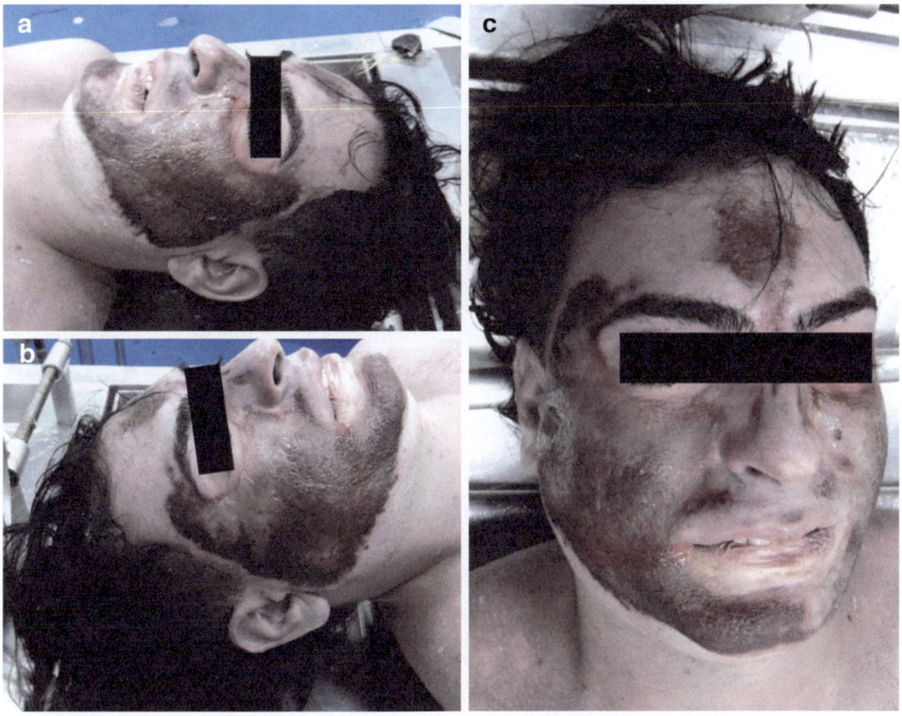

Fig. 4.5 Post-mortem images showing black necrotic eschar with clear demarcation in the malar, temporal, mental, and mid-forehead regions, consistent with high-concentration phenol exposure. Lighter areas of necrosis are observed in the perioral, nasal, malar, and lateral forehead regions. (**a**) Left lateral view. (**b**) Right Lateral view. (**c**) Near-frontal view, slightly angled to the right. *Source: Marçon CR* et al. *Fatal Phenol Peel by an Unlicensed Social Media Practitioner: A Forensic Medical Analysis. J Am Acad Dermatol.* 2025 Aug 5:S0190-9622(25)02555-1. *Reproduced with permission from the publisher*

severe cases, hepatic failure may occur, necessitating cautious use in therapeutic contexts.

4.2.2.6 Hematopoietic System

Cases of methemoglobinemia and intravascular hemolysis due to phenol exposure, in which oxygen transport was compromised, resulting in hypoxia and acidosis, have been described. These are severe conditions that require prompt identification and intervention.

4.2.3 What Is the Safe Dose of Phenol for Dermatological Use?

Although the literature lacks precise data on safe doses for cutaneous absorption of phenol, several studies demonstrate that its toxicity is considerable at the concentrations and volumes commonly used in dermatological procedures such as phenol-croton oil peels. Toxicological literature provides a range for the median lethal dose (LD50) of phenol in humans, varying from 50 to 500 mg/kg body weight, resulting in an estimated dose of 3.5–35 g for a 70 kg individual.

In validated preparations for deep peels, such as Hetter's formula, 10 ml contains approximately 3.5 g of phenol, while Baker's formula contains about 4.9 g of phenol in 10 ml, and an 88% phenol solution contains 8.8 g in 10 ml. Considering that up to 70% of topically applied phenol may be absorbed within 30 min, the absorbed amounts would approach lethal doses: 2.45 g, 3.4 g, and 6.6 g in 10 ml, respectively (Table 4.1).

The presence of ingredients such as croton oil and other additives commonly found in irregularly marketed ready-made formulations, such as olive oil, cresol, sodium salicylate, camphor, glycerin, and soaps, among others, may potentially increase the cutaneous penetration of phenol, exacerbating the risks of systemic toxicity. The total volume of phenol, application methods, and types of dressing are not standardized, representing an additional risk, especially when the procedure is performed by non-medical professionals.

4.2.4 Safety in Procedures with Phenol

The safe management of phenol requires strict protocols, including multiparametric monitoring, adequate room ventilation, and segmented application techniques. Recent studies, such as that by Rullan et al. (2024), indicate that complications are rare in settings with continuous monitoring and careful application. Other studies, such as that by Landau, demonstrate that factors such as intervals between applications and administration of intravenous hydration are key to minimizing the risk of adverse events, especially in patients with comorbidities.

Toxicity is closely related to the rate of excretion, area of application, and duration of phenol solution application. Various organs of the body, including the heart, apparently can tolerate very low levels of phenol in the blood for short periods of

Table 4.1 Estimated phenol toxicity in different formulations used in chemical peels

Formulation/ concentration	Phenol in 10 mL (g)	Phenol absorbed (70% in 30 min) (g)	Remarks
Human LD_{50} (literature)	3.5–35 g (70 kg)	–	Reported median lethal dose range in humans (50–500 mg/kg)
Hetter (approx. 35%)	3.5 g	2.45 g	Lower range close to minimum lethal dose
Baker (approx. 49%)	4.9 g	3.4 g	Reaches critical toxicity threshold
Phenol 88%	8.8 g	6.6 g	Above the estimated safety limit

Estimates based on average values for cutaneous absorption (70% within 30 min) and the median lethal dose (LD_{50}) of phenol in humans (50–500 mg/kg). The proximity between the absorbed amounts and the toxicity range described in the literature reinforces the potential risk of dermatological formulations when not used under strictly controlled conditions. *Source: Table prepared by the author (Dr Carolina Marçon)* time. It therefore seems essential not to allow phenol absorption into the bloodstream to occur more rapidly than natural processes can eliminate it.

4.2.5 Final Considerations

Given the potential for systemic toxicity of phenol, even when used topically, it is essential to adopt rigorous control and safety measures during dermatological procedures involving this substance. Although the literature shows that serious complications are rare when appropriate protocols are followed, the margin between therapeutic efficacy and toxicity is narrow. For this reason, the use of phenol requires in-depth technical knowledge, a controlled environment, and continuous monitoring. Specific recommendations regarding safe application strategies, clinical monitoring, formulation preparation, and management of complications will be detailed in a dedicated chapter of this book, exclusively addressing Good Practices and Safety Protocols for the Use of Phenol.

4.3 Systemic Toxicity of Croton Oil

4.3.1 Historical and Ethnopharmacological Introduction to *Croton tiglium*

Croton tiglium is a plant belonging to the Euphorbiaceae family, native to tropical regions of Asia, especially India, China, Indonesia, the Philippines, and New Guinea. Cultivated to a lesser extent as an ornamental plant in southern California and other tropical and subtropical regions, the species is widely recognized for its potent and controversial phytochemical profile.

In traditional Chinese medicine, it is known as ba dou (巴豆), and has been used for millennia as a drastic purgative, employed to expel phlegm, eliminate abdominal accumulations, and relieve severe intestinal obstructions. In Indian Ayurvedic medicine, the oil from its seeds, known as Jamal gota or kuchila taila, is mentioned in ancient texts as a purgative and antispasmodic substance, although its internal use was restricted to specific situations due to its potency and toxicity.

Throughout history, the use of *Croton tiglium* has been associated with ritual practices, purification, and the treatment of diseases which, in the absence of modern pharmacological resources, required intense physiological effects. However, due to its high toxic potential, both traditional systems and modern phytotherapy have always emphasized the need for purification of the seed (shodhana), a procedure intended to reduce its adverse effects prior to medicinal use.

In Asian ethnopharmacological compendia and herbals, references can be found to the use of Croton oil not only orally, but also topically, in cases of mycoses, infections, rheumatic pain, and dermatological disorders. Nevertheless, its topical use was also approached with caution, especially on mucous membranes or large areas of skin, given its tendency to cause severe irritation and systemic effects.

In the West, the first botanical and medical records date from the seventeenth and eighteenth centuries, when explorers and naturalist physicians reported the drastic properties of Croton oil as a violent purgative, sometimes referred to as "hell's oil." During the nineteenth century, its use was incorporated into some allopathic formulas for the relief of severe constipation, always with warnings regarding dosage and route of administration (Table 4.2).

The genus name Croton derives from the Greek krotón, meaning "tick," in reference to the rounded, dark shape of the seeds (Fig. 4.6). Despite its therapeutic potential, the plant's notoriety has always been accompanied by warnings regarding its complex toxicological profile, especially when administered without technical preparation or in empirical contexts.

This duality between therapeutic potency and toxicological risk has accompanied the history of *Croton tiglium*, which straddles the fields of pharmacognosy and toxicology, requiring particular caution in any modern therapeutic application, including contemporary dermatological formulations.

4.3.2 Chemical Composition and Bioactive Constituents of *Croton tiglium*

The seeds of *Croton tiglium* constitute a highly complex and biologically active phytochemical reservoir, recognized both for their therapeutic effects and for the risk of severe toxicity. The oil extracted from these seeds contains various

Table 4.2 Historical use of *Croton tiglium* in different traditions

Medical system/ region	Traditional name	Route of administration	Main indication	Reported risks
Traditional Chinese medicine	Ba dou (巴豆)	Oral and topical	Powerful purgative; expels phlegm; treats intestinal obstruction	Severe gastrointestinal irritation; systemic toxicity
Ayurvedic medicine (India)	Jamal gota; Kuchila taila	Oral and topical	Severe constipation; antispasmodic; ritual use	Vomiting, intense diarrhea, risk of cardiovascular collapse
Persian/Arab medicine	Croton oil	Oral	Purgative in severe cases of constipation and hepatic congestion	Gastroenteritis, intestinal hemorrhage, fatality at high doses
Modern Asian phytotherapy	Croton oil (purified)	Topical	Skin infections, mycoses, rheumatic pain	Contact dermatitis, dermal necrosis, systemic absorption
Western medicine (17th–19th centuries)	Croton oil	Oral	Violent purgative in allopathic formulas for constipation	Profuse diarrhea, dehydration, circulatory collapse

The use of *Croton tiglium* has historically been characterized by its intense purgative action, associated with a high risk of toxicity. All medical traditions emphasized the need for caution, seed purification, and strict dose limitation. *Source: Table prepared by the author (Dr Carolina Marçon)*

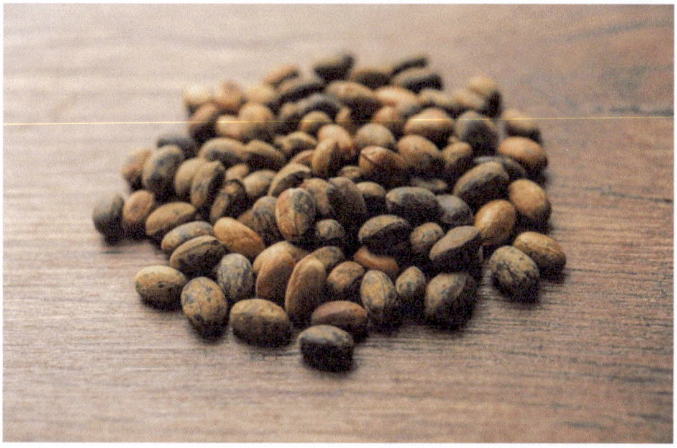

Fig. 4.6 Seeds of *Croton tiglium* (jamalgota), with a shape reminiscent of a "tick" (*Croton* in Greek). *Source:* Creative Commons Attribution-ShareAlike 4.0 International (CC BY-SA 4.0) license, available at Wikimedia Commons

compounds with relevant pharmacological properties, among which phorbol esters, phenolic compounds, bioactive proteins, and other secondary metabolites are noteworthy.

4.3.2.1 Diterpenes and Phorbol Esters

The main group of compounds responsible for the pharmacological and toxic effects of *Croton tiglium* is tigliane-type diterpenes, especially the phorbol esters. Among these, phorbol 12-myristate 13-acetate (PMA), also known as TPA (12-O-tetradecanoylphorbol-13-acetate), stands out as one of the most potent activators of the enzyme protein kinase C (PKC). Activation of PKC by these esters triggers complex intracellular cascades, with implications for processes such as cell proliferation, inflammation, apoptosis, and tumor promotion, depending on the physiological context and dose employed (Fig. 4.7).

Phorbol esters are widely used as tools in experimental models of tumorigenesis, due to their ability to promote uncontrolled cellular growth following exposure to initiating agents. Its lipophilic structure facilitates high penetration into biological membranes and intense interaction with intracellular targets, which accounts for its potent biological activity even at very low concentrations.

4.3.2.2 Phenolic Compounds, Tannins, and Flavonoids

Phytochemical analyses have shown that the oil of *Croton tiglium* also contains phenolic compounds, including flavonoids, tannins, and lignins, with potential antioxidant, anti-inflammatory, and antimicrobial effects. These components are recognized for their ability to modulate reactive oxygen species and interfere with pro-inflammatory signaling pathways. However, their actions do not neutralize the cytotoxic effects of diterpenes, especially when applied to mucous membranes or intact skin, highlighting the need for highly controlled formulations.

4.3.2.3 Bioactive Proteins

More recent studies, such as that by Shahid et al. (2008), have revealed the presence of a bioactive protein of approximately 50 kDa, isolated from the seeds of the plant, with strong antifungal and antibacterial activity. Designated Ct-50, this protein

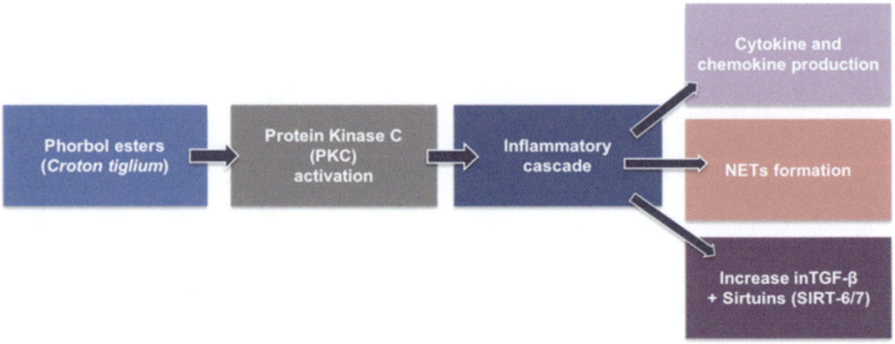

Fig. 4.7 Simplified diagram of the mechanism of action of phorbol esters present in *Croton tiglium*. These diterpenes activate protein kinase C (PKC), triggering inflammatory cascades that result in the production of cytokines and chemokines, formation of neutrophil extracellular traps (NETs), and stimulation of TGF-β and the sirtuins SIRT-6 and SIRT-7 expression. *Source: Figure prepared by the author (Dr Carolina Marçon)*

demonstrated inhibitory effects against strains such as *Bacillus subtilis, Pasteurella multocida, Mucor mucedo, and Aspergillus niger*, representing one of the first systematic reports of protein-based antimicrobial activity in *Croton tiglium*. Its purification involved successive steps of:

- Ammonium sulphate precipitation [$(NH_4)_2SO_4$].
- Gel filtration chromatography (Sephadex G-100 column), which separates proteins based on molecular size.
- Ion-exchange chromatography (DEAE-cellulose resin—diethylaminoethyl-cellulose), which separates proteins by electric charge.

The identity and purity of Ct-50 were confirmed by polyacrylamide gel electrophoresis in the presence of sodium dodecyl sulfate (SDS-PAGE), a technique that demonstrated a single band corresponding to a molecular mass of 50 kDa. Despite its promising in vitro activity, the absence of clinical trials in humans and the complexity of extraction and purification currently preclude its therapeutic use in conventional formulations.

4.3.2.4 Other Constituents

In addition to the aforementioned compounds, the oil of *Croton tiglium* contains unsaturated fatty acids, triterpenes, alkaloids, resins, volatile oils, and various enzymes, all of which contribute to its irritant and pharmacological profile. Toxicological studies have also identified mutagenic and genotoxic substances in crude extracts, further emphasizing the need for caution in the clinical use and handling of this plant. The presence of these substances also imposes important ethical and regulatory restrictions in the context of modern medical dermatology (Table 4.3).

Table 4.3 Main chemical and bioactive constituents of *Croton tiglium* and their effects

Chemical group	Example/compound	Pharmacological effect	Toxic effect
Diterpenes (phorbol esters)	12-O-tetradecanoylphorbol-13-acetate (TPA/PMA)	PKC activation; stimulation of cellular proliferation; inflammatory modulation	Tumor promotion; exacerbated inflammation; tissue necrosis
Phenolic compounds (flavonoids, tannins, lignins)	Flavonoids; condensed tannins	Antioxidant; anti-inflammatory; antimicrobial	Do not neutralize the toxic effects of diterpenes; risk of local irritation
Bioactive proteins	Ct-50 (≈ 50 kDa)	Antifungal and antibacterial activity (B. subtilis, P. multocida, A. niger, M. mucedo)	No clinical studies; immunogenic potential; risk of unassessed toxicity
Unsaturated fatty acids, resins, alkaloids, and triterpenes	Various (oleic, volatile, triterpenic)	Irritant profile; possible anti-inflammatory activity in related species	Dermatitis, cutaneous necrosis, hepatic and hematological toxicity in crude extracts

The constituents of *Croton tiglium* exhibit relevant pharmacological activities, but their clinical use is limited by toxicity, particularly that of phorbol-type diterpenes, which are responsible for the main adverse effects. *Source: Table prepared by the author (Dr Carolina Marçon)*

4.3.3 Pharmacological Effects Described in the Literature

Croton tiglium, although notorious for its toxicity, has a long history of use in traditional Indian (Ayurvedic), Chinese, and Persian medicine. Historically employed as a purgative, antispasmodic, and antimicrobial, its broad spectrum of pharmacological activities has been empirically explored for centuries. With advances in modern pharmacology, many of these effects have been experimentally confirmed, while others have revealed significant risks to human health. The available scientific data demonstrate a duality between therapeutic potential and severe toxicity, with the context of use (dose, route of administration, and formulation) being the main determinant of benefit versus risk.

4.3.3.1 Purgative and Gastrointestinal Irritant Action

The most traditional use of *Croton tiglium* oil was as a drastic purgative, due to the caustic action of its diterpenes, especially phorbol esters. Ingestion of the oil causes intense irritation of the gastrointestinal mucosa, leading to violent diarrhea, and it was traditionally used to treat severe constipation, hepatic congestion, and parasitic infections. However, the risks of intestinal perforation, dehydration, and cardiovascular collapse have rendered its oral use absolutely contraindicated in modern medicine.

4.3.3.2 Antimicrobial and Antifungal Activity

Laboratory studies have confirmed antimicrobial effects of *Croton tiglium* constituents, such as the protein Ct-50, isolated by Shahid et al. (2008), which showed significant activity against Bacillus subtilis, Pasteurella multocida, Aspergillus niger, and Mucor mucedo. This action supports the ethnomedicinal topical use of the oil in cutaneous infections and parasitic diseases. However, clinical application remains limited due to the risk of irritation, tissue necrosis, and systemic toxicity, especially when applied to mucous membranes or intact skin.

4.3.3.3 Immunomodulatory and Pro-inflammatory Effect

Phorbol esters, particularly 12-O-tetradecanoylphorbol-13-acetate (TPA) , are potent activators of the enzyme protein kinase C (PKC), triggering broad immune responses. This activation stimulates the release of cytokines, prostaglandins, and chemokines, promotes the formation of NETs (Neutrophil Extracellular Traps), and influences the expression of TGF-β and sirtuins, especially SIRT-6 and SIRT-7, as discussed in Chap. 2 of this book. Although this effect is explored in experimental models of inflammation, wound healing, and dermal modulation, the same mechanism can induce exacerbated inflammatory responses, edema, and tissue injury, and has also been implicated in tumor promotion in co-carcinogenesis studies.

4.3.3.4 Cytotoxic and Antiproliferative Activities

Croton tiglium has also been studied for its cytotoxic and antiproliferative effects, attributed to phorbol esters. In vitro assays have demonstrated inhibition of proliferation in tumor cell lines, indicating potential application in experimental oncology. However, the lack of selectivity and high toxicity currently preclude its therapeutic use in humans, and further structural refinement of these compounds is required to separate their desirable effects from their deleterious properties.

4.3.3.5 Antioxidant and Anti-inflammatory Properties in Other Croton Species

Although *Croton tiglium* is more closely associated with irritant and pro-inflammatory effects, other species of the same genus have demonstrated significant antioxidant and anti-inflammatory properties. *Croton lechleri* (known as "dragon's blood") and *Croton celtidifolius*, for example, have distinct phytochemical profiles, rich in proanthocyanidins and phenolic compounds with therapeutic potential in inflammatory and infectious processes. Such differences among Croton species highlight the importance of specific phytochemical characterization and controlled scientific use.

4.3.3.6 Considerations Regarding Dermatological Use

Several pharmacological effects of *Croton tiglium* are also observed in the dermatological context, particularly when its derivatives are applied topically in strictly calibrated concentrations. Modern formulations of phenol-croton oil peels, for example, exploit the controlled effects of phorbol esters on the epidermis and papillary dermis, inducing tissue remodeling, increased production of collagen and skin restructuring (Fig. 4.8). Nevertheless, such benefits are contingent upon correct handling of the substance, safe concentration, and exclusive medical administration.

The therapeutic potential of *Croton tiglium*, therefore, should not be dismissed, but must be carefully defined due to its narrow safety margin. Empirical use, improper handling, and extrapolation of in vitro data without adequate clinical validation pose significant risks, particularly when dealing with substances of such potent pharmacodynamic action.

4.3.4 Systemic Toxicity and Reports of Adverse Events

Croton tiglium is widely recognized as a highly toxic medicinal plant, with both historical and contemporary records of severe adverse effects in experimental models and humans. The primary agents responsible for its toxicity are phorbol esters, especially 12-O-tetradecanoylphorbol-13-acetate (PMA), which induce excessive activation of protein kinase C (PKC), triggering systemic inflammatory cascades and marked cytotoxicity.

Historically, oil extracted from the seeds—known as croton oil—was used in traditional medicine as a drastic purgative, but ingestion is associated with a range of potentially fatal adverse effects. Documented symptoms include nausea, vomiting, abdominal pain, profuse diarrhea, hemorrhagic colitis, hepatotoxicity, tremors, lethargy, headache, mental confusion, cardiovascular collapse, and death. Digestive toxicity is exacerbated by intestinal necrosis, hemolysis, and possible acute hepatic dysfunction.

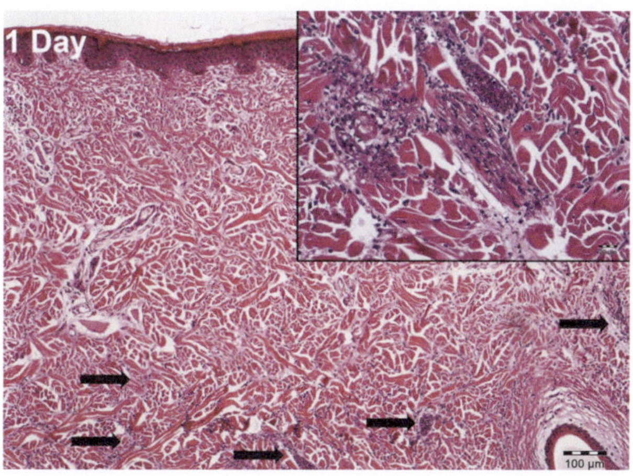

Fig. 4.8 First postoperative day following 35% phenol peel combined with 1.6% croton oil (Hetter's formula—*very heavy peel*). Notable findings include edema, deep coagulative necrosis, vascular ectasia, and a pronounced pericoagulative neutrophilic inflammatory band (black arrows). Inset: magnified detail showing neutrophilic infiltrate. Hematoxylin–eosin, ×100; inset ×400. *Source: Courtesy of Dr Aline Justo, Dr Flavio Beltrame, and Dr Carlos Wambier*

Toxicological studies have shown that oral administration of the oil causes hemorrhagic gastroenteritis, hepatic necrosis, neurological dysfunction, and hematological changes. Cutaneous exposure to high concentrations, or even accidental inhalation, may provoke systemic manifestations such as fever, tachycardia, chest pain, and hepatic alterations, even in the absence of ingestion. Cases of chemical dermatitis, burns, and systemic symptoms have been reported among professionals exposed to crude oil, particularly in settings lacking adequate protective measures.

Animal studies corroborate these findings. In research conducted by Justo et al. (2021), topical application of *Croton tiglium* oil at concentrations equivalent to Hetter's formula induced a marked cutaneous inflammatory response, with epidermal thickening, acanthosis, and increased fibroblast density. In the group treated with isolated croton oil (without phenol), focal necrosis of the deep reticular dermis was observed, indicating that dermal toxicity is dose-dependent and may compromise deeper skin structures. Despite the intensity of the local response, no histological changes were detected in the lungs, kidneys, liver, or heart of the animals, suggesting an absence of measurable systemic toxicity at the topical concentrations tested.

In humans, however, the scenario is more severe. Oral use, even in small doses, can trigger acute severe intoxication, with historical reports of death following ingestion of only a few drops of the oil. This severity led to the adoption of specific purification rituals in Eastern medical traditions, such as shodhana, described in Ayurvedic literature, which aims to reduce toxicity prior to any therapeutic use. In an experimental study, Pal et al. (2014) demonstrated that traditional Ayurvedic processing significantly reduces the toxicity of extracts, although it does not completely eliminate the risks.

From a toxicological perspective, the irritant potency of phorbol esters is considered equivalent to or greater than that of crotonaldehyde or mustard oil, compounds known for their ability to induce edema and necrosis in skin tests. This potency explains why use should be restricted to qualified professionals, with strict control over dosage, formulation, and route of administration.

Improper handling of croton oil, its seeds, or formulations containing its extracts poses a significant risk. Variability in chemical composition between different batches, combined with the lack of pharmacological standardization and the extreme potency of the active components, renders empirical use potentially dangerous. Even with topical use, percutaneous absorption over extensive or damaged areas may result in undesirable systemic effects.

Thus, although *Croton tiglium* contains bioactive principles with documented pharmacological applications, its clinical use requires stringent safety criteria, specialized knowledge, and standardized protocols, particularly in dermatological formulations (Table 4.4).

Table 4.4 Pharmacological effects of *Croton tiglium* in contrast with its toxic risks

Desired/pharmacological effect	Mechanism of action	Associated toxic risk
Gastrointestinal purgative action	Mucosal irritation by phorbol esters; increased intestinal motility	Severe diarrhea, hemorrhagic colitis, intestinal perforation, cardiovascular collapse
Antimicrobial/antifungal activity	Bioactive protein Ct-50 with effect against bacteria and fungi	Potential tissue irritation, lack of clinical studies in humans
Immunomodulation/ controlled inflammation	PKC activation; release of cytokines, NETs, TGF-β, SIRT-6/7	Exacerbated inflammatory response, edema, tissue necrosis, tumor promotion
Dermal remodeling in peels	Phorbol esters stimulate fibroblasts and collagen synthesis	Risk of deep dermal necrosis, chemical dermatitis, and systemic absorption
Cytotoxic and antiproliferative activity (in vitro)	Phorbol esters inhibit cell growth in tumor cell lines	High toxicity without selectivity; precludes therapeutic use in humans
Antioxidant effect (in related Croton species)	Flavonoids and tannins neutralize reactive oxygen species	In *Croton tiglium*, these effects do not appear to offset the toxicity associated with diterpenes

The duality between pharmacological effects and toxic risks of *Croton tiglium* highlights its narrow safety margin. The context of use (dose, route of administration, and formulation) is the main determinant between benefit and harm. *Source: Table prepared by the author (Dr Carolina Marçon)*

4.4 Final Considerations

The use of *Croton tiglium* oil in modern dermatology, particularly in deep peels, illustrates the fine line between clinical benefit and toxicological risk. Although advances in contemporary formulations, such as those by Hetter, have enabled safer and more effective application of the compound in combination with phenol, it is essential to recognize that its handling requires medical expertise, a controlled environment, and in-depth knowledge of its pharmacology and toxicity.

The increasing availability of croton-containing formulations in non-medical settings or with ingredients of dubious origin poses a real threat to patient safety. The lack of standardization in phorbol ester concentration, combined with individual response variability and lack of monitoring, can result in serious adverse reactions, both local and systemic (Box 4.1).

Box 4.1. Main Risks of Croton Oil

Narrow therapeutic margin—small dose variations shift from pharmacological action to toxicity.

Variable composition—phorbol ester concentration differs between batches, with no standardization.

High irritant potency—risk of chemical dermatitis, dermal necrosis, and systemic absorption.

Multisystem toxicity—reports of hemorrhagic gastroenteritis, hepatotoxicity, and cardiovascular collapse.

History of fatalities—ingestion of only a few drops has been associated with deaths in traditional records.

Although it contains bioactive principles of pharmacological interest, the oil of *Croton tiglium* presents serious risks when used without proper preparation and medical supervision. *Source: Box prepared by the author (Dr Carolina Marçon)*

For this reason, it is recommended that the use of croton oil be restricted exclusively to qualified medical professionals, with appropriate training, using validated formulations, in strictly controlled doses, and with adequate monitoring throughout the procedure. Procurement of the substance should comply with pharmaceutical quality standards, with certificates of composition and purity, avoiding crude extracts, homemade preparations, or uncontrolled mixtures.

The history of *Croton tiglium* demonstrates that its use demands respect, knowledge, and responsibility. In qualified hands, it can be a powerful therapeutic tool. Outside this context, it remains a potentially hazardous substance, the indiscriminate use of which poses a serious risk to public health.

Sources

1. Deichmann WB. Local and systemic effects following skin contact with phenol; a review of the literature. J Ind Hyg Toxicol. 1949;31:146–54.
2. Rullan P, Lin EM, Schaut E, Wambier CG. Cardiac safety in full-face phenol-croton oil peels: A 22-year retrospective study. J Am Acad Dermatol. 2024;91:762–3.
3. Deichmann WB, Miller T, Roberts JB. Local and systemic effects following application of dilute solutions of phenol in water and in camphor-liquid petrolatum on the skin of animals. AMA Arch Ind Hyg Occup Med. 1950;2:454–61.
4. Lucas RC, Lane WA. Two cases of carbolic acid coma induced by the application of carbolic compresses to the skin. Lancet. 1895;145:1362–4.
5. Turtle WRM, Dolan T. A case of rapid and fatal absorption of carbolic acid through the skin. Lancet. 1922;200:1273–4.
6. Miller FG. Poisoning by phenol. Can Med Assoc J. 1942;46:615–6.
7. Giri PP, Sinha R, Sikka S, Meur S. Acute carbolic acid poisoning: a report of four cases. Indian J Crit Care Med. 2016;20:668–70.
8. Cohen N, Modai D, Khahil A, Golik A. Acute resin phenol-formaldehyde intoxication. A life-threatening occupational hazard. Hum Toxicol. 1989;8:247–50.
9. Hassan AB, Seligmann H, Bassan HM. Intravascular hemolysis induced by pentachlorophenol. Br Med J (Clin Res Ed). 1985;291:21–2.

10. Todorović V. Acute phenol poisoning. Med Pregl. 2003;56:37–41.
11. Lewin JF, Cleary WT. An accidental death caused by the absorption of phenol through skin. A case report. Forensic Sci Int. 1982;19:177–9.
12. Griffiths GJ. Fatal acute poisoning by intradermal absorption of phenol. Med Sci Law. 1973;13:46–8.
13. Abrahams R. A fatal case of carbolic acid poisoning in an infant, due to absorption by the skin. Pediatrics. 1900;9:241–2.
14. Litton C. Observations after chemosurgery of the face. Plast Reconstr Surg. 1963;32:554–6.
15. Stagnone GJ, Orgel MG, Stagnone JJ. Cardiovascular effects of topical 50% trichloroacetic acid and Baker's phenol solution. J Dermatol Surg Oncol. 1987;13:999–1002.
16. Truppman ES, Ellenby JD. Major electrocardiographic changes during chemical face peeling. Plast Reconstr Surg. 1979;63:44–8.
17. Gross BG. Cardiac arrhythmias during phenol face peeling. Plast Reconstr Surg. 1984;73:590–4.
18. Matarasso SL. Phenol chemical peels. In: Wheeland RG, editor. Cutaneous surgery. 1st ed. Saunders; 1994. p. 491–508.
19. Wexler MR, Halon DA, Teitelbaum A, Tadjer G, Peled IJ. The prevention of cardiac arrhythmias produced in an animal model by the topical application of a phenol preparation in common use for face peeling. Plast Reconstr Surg. 1984;73:595–8.
20. Beeson WH. The importance of cardiac monitoring in superficial and deep chemical peeling. J Dermatol Surg Oncol. 1987;13:949–50.
21. Li Z, Zhang H, Li SH, Byard RW. Fatal phenol toxicity following attempted tattoo removal. J Forensic Sci. 2016;61:1143–5.
22. Seak CK, Lin CC, Seak CJ, Hsu TY, Chang CC. A case of black urine and dark skin - cresol poisoning. Clin Toxicol (Phila). 2010;48:959–60.
23. Foxall PJ, Bending MR, Gartland KP, Nicholson JK. Acute renal failure following accidental cutaneous absorption of phenol: application of NMR urinalysis to monitor the disease process. Hum Toxicol. 1989;8:491–6.
24. Rodgers GC, editor. Ellenhorn's medical toxicology: diagnosis and treatment of human poisoning. 2nd ed. Baltimore: Williams & Wilkins; 1997.
25. Soares ER, Tift JP. Phenol poisoning: three fatal cases. J Forensic Sci. 1982;27:729–31.
26. Fu HS, Chu YK, Liao SQ, Liu RS. Scintigraphic appearance in Lysol-induced lung toxicity. Clin Nucl Med. 2001;26:655–6.
27. Gupta S, Ashrith G, Chandra D, Gupta AK, Finkel KW, Guntupalli JS. Acute phenol poisoning: a life-threatening hazard of chronic pain relief. Clin Toxicol (Phila). 2008;46:250–3.
28. Ghosh S. Self-injection of intravenous carbolic acid and multiorgan failure. Indian J Crit Care Med. 2014;18:43–5.
29. Rendon MI, Berson DS, Cohen JL, Roberts WE, Starker I, Wang B. Evidence and considerations in the application of chemical peels in skin disorders and aesthetic resurfacing. J Clin Aesthet Dermatol. 2010;3:32–43.
30. Wambier C, [Internet]. Brown Dermatology Phenol-croton oil Peeling - Standard Operating Procedure v1.1; 2023 [cited 2024 Oct 15]. Available from: https://www.peelingsociety.com/fileadmin/user_upload/pdf/press/2024/Brown_SOP_Phenol-croton_oil_2023.pdf
31. Bruce RM, Santodonato J, Neal MW. Summary review of the health effects associated with phenol. Toxicol Ind Health. 1987;3:535–68.
32. Botta SA, Straith RE, Goodwin HH. Cardiac arrhythmias in phenol face peeling: a suggested protocol for prevention. Aesthetic Plast Surg. 1988;12(2):115–7.
33. Kadunc BV, Vanti AA. Evaluation of the systemic toxicity of phenol in facial peels. Surg Cosmet Dermatol. 2009;1:10–4.
34. Agency for Toxic Substances and Disease Registry (US). Relevance to public health. In: Toxicological profile for phenol. Atlanta, GA: ATSDR; 2008. Available from: https://www.ncbi.nlm.nih.gov/books/NBK599443/.
35. Piotrowski JK. Evaluation of exposure to phenol: absorption of phenol vapor in the lungs and through the skin and excretion of phenol in urine. Br J Ind Med. 1971;28(2):172–8.
36. Landau M. Cardiac complications in deep chemical peels. Dermatol Surg. 2007;33:190–3.

37. Hecker E, Schmidt R. Phorbol esters—the irritants and cocarcinogens of *Croton tiglium* L. Fortschr Chem Org Naturst. 1974;31:377–467.
38. Justo AS, Lemes BM, Nunes B, Antunes KA, Capote ACMO, Lipinski LC, Campagnoli EB, Emiliano J, Meurer EC, Ezemma O, Miot HA, Beltrame FL, Wambier CG. Characterization of the activity of *Croton tiglium* oil in Hetter's very heavy phenol-croton oil chemical peels. Dermatol Surg. 2021;47(7):944–6.
39. Van Duuren BL, Langseth L, Sivak A, Orris L. The tumor-promoting principles of *Croton tiglium* L. II. A comparative study. Cancer Res. 1966;26(8):1729–33.
40. Zhang T, Liu Z, Sun X, Liu Z, Zhang L, Zhang Q, Peng W, Wu C. Botany, traditional uses, phytochemistry, pharmacological and toxicological effects of *Croton tiglium* Linn.: a comprehensive review. J Pharm Pharmacol. 2022;74(8):1061–84.
41. Gupta DP, Park SH, Yang HJ, Suk K, Song GJ. Neuroprotective and anti-neuroinflammatory effects of a poisonous plant *Croton tiglium* Linn. extract. Toxins (Basel). 2020;12(4):261.
42. Wang J, Qin L, Zhao B, Cai L, Zhong Z, Liu Y, Zhou X. Crotonols A and B, two rare tigliane diterpenoid derivatives against K562 cells from *Croton tiglium*. Org Biomol Chem. 2018;17(1):195–202.
43. Yun JW, Kwon E, Kim YS, Kim SH, You JR, Kim HC, Park JS, Che JH, Lee SK, Jang JJ, Kim HH, Kang BC. Assessment of acute, 14-day, and 13-week repeated oral dose toxicity of Tiglium seed extract in rats. BMC Complem Altern Med. 2018;18(1):251.
44. Zhang XL, Wang L, Li F, Yu K, Wang MK. Cytotoxic phorbol esters of *Croton tiglium*. J Nat Prod. 2013;76(5):858–64.
45. Shahid M, Tayyab M, Naz F, Jamil A, Ashraf M, Gilani AH. Activity-guided isolation of a novel protein from *Croton tiglium* with antifungal and antibacterial activities. Phytother Res. 2008;22(12):1646–9.
46. Saputera MD, Raharja S, Kardono LB, Iswantini D. Characteristics, efficacy and safety testing of standardized extract of *Croton tiglium* seed from Indonesia as a laxative agent. Pak J Biol Sci. 2008;11(4):618–22.
47. Pal PK, Nandi MK, Singh NK. Detoxification of *Croton tiglium* L. seeds by the Ayurvedic Śodhana process. Anc Sci Life. 2014;33(3):157–61.
48. Klein DR, Little JH. Laryngeal edema as a complication of chemical peel. Plast Reconstr Surg. 1983;71(3):419–20.
49. Marçon CR, Coppinger AJ, Salomão C, Alves Dos Reis V, Alves Dos Reis VN, de Menezes Gomes JL, Gianvecchio VAP, Medeiros de Aquino E, de Seixas Alves MT, Canzian M, Coelho Frenkelis Brandão SA, Fusel de Ue RR, Ribeiro F, Bageorgou F, Wambier CG. International Peeling Society (IPS) and São Paulo's Legal Medical Institute (IML-SP). Fatal phenol peel by an unlicensed social media practitioner: A forensic medical analysis. J Am Acad Dermatol. 2025;93(6):e211–3.
50. Tyagi A, Tyagi S, Malik N, Chawla H. Phenol ingestion: a case report. Int J Forensic Med Toxicol Sci. 2017;2(1):22–3.

5 Indications and Contraindications

5.1 Introduction

Phenol-croton oil peel has well-established indications, supported by clinical studies, for the treatment of various dermatological conditions, mainly related to photoaging, but also for premalignant and pigmentary lesions.

The main classical indication is deep facial rejuvenation, especially in patients with advanced photoaging, deep rhytids, and marked solar elastosis. The procedure is particularly effective in areas such as the perioral and periorbital regions, where other modalities, such as medium-depth peels or lasers, often yield inferior results. Studies demonstrate significant and long-lasting clinical improvement in these conditions, with high patient satisfaction and an objective reduction in apparent age.

Another well-established indication is the treatment of constitutional periorbital hyperpigmentation, especially in patients with Fitzpatrick skin types III–IV. A multicenter series demonstrated that phenol-croton oil peel provides clinical improvement greater than 50% in nearly 90% of cases, with long-lasting results (median of 24 months) and a low complication rate, making it one of the preferred options for this patient profile.

A multicenter study demonstrated that phenol–croton oil peel provides clinical improvement greater than 50% in nearly 90% of cases, with long-lasting results (median of 24 months) and a low complication rate, making it one of the treatment options of choice for this patient profile.

Phenol–croton oil is also indicated for the treatment of premalignant lesions, such as actinic keratosis, Bowen's disease, and actinic cheilitis. Randomized clinical trials and prospective studies have demonstrated higher clinical and histological response rates compared to conventional topical therapies, such as imiquimod, with clinical and histological clearance in over 90% of actinic cheilitis cases and complete response in 85% of actinic keratosis and Bowen's disease cases, in addition to a significant reduction in histopathological markers of dysplasia and intraepithelial neoplasia.

C. Marçon, C. Wambier, *Phenol-Croton Oil Peel*,
https://doi.org/10.1007/978-3-032-25993-6_5

Phenol–croton oil peel may be considered for atrophic scars, such as those from acne, and in refractory melasma, although the literature is more limited in these contexts. Alternative techniques, such as spot application of 88% phenol, have also shown efficacy in areas of skin laxity and static wrinkles, with shorter downtime and lower cost.

Patient selection is crucial, as individuals with fair skin (Fitzpatrick I–III) have a lower risk of pigmentary complications, but recent studies have also demonstrated safety and efficacy in higher phototypes, provided that postoperative management and patient expectations are appropriately addressed.

In summary, the indications for phenol–croton oil peel include: deep facial rejuvenation, constitutional periorbital hyperpigmentation, actinic keratosis, Bowen's disease, actinic cheilitis, atrophic scars, and refractory melasma. The robustness of the results and the durability of the effects are supported by multiple clinical studies, which also highlight the importance of technique and careful patient selection to optimize outcomes and minimize risks.

This chapter will systematically address the classical and contemporary indications for phenol–croton oil peel, supported by clinical and histological studies, as well as the absolute and relative contraindications that must be strictly observed. Eligibility criteria, specific care for skin types at higher risk of post-inflammatory hyperpigmentation, and the ethical parameters that should guide medical decision-making will also be discussed (Table 5.1).

Table 5.1 Main indications for phenol–croton oil peel and strength of evidence

Indication	Scientific evidence	Level of evidence (OCEBM, 2011)
Advanced photoaging (deep rhytids, marked solar elastosis)	Prospective clinical studies, case series, systematic reviews	2b–3b
Constitutional periorbital hyperpigmentation	Multicenter retrospective study, clinical series	3b–4
Premalignant lesions (actinic keratosis, Bowen's disease, actinic cheilitis)	Randomized clinical trial, prospective studies	1b–2b
Atrophic acne scars	Classic studies, randomized clinical trial (phenol monotherapy), case reports	2b–4
Refractory melasma	Retrospective cohort, case reports	3b–4
Lip rejuvenation (lip peel)	Clinical series, case reports	4–5
Dark and Asian skin (selected indications)	Observational studies, case reports	4–5

Main indications for phenol–croton peel and corresponding levels of scientific evidence. Note: Level of evidence assigned according to the criteria of the *Oxford Centre for Evidence-Based Medicine* (OCEBM), 2011. (*Source: Table prepared by the author (Dr Carolina Marçon)*)

5.2 Indications

5.2.1 Photoaging

The indication of phenol–croton peel for skin rejuvenation is supported by a robust body of clinical and histopathological evidence, demonstrating significant improvement in rhytids, texture, and pigmentation of photoaged skin. The procedure is particularly effective in challenging areas such as the perioral and periorbital regions, resulting in high patient satisfaction and objective reduction in apparent age. The effects are long-lasting, with benefits maintained for several years, and their magnitude is directly related to the concentration of croton oil and the application technique, which allows modulation of depth and recovery time according to clinical need (Fig. 5.1).

The efficacy of the procedure results from the combined action of phenol and croton oil. Croton oil, in particular, is the main modulator of the depth of dermal injury, being responsible for inducing a strong inflammatory response and significant neocollagenesis. Varying the concentration of the oil allows adjustment of the peel depth according to facial topography and the degree of photoaging. Concentrations between 0.25% and 0.5% promote re-epithelialization in approximately 7 days, while concentrations above 1% are associated with a higher risk of hypopigmentation and delayed healing, especially in areas of thinner skin (Figs. 5.2 and 5.3).

Both classic and contemporary studies demonstrate that the phenol-croton oil combination provides superior rejuvenation compared to less aggressive techniques, such as trichloroacetic acid (TCA) peels, particularly in patients with severe solar elastosis and deep rhytids. The peel is also shown to be equivalent or superior to

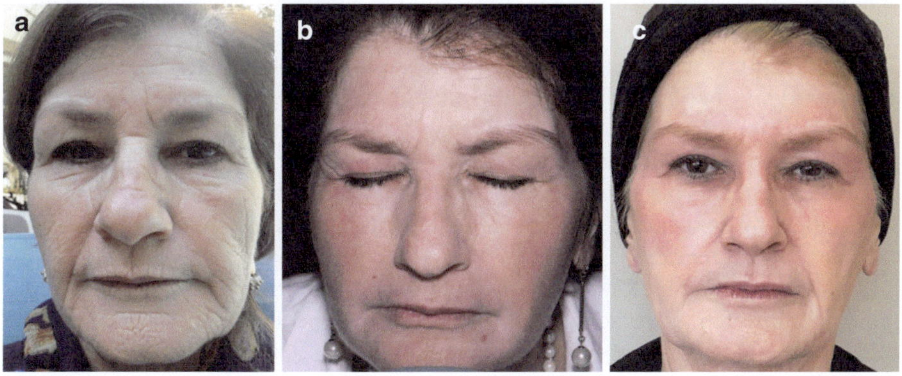

Fig. 5.1 Clinical progression after phenol–croton peel, demonstrating sustained improvement in skin texture, rhytids, and pigmentation: (**a**) before the procedure, (**b**) after full facial rejuvenation, and (**c**) 8 years after periocular retreatment, illustrating the long-lasting results. (*Source: Personal archive of Dr Carlos Wambier and Dr Carolina Marçon*)

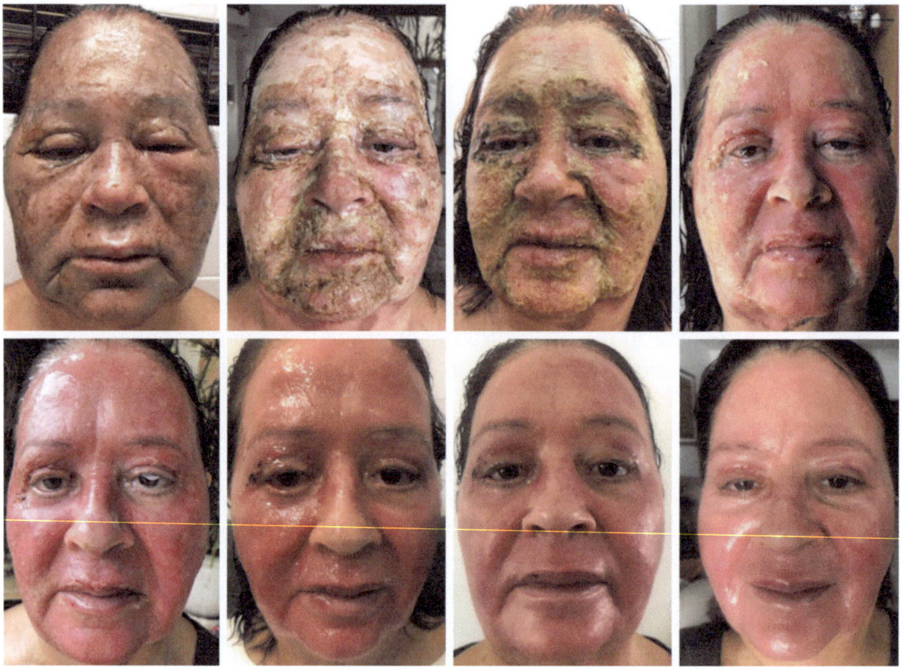

Fig. 5.2 Clinical sequence of the healing process following phenol-croton oil peel (Hetter, OC 1.2% full face). Complete removal of the outermost skin layers is observed, accompanied by significant edema in the first 36 h and intense inflammatory activity with exudation. The process culminates in the formation of new, homogeneous skin, free from signs of photoaging, with full recovery in 8–10 days. (*Source: Author's personal archive (Dr Carolina Marçon)*)

ablative technologies such as CO_2 laser, with the added advantage of being a more accessible and extensively tested procedure.

Hetter's study standardized formulas and application techniques with varying concentrations of croton oil, facilitating individualized treatment and clinical reproducibility (Fig. 5.4). In parallel, histological studies demonstrated that, without croton oil, phenol alone at concentrations below 50% does not produce a significant therapeutic effect. This scientific basis underpinned the development of segmental peels, allowing concentrations to be tailored to skin thickness and the sensitivity of each anatomical region.

The classic study by Fitzpatrick et al. compared the depth of action and healing process of different resurfacing methods. The phenol peel (Baker-Gordon formula) achieved the greatest depth of dermal ablation among all methods evaluated, even surpassing multiple-pass CO_2 laser. Although re-epithelialization was slower (up to 3 weeks), it was associated with deeper and more long-lasting tissue remodeling, without scar formation.

Experimental models support these findings. Lemes et al. compared, in a porcine model, the effects of three agents combined with croton oil (1.6%): phenol 35%, TCA 35%, and glycolic acid 35%. Phenol induced epidermal and deep dermal

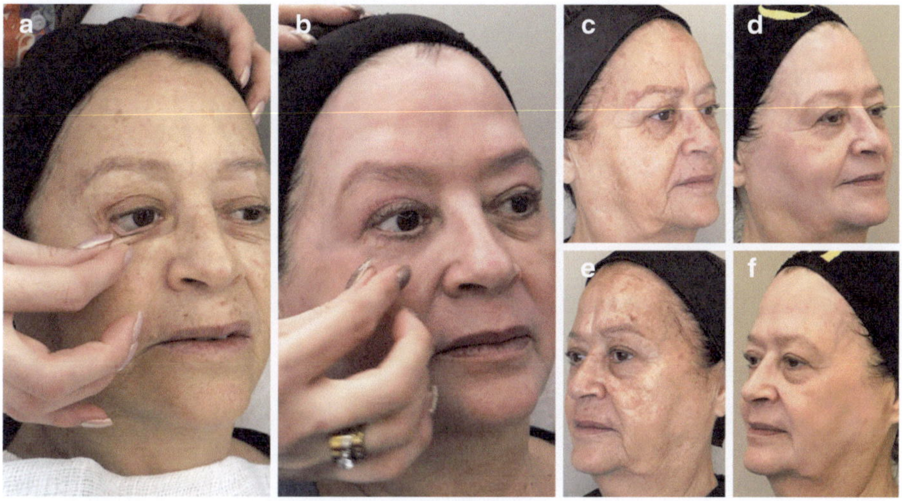

Fig. 5.3 Images showing the progress of the patient from Fig. 5.2, a 69-year-old woman treated with phenol-croton oil peel (Hetter 1.2%, full face). (**a**, **b**) After 1 month, demonstrating complete re-epithelialization and homogeneous texture. (**c**–**f**) After 6 months, renewed skin is evident, with improvement in rhytids, laxity, and pigmentation, as well as resolution of dyschromia. (*Source: Author's personal archive (Dr Carolina Marçon)*)

necrosis, with an intense inflammatory response, fibroblast proliferation, and type III collagen deposition in the reticular dermis. TCA showed limited action restricted to the papillary dermis, and glycolic acid, although it stimulated type I collagen, did not cause epidermal necrosis or deep alterations. These data reinforce the superiority of the phenol-croton oil combination for deep dermal remodeling.

The systematic review conducted by Wambier et al. consolidated clinical and histological evidence supporting the central role of croton oil as a modulator of lesion depth, with phenol acting predominantly as a penetration vehicle. The study confirms that the action of the phenol-croton oil peel occurs mainly in the reticular dermis, promoting intense neocollagenesis and reorganization of elastic fibers—effects essential for reversing severe solar elastosis. Compared to modern technologies such as fractional and ablative lasers, the phenol-croton oil peel demonstrated greater efficacy in correcting static rhytids, more durable results, and a lower risk of residual hypopigmentation, especially when using Hetter's standardized formulations. The review also highlights the importance of precise croton titration, segmented application, and prior skin preparation as key determinants for clinical safety and predictability (Fig. 5.5).

Kass, in his retrospective analysis of 15 years' experience with the method, advocates the renewed use of phenol-croton oil as a safe and effective alternative to ablative technologies. The author highlights that personalizing treatment with variable concentrations of croton oil according to anatomical zone (zones 1–4) yields individualized and harmonious results. Segmented application enables effective treatment of critical areas such as the perioral region (0.7–1.1% croton) and eyelids

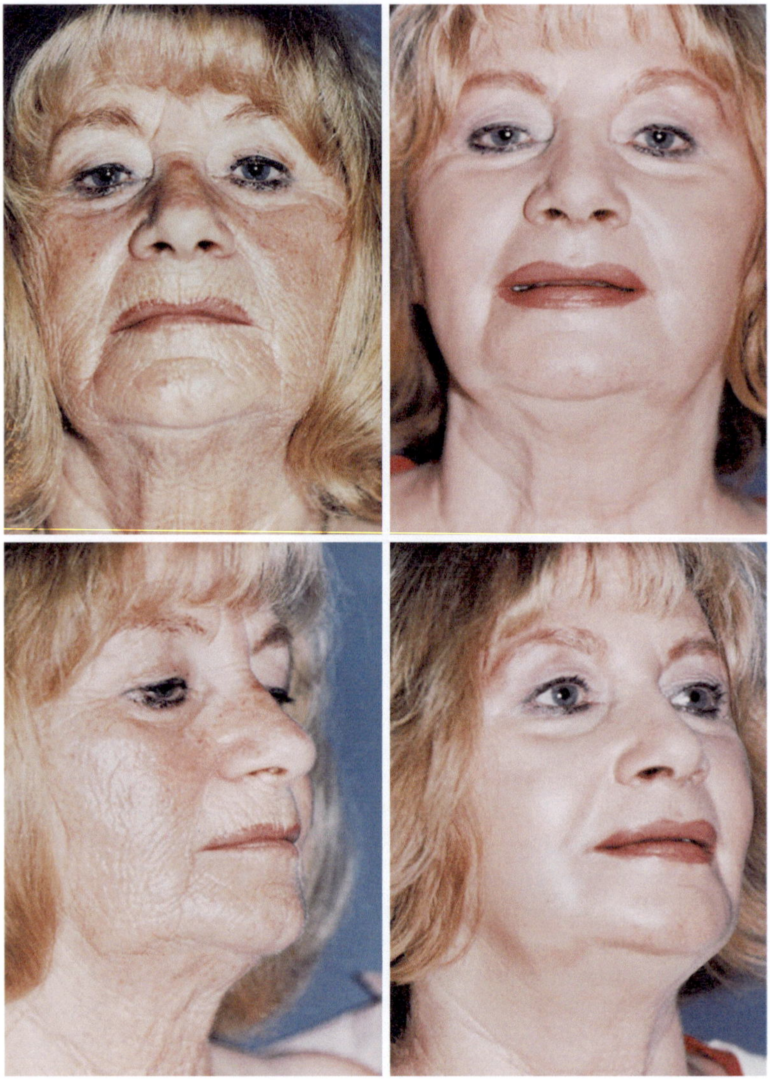

Fig. 5.4 Long-term results (33 months) of the phenol-croton oil peel as described by Hetter, demonstrating lasting facial rejuvenation with marked improvement of deep rhytids, chin wrinkles, and irregular pigmentation. A classic case that established the serial dilution formulas and demonstrated the durability of the method. (*Source: Adapted from Hetter GP. An examination of the phenol-croton oil peel: part IV. Face peel results with different concentrations of phenol and croton oil. Plast Reconstr Surg. 2000 Mar;105(3):1061–83; discussion 1084–7. doi:10.1097/00006534-200003000-00035. PMID: 10724270. Reproduced with permission from the publisher*)

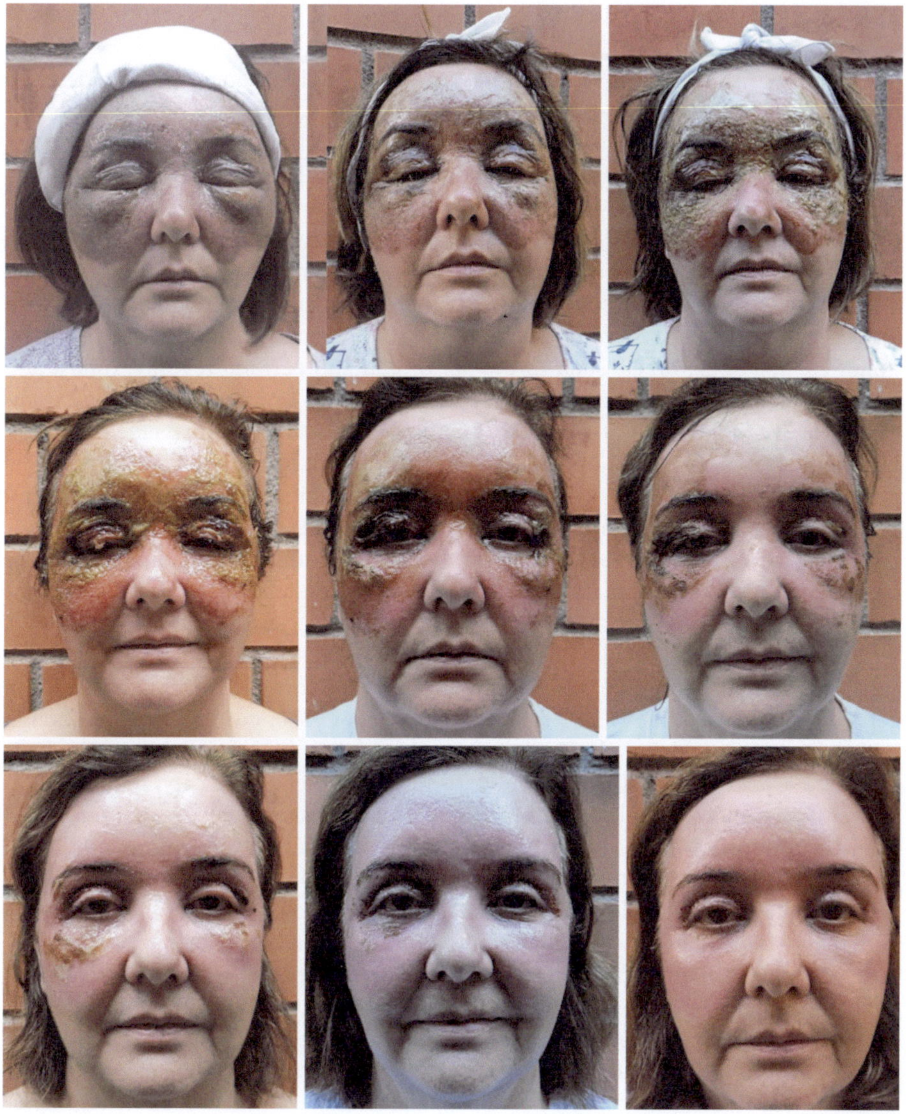

Fig. 5.5 Evolutionary sequence following deep facial peeling with 1.6% croton oil in 35% phenol and occlusion with petroleum jelly. An intense initial inflammatory response is observed, with edema and exudation in the first days, followed by crust detachment and complete re-epithelialization by day 14. At 12 months, there is a significant and sustained improvement in deep rhytids and the overall appearance of photoaging. (*Source: Personal archive of the author (Dr Carolina Marçon)*)

(0.1–0.35%), with excellent clinical response, minimal hypopigmentation, and uniform recovery within up to 10 days.

Contemporary advances in the application of phenol-croton oil peel, as detailed by Larson, have enabled an even more effective and safer approach to the treatment of advanced photoaging. Based on a carefully structured experimental model, the author demonstrated that small variations in croton oil concentration induce substantial histological changes in the depth of dermal injury, allowing precise modulation of the procedure's effects according to the severity of solar damage and skin thickness. Clinical analysis of patients treated with segmented formulations showed marked improvement in deep rhytids, texture, tone, and skin pigmentation, with long-lasting results and high satisfaction. The study demonstrated that even in traditionally challenging areas, such as the periorbital and perioral regions, robust and harmonious rejuvenation was achieved without residual hypopigmentation—a complication frequently observed with classic phenol or ablative technologies. Histologically, deep and homogeneous necrosis of the mid-reticular dermis was observed, with stimulation of neocollagenesis, reorganization of elastic fibers, and structured tissue regeneration. These findings reinforce the superiority of phenol-croton oil as the technique of choice for the treatment of severe photoaging, especially when the formulation is tailored to the facial anatomy and clinical needs of each patient.

A small but methodologically relevant study by Vasconcelos et al. employed a split-face model to compare the classic Baker-Gordon formula (phenol 49%, croton 2.1%) with the modified Hetter formulation (phenol 35%, croton 1.4%). Although both promoted significant clinical improvement in rhytids, the Hetter formula demonstrated a better tolerability profile, with lower erythema intensity, reduced incidence of post-inflammatory hyperpigmentation, and a shorter recovery time. These findings reinforce that reduced concentrations of phenol and croton oil, when applied with an appropriate technique, maintain the desired clinical efficacy in deep skin rejuvenation, with additional advantages in safety and recovery profile.

Recent studies have also highlighted additional molecular mechanisms associated with rejuvenation. Cardoso et al. demonstrated an increase in type I and III collagen and elevated expression of sirtuins SIRT-6 and SIRT-7 following phenol–croton oil peel, suggesting the involvement of epigenetic pathways in cellular regeneration, in addition to mechanical remodeling of the dermal matrix (Fig. 5.6).

Historical studies, such as that by Gross and Maschek, which documented clinical experience with over 3000 patients undergoing full-face peeling with a phenol formulation combined with croton oil, corroborate contemporary findings regarding the efficacy of this method in the treatment of severe photoaging. The described technique involved the use of an occlusive mask with adhesive tape (Maskentechnik), applied immediately after the chemical solution, with the aim of enhancing the penetration of the exfoliating agent and standardizing the tissue response. Histologically, the authors observed controlled necrosis of the epidermis and superficial dermis, followed by a regeneration phase with deposition of new collagen and reorganization of the dermal matrix. Clinically, improvement in skin contour, texture, and

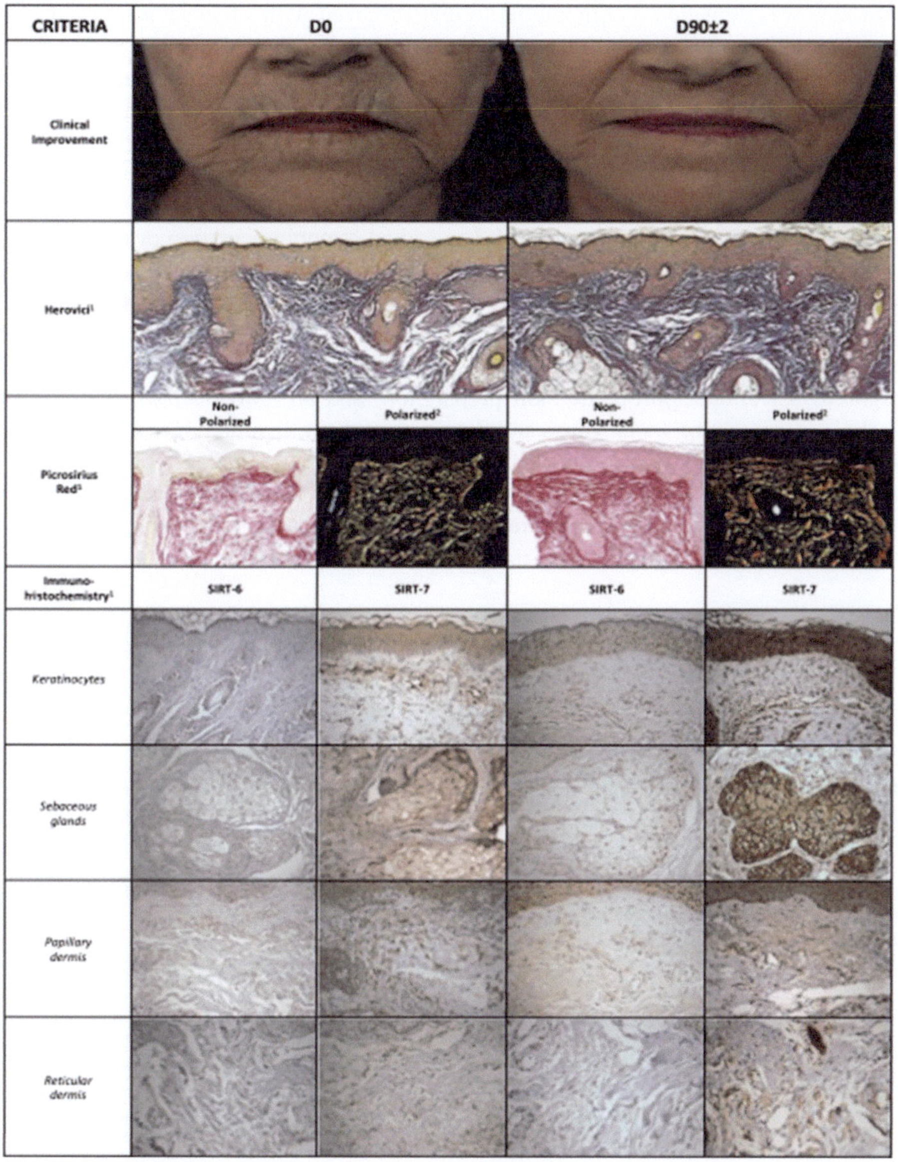

Fig. 5.6 Clinical, histochemical, and immunohistochemical improvement before (D0) and after 90 ± 2 days (D90 ± 2) of phenol–croton oil peel. Notable findings include increased papillary and reticular collagen (Herovici and Picrosirius Red under polarized light) and greater expression of SIRT-6 and SIRT-7 in keratinocytes, sebaceous glands, and dermis. (*Source: Adapted from Cardoso FAMES, Moura RD, Pilar EFS, Moura ICG, Miot HA, da Costa A. Phenol–croton oil peel enhances type-1 and type-3 collagen amounts by stimulating SIRT-6 and SIRT-7. Int J Dermatol. 2021;60:1234–1244, reproduced with permission from the publisher*)

firmness was considered comparable to that achieved with superficial surgical lifting, but with greater durability, especially in patients with marked solar elastosis.

The patients who benefit most from phenol–croton oil chemical peeling are those with advanced photoaging, characterized by deep rhytids, pronounced solar elastosis, irregular texture, and marked facial dyschromia, particularly in the periorbital and perioral regions (Fig. 5.7). Individuals with fair skin (Fitzpatrick phototypes I–III) have traditionally shown greater safety and better aesthetic outcomes, with a reduced risk of pigmentary complications such as residual hypopigmentation or post-inflammatory hyperpigmentation, as evidenced in clinical series and historical reviews. However, contemporary modifications in formulations and a better understanding of anatomical and pharmacological parameters have also increased the safety of the method in patients with higher phototypes and in Asian populations, provided there is rigorous selection, appropriate skin preparation, and an individualized application technique, respecting facial zones and the limits of the inflammatory response.

In summary, phenol-croton oil peel remains the gold standard for deep facial rejuvenation. Its clinical efficacy, durability, and robust histological basis set it apart from other modalities, although it requires careful assessment, appropriate preparation, and technical expertise from the practitioner.

5.2.2 Acne Scars

The application of phenol in acne scars dates back to classic studies, such as that conducted by MacKee and Karp, one of the first systematic reports on the therapeutic use of this caustic agent in atrophic lesions. In the study, 112 patients underwent more than 540 facial applications of liquefied USP phenol, resulting in significant clinical

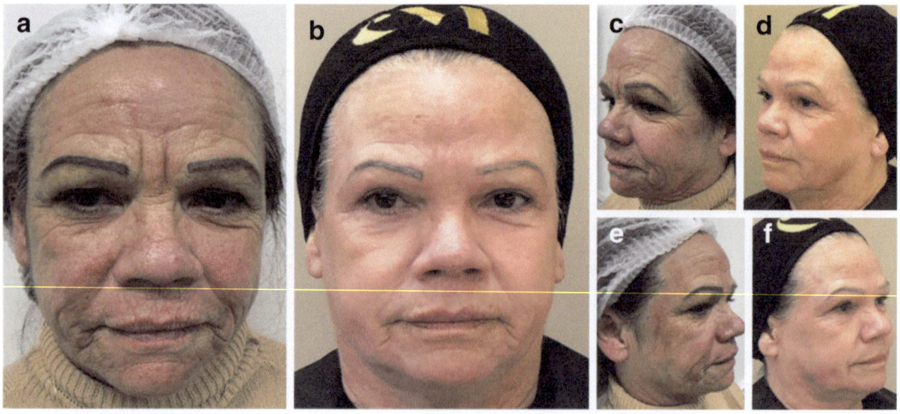

Fig. 5.7 55-year-old patient with severe photoaging, who underwent phenol–croton oil peel in stages: initially the perioral region, followed by the periocular area and, subsequently, the entire face. Comparative photographs (**a**, **c**, **e**) before treatment and (**b**, **d**, **f**) 2 years after completion demonstrate significant improvement in deep rhytids, skin laxity, and texture, with long-lasting results. (*Source: Author's personal archive (Dr Carolina Marçon)*)

improvement in nearly all cases, with an average response exceeding 80% after 2–4 sessions. Histological changes observed included denser collagen, reorganization of collagen fibers in a horizontal orientation, reduction of elastic fibers, and increased fibroblast density, indicating intense dermal remodeling. The epidermis became thicker and more organized, and clinical results were maintained for over 10 years. No significant complications, such as infection, keloids, or neoplasms, were reported, supporting the use of phenol as an effective and safe option, especially in fair skin.

More recently, Lee and Rullan described an effective combined approach for acne scars in all skin phototypes, associating the CROSS technique with 88% phenol (carbolic acid), subcision with a blunt cannula in two planes, and motorized microneedling. The protocol proved safe and highly effective for different types of scars (ice pick, boxcar, and rolling), including in patients who had not responded to fractional CO_2 laser. Phenol demonstrated better control of dermal vesiculation and a lower risk of scarring than TCA, and was well tolerated even in higher phototypes when applied in a segmented and judicious manner.

In a randomized clinical trial, Leheta et al. compared deep phenol peeling with the combination of microneedling and 20% TCA in atrophic acne scars in phototypes III and IV. The group treated with phenol (single session) achieved a mean reduction of 75.1% in scar severity scores, while the PCI-TCA 20% group (4 sessions) showed an improvement of 69.4%. Although statistically similar, phenol demonstrated superior performance in terms of individual response and durability, at the cost of longer downtime and a higher incidence of mild adverse effects such as hyperpigmentation and prolonged erythema. The PCI-TCA group, in turn, showed better tolerability and a more pronounced response in rolling-type scars, with minimal side effects.

Despite the lack of controlled clinical trials specifically investigating the efficacy of phenol-croton oil peel in the treatment of atrophic acne scars, there are numerous anecdotal reports and clinical observations described in the literature by experienced authors suggesting significant improvement in skin texture and contour in areas with residual scarring (Fig. 5.8). In publications focused on facial rejuvenation, this additional benefit is often mentioned, even if not assessed as a primary outcome. The deep action of phenol-croton oil in the reticular dermis, with intense neocollagenesis, reorganization of collagen fibers, and three-dimensional tissue regeneration, provides a plausible histological basis for its use in this indication. In patients with extensive scarring, mature skin, and lower phototypes, the technique may represent a strategic and effective approach, provided that strict selection criteria are applied and the procedure is performed by qualified professionals. Nevertheless, the scarcity of formal evidence highlights the importance of developing prospective controlled studies to validate this practice with robust scientific support.

5.2.3 Dark Circles

Dark circles, especially those of constitutional origin, represent a significant therapeutic challenge in aesthetic dermatology due to their multifactorial etiopathogenetic, chronic nature, and generally unsatisfactory response to conventional

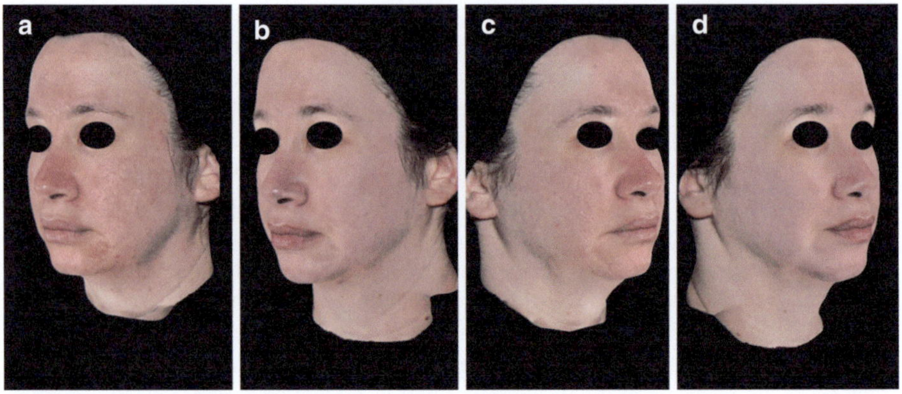

Fig. 5.8 A 38-year-old patient with acne scars unresponsive to previous treatments (dermabrasion/CO_2 laser) underwent phenol-croton oil peel (Hetter OC 1.2%). Serial images demonstrate progressive improvement in skin texture and quality before and after 1 year: (**a**, **b**) (left hemiface); (**c**, **d**) (right hemiface). (*Source: Author's personal archive (Dr Carolina Marçon)*)

treatments. Among the contributing factors are dermal hyperpigmentation, cutaneous transparency with visualization of underlying vessels, eyelid laxity, pronounced grooves, and anatomical shadowing. In the refractory pigmented component, the main histological alteration is the presence of dermal melanophages without proliferation of epidermal melanocytes, which limits the therapeutic success of topical lightening agents, lasers, and intense pulsed light.

In this context, phenol-croton oil peel has been explored as a promising and long-lasting alternative for constitutional pigmented dark circles. A multicenter retrospective study conducted by the International Peeling Society, published by Soon et al. gathered data from 55 procedures performed in 52 patients, with over three decades of accumulated experience. The sample was predominantly female (92%), with phototypes III (54%) and IV (35%), and a mean age of 40 years. The formulations used contained phenol at 60–65% and croton oil at 0.6–0.7%, applied exclusively to the lower eyelid.

Clinical results showed an improvement of over 50% in hyperpigmentation in 89% of cases, as well as improvement in the texture of the lower eyelid skin. In some patients, the effects persisted for more than a decade, with a mean duration of 24 months. Histological findings corroborated the observed efficacy: reorganization of collagen and elastic fibers, thickening of the reticular dermis, and reduction of melanophages—changes that promote lightening and reduce the visibility of underlying vessels (Fig. 5.9).

With regard to safety, adverse effects were mostly mild and self-limiting. Post-inflammatory hyperpigmentation was observed in 45% of cases, but resolved with or without depigmenting treatment. Persistent erythema occurred in 4%, and permanent dyschromia or scarring was rare. The absence of serious events is directly related to technical mastery of the procedure, respect for the anatomical boundaries of the eyelid, and limitation of the treated area—generally less than 1.5% of total body surface area, which obviates the need for intravenous hydration and cardiac

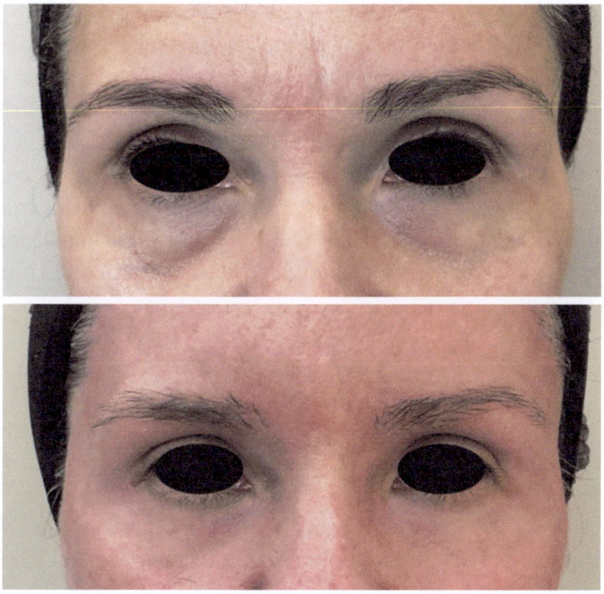

Fig. 5.9 Clinical appearance before (above) and after phenol 35% peel combined with 1.2% croton oil (below), demonstrating significant improvement in dark circles, with reduced pigmentation, increased skin density and texture, and decreased dermal transparency. (*Source: Author's personal archive (Dr Carolina Marçon)*)

monitoring. Careful application, avoiding the inner canthus and ensuring a smooth transition with adjacent skin, is essential to prevent demarcation lines.

Additionally, Platsidaki et al. evaluated the efficacy and safety of a combined peel containing 10% phenol and 20% trichloroacetic acid (TCA) for the treatment of dark circles (periorbital hyperpigmentation) in 31 women aged 43 to 75 years, predominantly Fitzpatrick skin phototypes III and IV. After pretreatment with 8% glycolic acid, three layers of the peel were applied to the periorbital area until homogeneous frosting was achieved. Nearly all patients demonstrated aesthetic improvement, with physician assessment rating approximately 71% of cases as good or excellent, while about 70% of patients reported good or excellent outcomes. Better responses were observed in younger individuals and in patients with fairer skin phototypes. The procedure was well tolerated, with no ocular complications reported; adverse effects were limited mainly to transient erythema, mild edema, and temporary scaling. The authors concluded that the combination of low-concentration phenol and TCA produces a medium-depth peel capable of reducing pigmentation and promoting dermal remodeling with a favorable safety profile, representing a promising, safe, and cost-effective option for the treatment of dark circles.

Although not specifically designed for the treatment of dark circles, the multicenter study published by Lee et al. on behalf of the International Peeling Society reinforces the potential of segmental phenol-croton oil peel application in the eyelid region. A total of 639 patients underwent deep peels in restricted facial aesthetic areas (periorbital and perioral), using phenol at 27.5–33% and croton oil between 0.1% and 1.6%, according to skin thickness and location. For the lower eyelid, formulations with 0.1% croton oil were applied, resulting in visible rejuvenation, improved texture, and smoothing of rhytids, without significant adverse events. Histologically, durable formation of a new functional dermal band was observed even decades after the procedure. Although the main focus was wrinkle treatment, the data suggest that segmental peeling may also benefit patients with dark circles associated with laxity, hyperpigmentation, and dermal irregularities.

In light of this evidence, phenol peeling is established as a relevant tool in the management of constitutional pigmented dark circles, particularly in refractory cases. The durability of its effects, histological correction of pigmentary and structural changes, and its applicability in higher phototypes when performed with technical expertise, place this method among the most promising approaches for this highly prevalent and challenging aesthetic concern (Figs. 5.10, 5.11, and 5.12).

5.2.4 Premalignant Lesions and Cutaneous Neoplasms

A prospective study conducted by Kaminaka et al. evaluated the clinical, histological, and immunohistochemical efficacy of 100% phenol in the treatment of premalignant cutaneous lesions, including actinic keratoses (AK) and Bowen's disease (BD). The study included 46 Japanese patients (32 with AK and 14 with BD), treated with monthly applications of phenol for up to eight sessions. The complete clinical response (CR) rate was 84.8% (39 patients), with sustained control for at least 1 year in the majority of cases. Therapeutic efficacy showed a significant correlation with tumor thickness and with cyclin A expression, a marker of cellular proliferation. Lesions with a thickness greater than 400 µm and a higher cyclin A index required more treatment sessions or exhibited disease progression, whereas markers such as PCNA, p53, and TUNEL did not demonstrate a statistical correlation with clinical response. Post-treatment histopathology revealed a marked reduction in tumor thickness in responsive lesions. No serious systemic adverse events were observed, and local side effects were mild and self-limiting. This study represents the first systematic analysis of the clinical, histological, and molecular

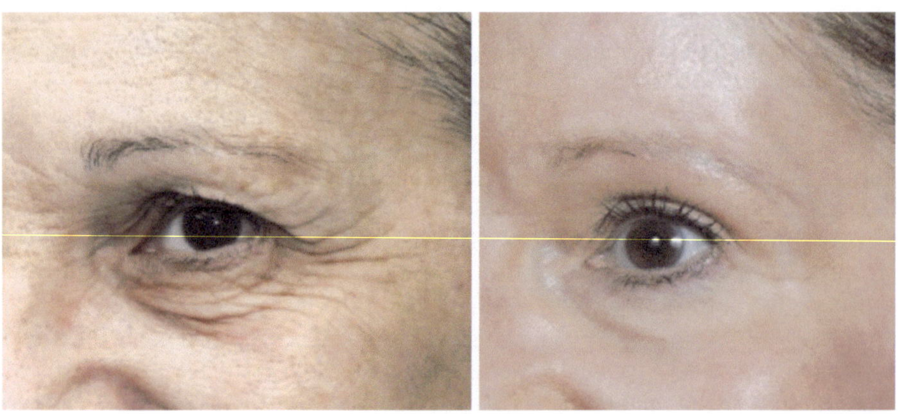

Fig. 5.10 Results of phenol-croton oil peel in the periorbital region of a 67-year-old patient. After 20 months, there is evident rejuvenation, with softening of deep rhytids and improvement in the color and quality of the eyelid skin. (*Source: Courtesy of Dr Tereza Cristina Celidonio*)

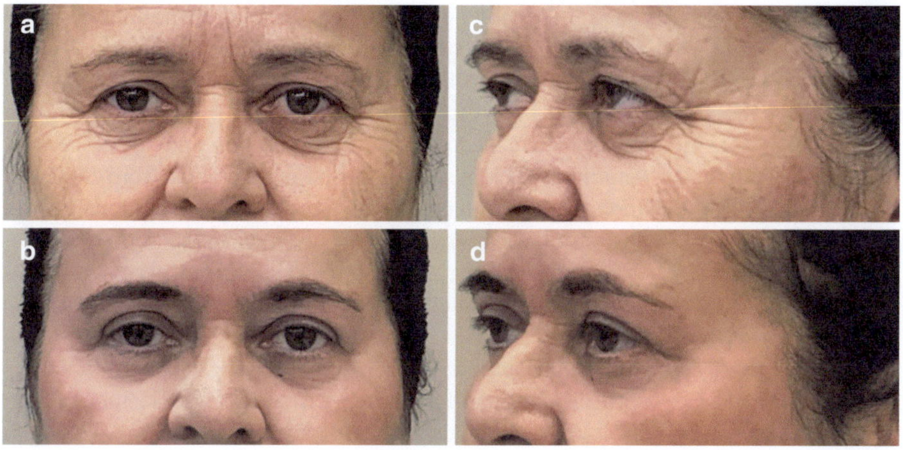

Fig. 5.11 Fifty-nine-year-old patient, before (**a**, **c**) and after (**b**, **d**) 6 months following 35% phenol/1.2% croton oil peel for periocular rejuvenation. (*Source: Author's personal archive (Dr Carolina Marçon)*)

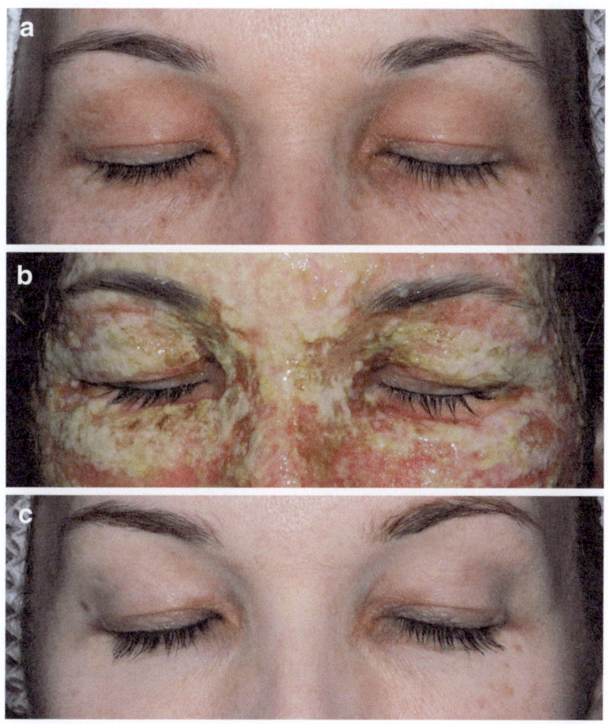

Fig. 5.12 Treatment of periorbital hyperpigmentation with phenol-croton oil peel (Hetter, 1.2% croton oil in 35% phenol). (**a**) Pre-treatment, showing hyperpigmentation and fine lower eyelid rhytids. (**b**) Fourth postoperative day, characterized by intense inflammatory reaction, exudate, and crust formation. (**c**) Result after 1 year, with lightening of the periorbital region and improvement in skin texture. Note the persistence of pigment at the medial canthus, where the skin was deliberately untreated due to the risk of scarring. (*Source: Personal archive of Dr Carlos Wambier*)

response to phenol peeling in intraepidermal neoplastic lesions, supporting its therapeutic utility in patients with surgical contraindications or those who opt for less invasive approaches.

In addition to this discussion, Wambier et al. published a letter in the Journal of the American Academy of Dermatology suggesting pharmacodynamic similarities between ingenol mebutate and deep peels based on phenol and croton oil. Both share mechanisms mediated by diterpenoid esters with the potential to activate protein kinase C (PKC), inducing selective necrosis of the epidermis and upper dermis, destruction of mutated keratinocyte clones, and dermal regeneration from follicular niches. However, the authors highlight that, while ingenol mebutate (extracted from *Euphorbia peplus*) reaches only the papillary dermis at topical concentrations, phenol-croton oil peels penetrate more deeply, reaching the reticular dermis and promoting more extensive regenerative effects, such as cellular apoptosis, remodeling of the dermoepidermal junction, elimination of solar elastosis, and stimulation of collagen synthesis. Despite these effects, the authors note a lack of randomized controlled trials evaluating the efficacy of phenol-croton oil peeling in the treatment of lesions such as AK and cutaneous neoplasms, indicating a significant gap in the literature.

The response from the authors of the original study on ingenol mebutate confirms its structural similarity to phorbol esters and acknowledges the superiority of phenol-croton oil peeling in eliminating mutated keratinocyte clones, dermal remodeling, and sustained tissue regeneration. They cite their own data demonstrating that ingenol mebutate regulates pro-apoptotic factors (such as p53, BCL2, and EDR1), but admit that its limited cutaneous penetration restricts its therapeutic potential when compared to deep peeling. They also warn of a higher risk of post-inflammatory hyperpigmentation and hypertrophic scarring in Asian patients (phototypes III–IV), indicating the need for rigorous preparation and recovery protocols in these groups.

Another study by Kaminaka et al. investigated the use of 100% phenol as a therapeutic modality in three patients with cutaneous angiosarcoma (AS). Treatment consisted of localized applications with subsequent histological monitoring. Biopsies revealed extensive tumoral and endothelial cellular degeneration in the dermis, with apoptosis confirmed by positive staining using the TUNEL (terminal deoxynucleotidyl transferase dUTP nick end labeling) method. The authors report that the procedure was well tolerated, rapid, accessible, with manageable pain and sustained efficacy, suggesting that phenol may represent a promising complementary alternative for the local management of AS, especially in patients who do not tolerate conventional aggressive therapies.

Finally, a randomized controlled clinical trial, registered on ReBEC (RBR-1044sz68), compared the efficacy of 1.6% phenol-croton oil peel (Hetter's formula) with the topical application of 5% imiquimod for 30 days in the treatment of actinic cheilitis. Thirty-six patients with biopsy-confirmed diagnosis were randomized into two groups (1:1). The group treated with phenol-croton oil underwent a single peeling session, while the control group used imiquimod three times per week for 1 month. At 56 days, 94% of patients in the phenol-croton oil group achieved complete clinical remission, compared to no response in the imiquimod group ($P < 0.01$). Histological normalization was achieved in 72% of patients in the phenol-croton oil group versus 17% in the control group ($P < 0.01$). Furthermore, clinical improvement and regression of epithelial atypia (KIN score), solar elastosis, and hyperkeratosis were statistically significant only in the group treated with peeling ($P < 0.05$). Adverse effects were more intense on day 7 in the phenol-croton oil group, but persisted longer in the imiquimod group, up to day 21. The study was terminated early after the interim analysis due to the clear superiority of the peeling treatment. The authors conclude that phenol-croton oil peeling represents an effective, safe, and rapidly recoverable intervention for the treatment of actinic cheilitis, overcoming the limitations of conventional topical treatments (Fig. 5.13).

5.2.5 Melasma

Melasma is a chronic, recurrent, and multifactorial dermatosis characterized by symmetrical hyperpigmentation of the face and strongly influenced by hormonal factors, sun exposure, genetic predisposition, and degradation of the dermal matrix. Recent studies have highlighted the role of solar elastosis and dysfunction of the dermoepidermal junction as key structural components in the perpetuation of the disease, suggesting that therapies with profound restorative action may offer more lasting responses.

To date, there is only one published study specifically evaluating the use of phenol-croton oil peel in the treatment of melasma. This is a retrospective cohort (2024) comparing two formulations: one with moderate concentrations of croton oil (CO) (0.7–0.9%) and another with higher concentrations (1.1–1.6%). Both demonstrated significant improvement in the modified Melasma Area and Severity Index (mMASI) and high scores on the Global Aesthetic Improvement Scale. The group treated with CO <1% showed a more pronounced reduction in mMASI, suggesting that milder concentrations may be sufficient for effective and long-lasting results. The sustained remission rate exceeded 85% after 1 year in both groups, attributed to the prolonged resolution of dermal elastosis—a pathogenic substrate increasingly recognized in the chronicity of melasma (Fig. 5.14).

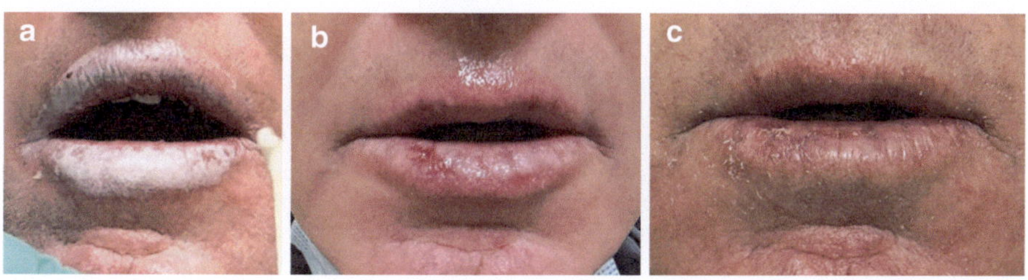

Fig. 5.13 Refractory actinic cheilitis, with no satisfactory response to multiple previous sessions of photodynamic therapy, imiquimod, cryotherapy, and 5-fluorouracil. The patient underwent a single session of phenol-croton oil peel with approximately 90% clinical improvement. (**a**) Immediately during application, showing initial frosting; (**b**) seventh postoperative day, with ongoing re-epithelialization; (**c**) 3 months after the procedure, demonstrating clinical normalization and significant improvement in the texture and color of the vermilion. (*Source: Personal archive of Dr Carlos Wambier*)

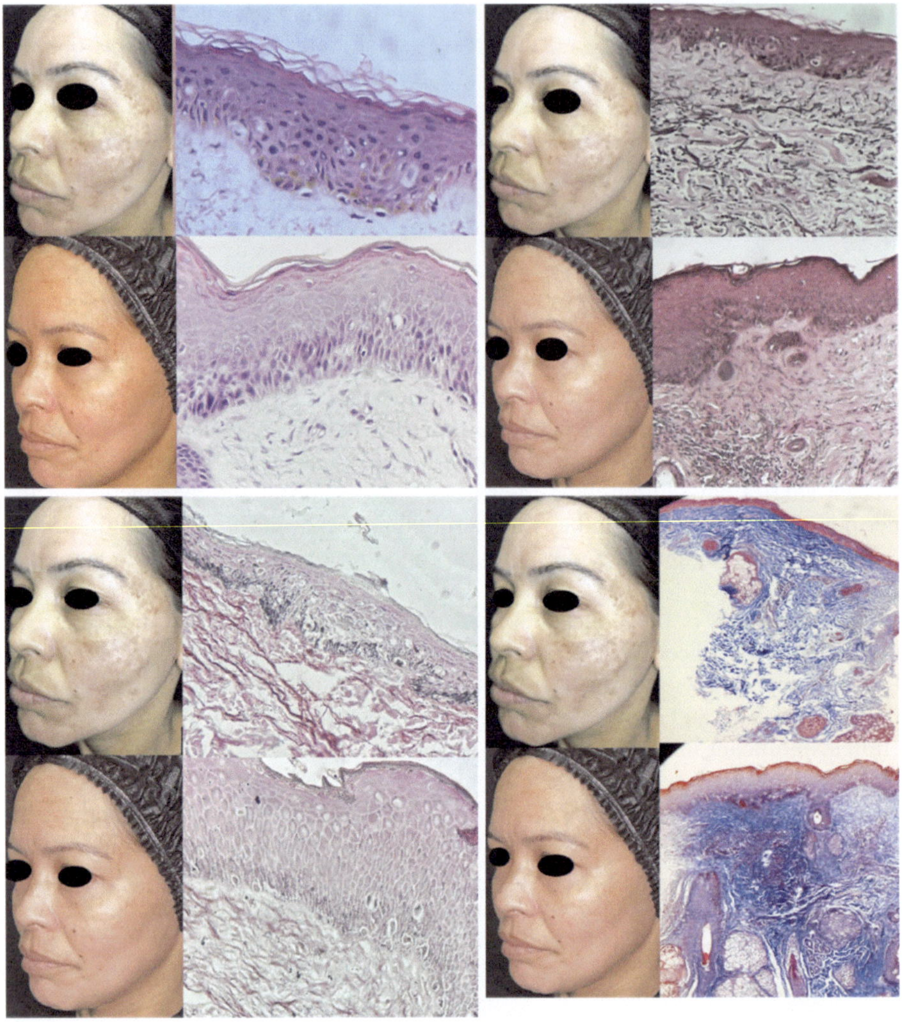

Fig. 5.14 Clinical and histological assessment of a 47-year-old patient, phototype IV, with persistent melasma, before (top row) and 120 days after (bottom row) treatment with 35% phenol peel combined with 0.8% croton oil (Hetter's formulation). Biopsies of the left zygomatic region demonstrate: reduction of basal layer hyperpigmentation (Hematoxylin-Eosin, 20×); decreased melanin deposition (Fontana-Masson, 20×); reduction of solar elastosis (Verhoeff, 20×); and increased collagen deposition (Masson's Trichrome, 10×). (*Source: Adapted from Maymone MBC, Mirza FN, Steiner D, Ribeiro F, Landau M, Marçon C, Celidonio T, Soon SL, Wambier CG. Comparative long-term efficacy of phenol-croton oil chemical peels for persistent melasma at varied Croton tiglium oil concentrations. J Am Acad Dermatol. 2024. doi:10.1016/j.jaad.2024.03.034. Reproduced with permission from the publisher*)

Despite the scarcity of formal studies, the accumulated experience of the authors and other specialists with extensive backgrounds in the use of phenol-croton oil peels points to even more remarkable results, with sustained clinical remission for several years—a result rarely observed with currently available treatments. These findings position the phenol-croton oil peel as a promising therapeutic approach for long-term control, and possibly prolonged remission, of a historically challenging and refractory condition such as melasma (Figs. 5.15 and 5.16).

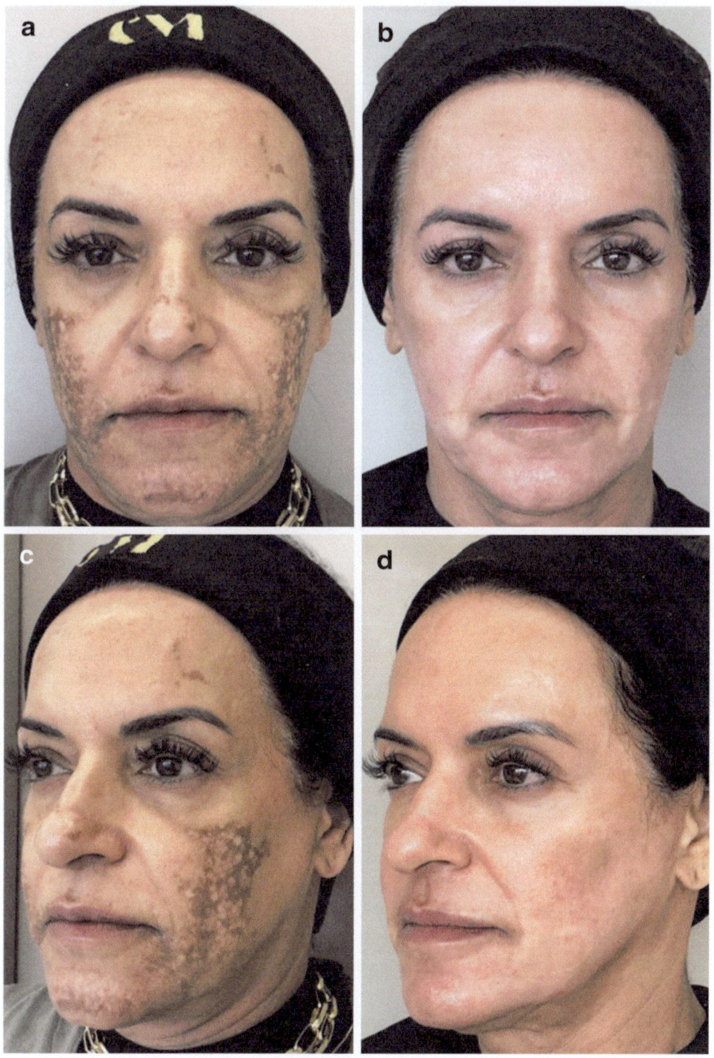

Fig. 5.15 Sixty-three-year-old patient with refractory melasma, before and after 6 months: (**a**, **b**) (frontal view); (**c**, **d**) (left hemiface), phenol-croton oil peel 35%/1.2%. (*Source: Personal archive of the author (Dr Carolina Marçon)*)

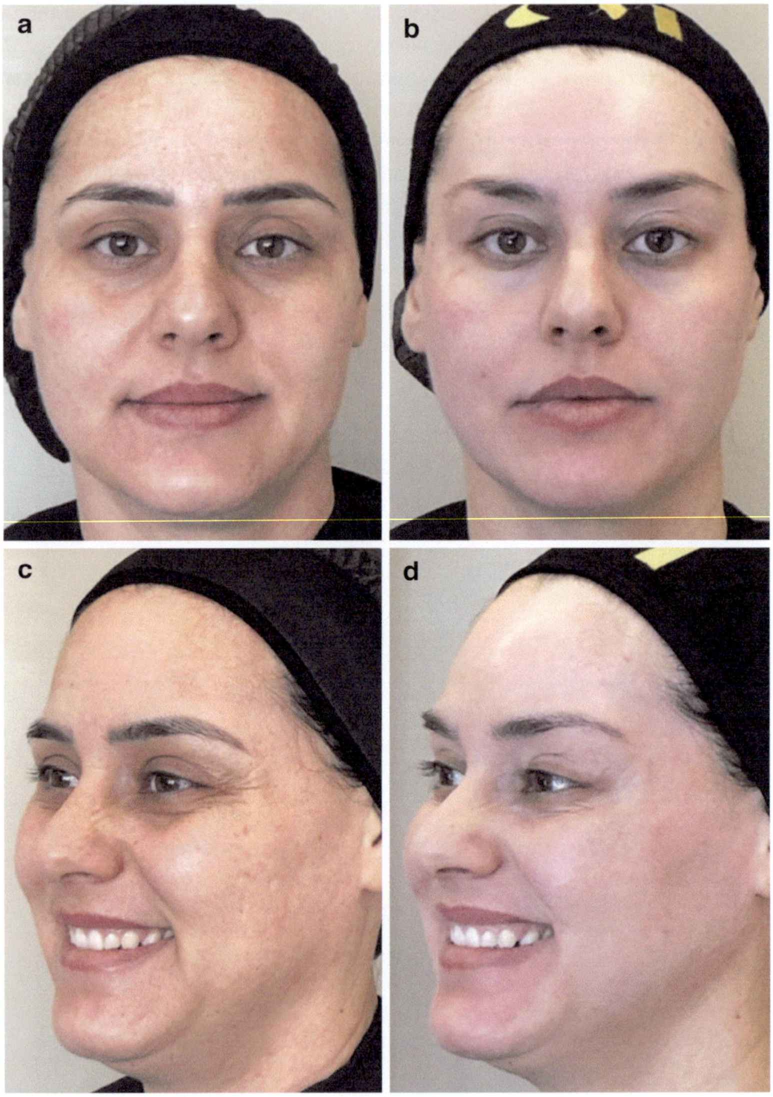

Fig. 5.16 Sixty-three-year-old patient with refractory melasma, atrophic acne scars and periorbital hyperpigmentation. Treated with phenol-croton oil peel (Hetter, 1.2%). (**a**, **c**) Pre-treatment. (**b**, **d**) Six months after the procedure, showing significant lightening of melasma, improvement of acne scars, reduction of dark circles and overall facial rejuvenation, with more even and radiant skin. (*Source: Author's personal archive (Dr Carolina Marçon)*)

5.2.6 Lip Rejuvenation (Lip Peel)

Lip aging is characterized by loss of volume, blurring of the contour, inversion of the vermilion border and accentuation of vertical wrinkles, often worsened by photodamage and structural changes of the labial mucosa. Traditionally, treatment of these changes involves the use of hyaluronic acid-based fillers, which provide immediate volumization but have limited efficacy in reversing actinic damage and in structural tissue remodeling.

Chemical peeling with phenol combined with croton oil—known as *lip peel*—has become established as an effective and safe approach for non-injectable lip rejuvenation (Fig. 5.17). The procedure promotes deep dermal restructuring, with neocollagenesis, reorganization of the dermoepidermal junction and dermal contraction, resulting in improved texture, color and lip projection, as well as eversion of the vermilion. The technique has proven particularly useful in patients with significant lip aging, pronounced vertical wrinkles and actinic cheilitis.

The durability of the results is remarkable, with clinical and photographic evidence of sustained improvement up to 2 years after a single application. There is restoration of the natural lip contour, elevation of the Glogau-Klein point, homogenization of color and redefinition of the vermilion border, resulting in a rejuvenated and natural appearance (Fig. 5.18).

In addition, *lip peel* can be used as a stand-alone procedure or combined with perioral or facial peels (Fig. 5.19). In cases requiring greater volumization, its combination with hyaluronic acid fillers allows for even more comprehensive and

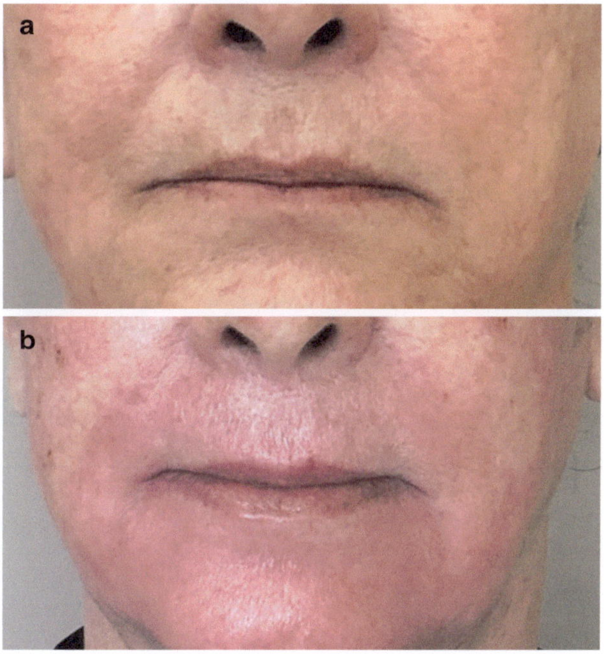

Fig. 5.17 Lip volumization and eversion achieved with phenol-croton oil peel ("lip peel"). (**a**) Before treatment, reduced volume and definition of the lip contour are noted. (**b**) Two months after the procedure with Hetter 1.2% phenol-croton oil in the perioral region and 0.8% on the lips, there is a natural increase in volume, restoration of the contour and elevation of the Glogau-Klein point. (*Source: Author's personal archive (Dr Carolina Marçon)*)

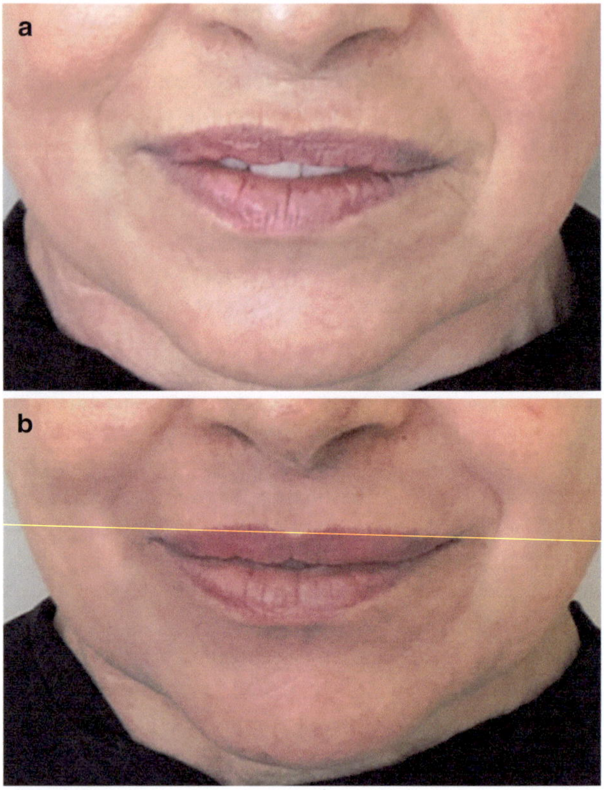

Fig. 5.18 Lip volumization and definition achieved with phenol-croton oil peel (Hetter 1.2%). (**a**) Before treatment, loss of lip contour and volume is observed. (**b**) (Below) After 6 months, there is a natural increase in volume, restoration of the contour and elevation of the Glogau-Klein point, with a harmonious result and without the use of fillers. (Source: Author's personal archive (Dr Carolina Marçon))

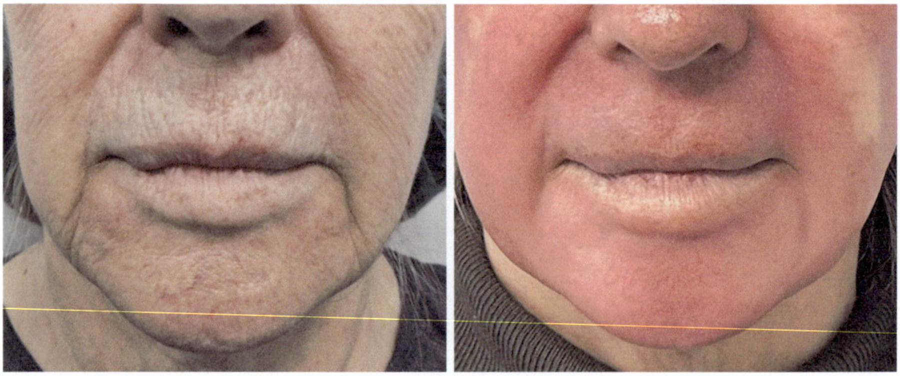

Fig. 5.19 Clinical aspect before (left) and 1 month after (right) phenol-croton oil peel (Hetter 1.2%), using the *feathering* technique for the cheeks. Despite the intense erythema still present, there is significant improvement in perioral rhytids, skin color and texture. (*Source: Author's personal archive (Dr Carolina Marçon)*)

natural results, promoting three-dimensional harmonization of the lip region and expanding the therapeutic reach of the approach.

The technique is considered low-cost and highly predictable, with an excellent safety profile and high patient satisfaction, provided it is performed by properly trained professionals. Standardization of croton oil concentration and careful case selection are essential to achieve effective, long-lasting and safe results.

5.3 Special Considerations: Dark and Asian Skin

The use of chemical peels in patients with dark skin (phototypes IV–VI) and Asian skin represents a technical and biological challenge that requires in-depth knowledge of skin physiology, rigorous therapeutic planning and specialized execution. These skin types have structural and functional characteristics that make them highly reactive to inflammatory and abrasive stimuli, with a higher risk of pigmentary changes—especially post-inflammatory hyperpigmentation (PIH) and permanent hypopigmentation.

The greater density and activity of melanocytes, the predominance of eumelanin, the deeper and more compact distribution of melanosomes, and the higher reactivity of the enzyme tyrosinase confer increased natural photoprotection to these skin types. On the other hand, such characteristics increase the propensity for exaggerated pigmentary reactions in response to chemical, thermal, or mechanical injuries. Additionally, the cutaneous barrier function may be compromised by reduced cohesion between corneocytes and increased transepidermal permeability, facilitating the penetration of chemical agents and the subsequent inflammatory response.

The main complication of chemical peels performed on dark and Asian skin is post-inflammatory hyperpigmentation (PIH), which is directly related to the depth of the chemical injury and the magnitude of the inflammatory response. Prior skin preparation with topical depigmenting agents (such as hydroquinone, kojic acid, azelaic acid, and retinoids), in combination with strict photoprotection for at least 2–4 weeks, is considered essential to minimize this risk.

Another relevant complication is hypochromia, which occurs when there is partial or total destruction of basal melanocytes or their regenerative niches, such as cutaneous appendages. Traditionally considered irreversible, this condition has been re-evaluated in light of more recent evidence.

Paiva et al. documented spontaneous repigmentation of hypochromic areas in dark-skinned pigs and in humans with phototypes V and VI following application of the Hetter peel (phenol 35% + croton oil 1.6%). Complete repigmentation was observed within 21 days in animal models and between 14 and 21 days in humans, except in one area subjected to overlapping chemoabrasion. Histological findings included epidermal regeneration, presence of melanophages, and type III collagen deposition. These data suggest that preservation of hair follicles and control of chemical aggression are fundamental to enable regeneration of the melanoepidermal unit and to prevent permanent sequelae.

In the case of Asian skin, the risks associated with PIH are shared, but there is a greater tendency towards dermal melasma and cutaneous sensitivity. This susceptibility requires greater care in the selection of chemical agents, avoiding traditional medium and deep peels in favor of superficial alternatives such as mandelic, lactic, glycolic acids, and modified Jessner's solution. Nevertheless, there is growing evidence that phenol can be used safely in Asian patients, provided that modified formulations and well-controlled protocols are employed.

Sun et al. reported a large case series involving 896 Asian patients treated with a modified crystalline phenol solution, specifically developed to reduce systemic toxicity and pigmentary risks associated with deep chemical peels. The formulation excluded classic components of the Baker-Gordon and Hetter solutions, such as croton oil and hexachlorophene, and consisted of crystalline phenol (818 g), dyclonine (16 g), camphor (2 g), anhydrous alcohol (82 mL), and glycerin (50 mL), completed with distilled water to a final volume of 1000 mL. The solution was then divided into opaque 5 mL vials and stored protected from light, with the final concentration adjusted between 73.6% and 90%. Application followed a strict technical protocol, including systemic analgesia, continuous cardiac monitoring, and Ringer's lactate infusion to accelerate phenol excretion. The clinical endpoint was defined by the degree of frosting achieved, ranging from translucent frosting (indicative of papillary dermal penetration) to thick white-grey frosting (indicating penetration to the mid-reticular dermis). The total amount of solution applied per patient ranged from 2 to 3 mL. The clinical outcomes were remarkable: 99.66% of patients showed improvement of 51% or greater in the appearance of facial freckles, with a mean score of 3.71 on a 0–4 scale (excellent). The most common complication was post-inflammatory hyperpigmentation, observed in 6.58% of patients, with spontaneous resolution within 4–6 months. There were no cases of persistent hypopigmentation, hypertrophic scarring, or systemic toxicity. These findings suggest that, even in highly reactive Asian skin, phenol can be used safely and effectively, provided that adapted formulations and rigorous technical control are employed.

Similar results were reported by Park et al. using another modified phenol formulation composed of phenol, resorcinol, citric acid, glycerin, vegetable oils, and buffering agents. The study included 46 Asian patients with Fitzpatrick skin types IV and V and demonstrated excellent outcomes in the treatment of wrinkles, acne scars, and melasma, with only 2% persistent hypopigmentation and 74% transient post-inflammatory hyperpigmentation (PIH), which was managed with topical lightening agents.

The depigmenting effect of phenol in pigmented skin appears to be associated with the removal of epidermal melanin, inhibition of melanocytic activity, modulation of inflammation, and reorganization of the basal layer. However, this same therapeutic effect may become detrimental if the injury exceeds the regenerative capacity of the melanoepidermal unit, resulting in long-lasting hypopigmentation.

The systematic review conducted by Handog et al. reinforces the high risk of post-inflammatory hyperpigmentation (PIH) in Asian patients, even when using chemical peels considered safe and of superficial to medium depth. Assessing 14 clinical studies on the use of peels for the treatment of acne and acne scars in Asian skin (phototypes III–V), the authors observed that acids such as glycolic (20–70%), salicylic (20–30%), mandelic, and modified Jessner produced significant clinical results, though not without adverse effects. Glycolic acid, widely used, was associated with cases of PIH, particularly at higher concentrations. In contrast, salicylic acid demonstrated greater tolerability, with a lower incidence of residual pigmentation.

Trichloroacetic acid (TCA) , particularly at concentrations between 25% and 35%, proved effective for atrophic scars but carries a high risk of dyschromia and even permanent scarring, and is therefore recommended only for focal applications (such as the CROSS technique) or in patients with lower phototypes. The need for strict protocols—including prior preparation with topical depigmenting agents, intensive photoprotection, and meticulous technique—was reiterated as a critical factor for therapeutic success in Asian skin.

Although phenol-croton oil was not directly addressed in the review, the data presented allow us to infer that the use of deep peels in Asian patients requires significant adaptations in formulation and technique to mitigate risks. The high frequency of PIH even with moderate agents highlights the melanocytic reactivity of this group, underscoring the need for utmost caution when considering phenol as a therapeutic option. Thus, extrapolation of the findings from Handog et al.'s review supports the importance of personalized formulation, strict control of penetration, and performance by experienced professionals when managing highly reactive skin types such as Asian skin.

In addition to the risk of post-inflammatory hyperpigmentation, patients with more pigmented skin—including Black and Asian skin—are more prone to the development of hypertrophic scars and keloids. This predisposition is related to structural and cellular differences in the skin, such as a higher density of fibroblasts, which modulate both the inflammatory response and tissue repair mechanisms. Studies show that fibroblasts in higher phototypes exhibit increased collagen synthesis activity and greater expression of TGF-β, factors that promote aberrant scarring and excessive extracellular matrix deposition, especially after deep injuries. Such characteristics demand strict control of the depth of chemical injury and careful patient selection, as even poorly performed medium-depth peels can trigger disproportionate scarring responses with significant functional and aesthetic impact.

In light of this, the use of phenol-croton oil peel in dark and Asian skin types should be reserved for well-selected cases, with individualized protocols, rigorous skin preparation, and absolute technical expertise on the part of the practitioner. Recommended strategies include: segmental application (for example, perioral or malar areas), use of formulations with lower croton oil concentration, and close clinical monitoring in the postoperative period.

Continuous photoprotection, maintenance of topical depigmenting agents, and, when indicated, the use of topical corticosteroids complement post-procedure management. Informed consent should be detailed and include a clear discussion of the risks of PIH and hypopigmentation.

In conclusion, although patients with dark and Asian skin types have an increased risk of pigmentary complications, they should not be systematically excluded from therapies with the potential for profound remodeling and effective rejuvenation. With technical expertise, appropriate modifications to the formula and technique, and rigorous monitoring, phenol-croton oil peel can be performed safely and effectively in these groups, respecting their biological particularities and maximizing both aesthetic and functional benefits.

5.4 Contraindications to Phenol-Croton Oil Peel

5.4.1 Absolute Contraindications

Phenol-croton oil peel is a deep ablative procedure with significant potential for systemic toxicity and local complications. Therefore, careful identification of absolute contraindications is essential to ensure patient safety. The main clinical conditions that categorically contraindicate the procedure are listed below (Table 5.2):

5.4.1.1 Unstable or Uncontrolled Cardiovascular Disease

Phenol has a myocardial depressant effect and may trigger severe arrhythmias, conduction blocks, bradycardia, and even cardiac arrest. Patients with a history of myocardial infarction, heart failure, atrioventricular blocks, cardiomyopathies, unstable angina, or any uncompensated cardiovascular condition must be excluded. A QTc interval >475 ms is a formal contraindication due to the risk of torsades de pointes. Prior cardiological assessment and continuous monitoring during the procedure are mandatory for procedures involving a body surface area greater than 1.5%.

5.4.1.2 Uncontrolled Cardiac Arrhythmias or Use of Class I/III Antiarrhythmics

Even in stable patients, phenol may precipitate fatal arrhythmic events. Previously unstable arrhythmias, such as atrial fibrillation with rapid ventricular response, frequent ventricular extrasystoles, or supraventricular tachyarrhythmias, should be considered absolute contraindications.

5.4.1.3 Uncontrolled Systemic Arterial Hypertension

Decompensated hypertension increases myocardial vulnerability to the toxic effects of phenol and predisposes to hypertensive crises, arrhythmias, and intraoperative hemodynamic complications. Strict blood pressure control is essential before indicating the peel.

5.4.1.4 Decompensated Obstructive Pulmonary Diseases (e.g., Moderate/Severe COPD)

Patients with reduced ventilatory reserve, especially in the presence of hypercapnia, cor pulmonale, or need for oxygen therapy, are at increased risk of respiratory decompensation induced by stress and systemic absorption of phenol. Recent onset dyspnea is also a contraindication.

Table 5.2 Absolute contraindications to phenol–croton peel

Condition	Rationale/main risk	Objective criterion/ examples	Management
Unstable/ uncontrolled cardiovascular disease	Phenol is a cardio depressant → arrhythmias, conduction blocks, bradycardia, asystole	Recent MI, decompensated heart failure, unstable angina, advanced AV block; QTc > 475 ms	Contraindicated; requires cardiology assessment and, in future segmental cases, continuous monitoring
Uncontrolled arrhythmias or use of class I/III antiarrhythmic drugs	Risk of precipitating fatal arrhythmias	AF with rapid ventricular response, frequent PVCs, unstable SVT; use of class I/III drugs	Contraindicated
Uncontrolled systemic arterial hypertension	Hypertensive crises and intraoperative arrhythmias	Persistently elevated/ variable BP without control	Postpone until strict control is achieved
Decompensated COPD/recent onset dyspnea	Reduced ventilatory reserve; risk of respiratory decompensation	Hypercapnia, cor pulmonale, oxygen requirement; recent onset dyspnea	Contraindicated until clinical stabilization
Severe/ decompensated liver disease	Impaired hepatic metabolism of phenol → systemic toxicity	Cirrhosis, active hepatitis, hepatic failure	Contraindicated
Severe/ decompensated hepatic or renal disease	Reduced renal excretion of phenol → systemic accumulation	CrCl <30 mL/min, nephrotic syndrome, advanced CKD	Contraindicated
Decompensated diabetes mellitus	Impaired angiogenesis, epithelialization and collagen deposition	HbA1c ≥7% or persistent hyperglycemia	Postpone until adequate glycemic control
Severe immunosuppression or AIDS	Impaired inflammatory/ scarring response; increased risk of infection	Chronic use of immunosuppressants/ biologics; CD4 <200	Contraindicated
Severe autoimmune diseases	Risk of unpredictable cutaneous reactions/ necrosis/exacerbation	SLE, pemphigus vulgaris, dermatomyositis, scleroderma, pyoderma gangrenosum, sarcoidosis	Contraindicated
History of abnormal scarring/extensive keloids	Disorganized fibrosis (TGF-β/SMAD axis ↑; MMP/TIMP ↓) and poorer aesthetic outcome	Extensive keloids; high-tension areas (jaw, chin, preauricular)	Contraindicated; exception only with justification, test area, and extended consent
Frontal fibrosing alopecia (FFA)	Loss of pilosebaceous units/stem cells → failure of dermal regeneration	Diagnosis of FFA	Contraindicated
Active cutaneous or systemic infection	Risk of dissemination, necrosis, and sepsis	Active HSV, impetigo, mycoses; fever	Postpone until complete clinical resolution

(continued)

Table 5.2 (continued)

Condition	Rationale/main risk	Objective criterion/ examples	Management
Pregnancy or breastfeeding	Precautionary principle due to the potential systemic toxicity of phenol	Pregnant/breastfeeding women	Contraindicated
Severe/ decompensated psychiatric conditions	Poor adherence, psychosocial/litigious risk, and worse prognosis	Untreated major depression, psychosis, severe BDD; suicidal ideation	Contraindicated until stabilization with specialist assessment
Malnutrition	Interferes with all phases of wound healing (inflammation, proliferation, and remodeling), increases risk of infection, dehiscence, atrophic or hypertrophic scars	Low BMI, rapid weight loss, severe restrictive diets, protein and micronutrient deficiency, use of GLP-1 agonists	Contraindicated until nutritional status is optimized; consider supplementation and postponement of the procedure
Skin previously compromised by surgery or specific anatomical conditions	Permanent vascular compromise → isquemia/necrosis	History of lifting/flaps in the area to be treated	Contraindicated in the area; consider alternatives
Smoking	Vasoconstriction, tissue hypoxia, and impairment of healing (high risk of cutaneous necrosis, dehiscence, and infection)	Current use of cigarettes, electronic cigarettes, vapes, heated tobacco, or hookah; positive cotinine test	Contraindicated; only to be performed after a minimum cessation period of 4 weeks before and 4 weeks after the procedure
Active cutaneous neoplasm in the area (melanoma or NMSC)	Diagnostic masking; pro-tumoral microenvironment; interferes with therapies	Active/suspected lesion in the treatment area	Contraindicated; prioritize specific oncological management

Contraindications that preclude the procedure regardless of aesthetic indication; consider only after resolution/stabilization and with complete clinical documentation. (*Source: Table prepared by the author (Dr Carolina Marçon)*)

5.4.1.5 Severe or Decompensated Hepatic or Renal Disease

The hepatic metabolism of phenol via conjugation (glucuronidation and sulphation) and its renal excretion make proper liver and kidney function essential. Patients with cirrhosis, active hepatitis, nephrotic syndrome, or chronic renal failure (clearance <30 mL/min) are at significantly increased risk of systemic toxicity.

5.4.1.6 Decompensated Diabetes Mellitus

Persistent hyperglycemia impairs angiogenesis, neutrophil chemotaxis, epithelialization, and collagen deposition, increasing the risk of necrosis, infection, and pathological scarring. Glycemic control should be strict, ideally with HbA1c <7%.

5.4.1.7 Severe Immunosuppression or AIDS

States of immunosuppression, whether due to chronic use of corticosteroids, immunobiological agents, chemotherapy, or immunodeficiencies such as AIDS (CD4 <200), impair the inflammatory response, increase susceptibility to infections, and hinder tissue regeneration.

5.4.1.8 Severe Autoimmune Diseases

Conditions such as systemic lupus erythematosus, pemphigus vulgaris, dermatomyositis, scleroderma, pyoderma gangrenosum, and sarcoidosis are associated with immune dysregulation and a high risk of unpredictable cutaneous reactions, necrosis, or exacerbation of the underlying disease.

5.4.1.9 History of Abnormal Scarring or Extensive Keloids

The presence of extensive keloids or a history of abnormal scarring, such as hypertrophic scars, fibrotic contractures, or poor scar evolution following previous procedures, constitutes a significant contraindication to phenol-croton oil peel. Although the procedure primarily affects the epidermis and papillary dermis, its depth and inflammatory potential render predisposed patients more vulnerable to disorganized fibrosis and unfavorable aesthetic outcomes, particularly in the mandibular, mental, and preauricular regions, where scar tension is greatest.

5.4.1.10 Pathophysiology of Abnormal Scarring

Hypertrophic scars and keloids represent manifestations of exuberant wound healing, characterized by excessive deposition of collagen (mainly types I and III), fibronectin, TGF-β1, and other pro-fibrotic cytokines, as well as persistent proliferation of fibroblasts and myofibroblasts. In the case of keloids, collagen forms thick, hyalinized bundles with irregular orientation, which extend beyond the boundaries of the original lesion and show no tendency for spontaneous regression.

From a molecular perspective, there is hyperactivity of the TGF-β/SMAD pathway, reduced expression of MMPs (matrix metalloproteinases), and increased levels of their inhibitors (TIMPs), resulting in disorganized remodeling of the extracellular matrix. Persistent production of inflammatory mediators and growth factors following trauma is considered a key factor, especially in patients with a genetic predisposition or epigenetic regulatory alterations.

5.4.1.11 Clinical and Genetic Risk Factors

Patients with a personal or family history of keloids, particularly in areas subjected to trauma, surgery, vaccination, or inflamed acne, should be considered high risk. Anatomical location is a critical factor: regions such as the chest, back, shoulders, ears, and jaw are more susceptible, but facial keloids are also reported, especially in areas of tension or repetitive injury.

Ethnicity is another relevant factor: individuals with skin phototypes IV–VI, particularly those of African or Asian descent, have a higher risk of abnormal scarring. A population-based study demonstrated a keloid incidence of between 4.5% and 16% in people of African descent, compared to less than 1% in

Caucasians. These differences are attributed to genetic variants in the TGF-β1, SMAD3, and p53 genes, as well as differences in inflammatory response profiles and dermal biomechanics.

5.4.1.12 Implications for Phenol-Croton Oil Peel

Phenol-croton oil peel induces coagulative necrosis of the epidermis and upper dermis, with intense inflammatory activation in the first 48 h, followed by profound dermal remodeling in the subsequent weeks. Although this process normally results in harmonious reorganization of the extracellular matrix, patients predisposed to disorganized fibrosis may develop skin thickening, raised scars, contractures, or permanent irregularities.

Furthermore, transition zones between aesthetic units (such as the jawline and nasolabial folds) are particularly susceptible to abnormal scarring behavior, whether due to mechanical tension or heterogeneity in solution penetration.

5.4.1.13 Recommended Management

Phenol-croton oil peel should not be performed in patients with active keloids on the face or with a history of severe keloids at any site, except under exceptional justification and with informed consent.

In cases with a limited history of abnormal scarring, the procedure may be considered with:

- Prior test on a restricted area (test spot).
- Avoidance of anatomically high-risk areas.
- Reduction of croton concentration.
- Careful application with reduced depth.

Strict and prolonged follow-up.

The use of prophylactic measures, such as topical or intralesional corticosteroids (if there are early signs of scar thickening), may be considered in borderline cases, always under specialist guidance.

In summary, assessment of the patient's previous scarring should be a mandatory part of the medical history and pre-procedure documentation, especially in high-risk individuals. The decision must be individualized, weighing the potential aesthetic benefit against the possibility of permanent complications.

5.4.1.14 Frontal Fibrosing Alopecia (FFA)

Patients with FFA should be excluded from deep chemical peels. The condition is characterized by progressive loss of pilosebaceous units and follicular stem cells in the frontotemporal region, significantly impairing dermal regeneration. The absence of stem cells hinders wound healing and increases the risk of necrosis, atrophy, and unsightly scarring. Recent reports have documented severe cutaneous complications following phenol-croton oil peels in patients with FFA, leading to a growing consensus regarding its absolute contraindication (Fig. 5.20).

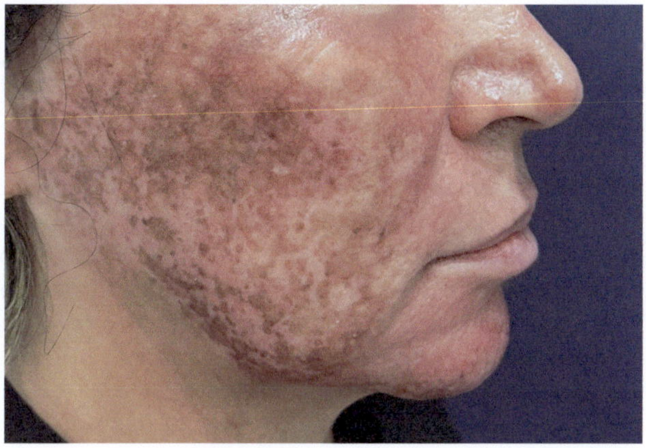

Fig. 5.20 Abnormal healing 1 month after phenol-croton oil peel (Hetter 1.2%) in a patient with frontal fibrosing alopecia. (*Source: Courtesy of Dr Felipe Ribeiro*)

5.4.1.15 Active Infection (Cutaneous or Systemic)

The presence of active viral (e.g. herpes simplex), bacterial or fungal infection at the treatment site or systemically increases the risk of infectious dissemination, tissue necrosis, and septicemia. The procedure should be postponed until complete clinical resolution.

5.4.1.16 Pregnancy or Lactation

The available medical literature does not report any formal or specific contraindications for the use of phenol in chemical peels during pregnancy or lactation, either for patients or for professionals handling the product. However, observational studies suggest that phenolic compounds in general may act as endocrine disruptors and, in animal models, are associated with reproductive and developmental effects. In humans, there are limited and inconclusive data regarding exposure to low levels of phenols during pregnancy, with some findings indicating possible changes in neonatal anthropometric measures, but without a clear association with major adverse outcomes.

There are no reports in the literature of serious adverse events related to occupational exposure of healthcare professionals to phenol during dermatological procedures, nor are there formal contraindications for pregnant or breastfeeding women acting as applicators of the product. Nevertheless, given the potential toxicity of phenol in cases of systemic exposure and the lack of robust safety data for pregnant and breastfeeding women, caution is advised and measures should be taken to minimize exposure, in accordance with the precautionary principle.

The medical literature demonstrates that occupational exposure of healthcare professionals to phenol during dermatological procedures, such as chemical matricectomy, results in exposure levels well below environmental safety limits, even when using high-concentration phenol solutions and exposures of up to 20 min. There is no evidence of significant risk for breastfeeding professionals under these conditions, and urinary phenol levels following such procedures remain within parameters considered safe.

Nevertheless, it is recommended to adopt standard precautions when handling phenol, such as the use of gloves, eye protection, and adequate room ventilation, to minimize dermal absorption and inhalation of vapors. Furthermore, product labels containing phenol in the United States advise that pregnant and breastfeeding women consult a healthcare professional before use, reflecting a precautionary approach in the absence of robust safety data for these populations.

Thus, given the scarcity of robust data and the potential toxicity of phenol in cases of systemic exposure, phenol–croton oil peels should be considered contraindicated during pregnancy and lactation. In addition, physicians and technical staff who are pregnant or breastfeeding should exercise extreme caution, even in the absence of formal contraindications. Strict use of personal protective equipment is recommended, including:

- Nitrile gloves resistant to chemical compounds.
- Heavyweight, long-sleeved gown, preferably impermeable.
- Protective goggles or full-face shield.
- Mask with chemical filter for organic vapors of the PFF3 type or combined cartridge class A1 (for organic vapors) + P3 (particulates), with full facial seal, in accordance with NIOSH or EN 14387 specifications—as surgical masks or PFF2/N95 do not provide adequate protection against phenolic vapors.
- An environment with effective local exhaust or a ventilation system with adequate air renewal, minimizing inhalation of volatile vapors.

Such precautions are especially mandatory for pregnant or breastfeeding professionals, even if they are not directly applying the product, in order to ensure occupational safety and prevent inadvertent exposures.

5.4.1.17 Severe or Decompensated Psychiatric Conditions

Patients with severe or decompensated psychiatric disorders—such as untreated major depression, suicidal ideation, psychosis, dementia, borderline or narcissistic personality disorders in crisis, or severe anxiety with functional impairment—should be excluded from undergoing phenol-croton oil peel.

These conditions negatively affect the patient's ability to understand the risks of the procedure, to follow postoperative instructions appropriately, to tolerate the re-epithelialization and healing process (which may be lengthy and emotionally challenging), and to maintain realistic expectations regarding the outcomes.

Studies in aesthetic surgery show that decompensated psychiatric disorders are associated with a higher risk of psychosocial complications, such as extreme dissatisfaction, regret, body image distortion, and litigious behavior. Furthermore, poor adherence to self-care and the impulsivity common to certain psychiatric conditions increase the risk of infections, wound dehiscence, premature manipulation of re-epithelialized skin, formation of abnormal scars, and worsening of the overall clinical picture.

Active or recent suicidal ideation, in particular, is an absolute contraindication, as invasive procedures with significant physical and emotional impact may act as precipitating factors for fatal outcomes. Cases of mild or moderate depression, controlled with psychiatric follow-up and medication stability, should be assessed individually, with a documented specialist opinion.

Therefore, thorough psychiatric screening is essential prior to deep ablative procedures, with particular attention to a history of:

- Mood disorders (depression, bipolar disorder).
- Personality disorders.
- Current or previous psychosis.
- Eating disorders.
- Body dysmorphic disorders (BDD).
- Dependence on psychoactive substances (including alcohol, benzodiazepines, opioids, and stimulants).
- Cognitive disorders (dementia, mild cognitive impairment).

The presence of body dysmorphic disorder (BDD), even when not severe, requires special attention, as these patients tend to have unrealistic expectations, obsessive focus on minor imperfections, and a high rate of dissatisfaction with aesthetic outcomes, regardless of the technical quality of the procedure. The literature indicates that BDD is present in up to 15% of candidates for cosmetic surgery and is often underdiagnosed.

In cases of diagnostic uncertainty or lack of clinical stability, the procedure should be postponed until a formal psychiatric assessment and documented control of the condition. Careful documentation of this assessment is recommended for patient safety and medico-legal protection of the practitioner.

5.4.1.18 Smoking

Smoking represents a critical risk factor for complications in deep dermatological procedures, including phenol–croton oil peels. Nicotine and its metabolites exert direct vasoconstrictive effects, reduce tissue oxygenation, impair fibroblast function, and inhibit collagen synthesis, all of which are essential for effective wound healing. In addition, carbon monoxide present in cigarettes binds to hemoglobin, further reducing oxygen transport capacity and exacerbating post-procedural tissue hypoxia (Fig. 5.21).

Several studies have shown that smokers have higher rates of complications such as skin necrosis, wound dehiscence, infections, delayed healing, and unsightly scarring. Even in less invasive procedures, such as nail phenolization, healing time is significantly prolonged in smokers, suggesting that the risk is even greater in deep facial peels, which involve large areas and require a high regenerative demand.

Studies in facial plastic surgery demonstrate that smoking is one of the main predictors of skin flap necrosis, often requiring corrective interventions. The risk of tissue loss is particularly relevant in regions such as the perioral area, malar region, and eyelids, with reports of partial or total necrosis of the treated skin in patients who continued nicotine use during the perioperative period.

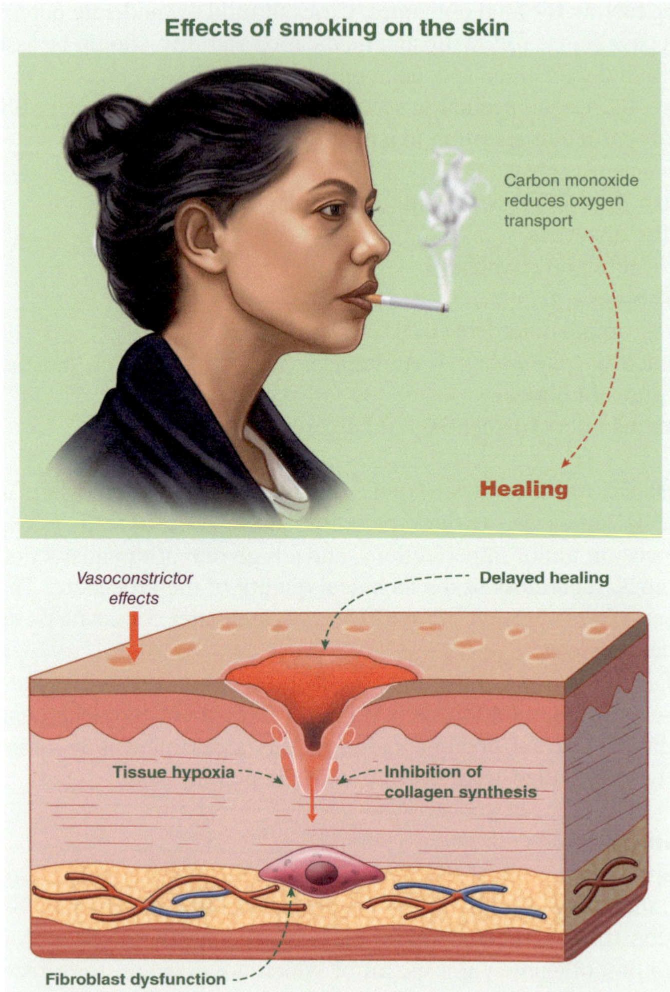

Fig. 5.21 Mechanisms of smoking in the skin and wound healing. Nicotine promotes vasoconstriction and reduced tissue perfusion; carbon monoxide binds to hemoglobin, worsening hypoxia; fibroblasts become dysfunctional with reduced collagen and elastin synthesis; and there is an increase in reactive oxygen species and chronic inflammation. The end result is a higher risk of necrosis, delayed healing, infections, and hypertrophic scarring in smokers undergoing deep dermatological procedures. (*Source: Figure created by the author (Dr Carolina Marçon)*)

In this context, smoking should be considered an absolute or relative contraindication, depending on the degree of nicotine dependence, the presence of associated comorbidities, and the inability to cease smoking. The literature strongly recommends that patients completely stop smoking at least 4 weeks before and 4 weeks after the procedure to minimize risks. This guidance applies to traditional cigarettes as well as electronic cigarettes, vaporizers, heated tobacco, and waterpipes, all of which are associated with vascular and inflammatory effects detrimental to wound healing.

Underreporting of smoking is common, which is why urinary or salivary cotinine measurement may be considered in at-risk patients, especially those who deny smoking but present clinical signs suggestive of chronic nicotine exposure.

Therefore, active smoking must be rigorously assessed and proactively addressed when selecting candidates for phenol–croton oil peel. Complete cessation is mandatory to reduce risks and optimize outcomes. If cessation is not possible, the procedure should be postponed or even contraindicated, especially in the presence of additional risk factors for impaired wound healing.

5.4.1.19 Malnutrition

A prior nutritional assessment is mandatory before performing deep chemical peels, such as phenol–croton oil, especially in elderly patients, those with low BMI, chronic diseases, a history of delayed wound healing, or restrictive eating behaviors. Malnutrition adversely affects all phases of the healing process, impairing the inflammatory response, cellular migration and proliferation, collagen synthesis, and tissue remodeling. Protein–calorie deficiency reduces collagen deposition, wound tensile strength, and immunocompetence, increasing the risk of infection, dehiscence, and the formation of atrophic or hypertrophic scars. Carbohydrate deficiency compromises the energy production required for cellular proliferation and fibroblast migration. Micronutrients such as zinc, iron, vitamins A, C, D, and B complex are essential for angiogenesis, modulation of inflammation, re-epithelialization, and organization of the extracellular matrix. Deficiency of these elements is associated with a higher incidence of chronic wounds, pressure ulcers, delayed healing, infections, and abnormal scarring.

In addition to overt malnutrition, states of functional undernutrition are also relevant and frequently underdiagnosed. Restrictive diets for aesthetic purposes, such as ketogenic, extreme low-carb regimens, prolonged intermittent fasting, or severe caloric restriction, have become increasingly common, particularly among patients seeking facial rejuvenation. Even in individuals with an appropriate body weight, these practices can deplete reserves of amino acids and micronutrients essential for tissue regeneration, thereby impairing wound healing and the immune response following peeling procedures.

Another emerging factor is the use of GLP-1 receptor agonists, such as semaglutide (Ozempic®, Wegovy®), tirzepatide (Mounjaro®), and liraglutide (Saxenda®), which are widely prescribed for the management of type 2 diabetes and weight loss. Although these drugs improve metabolic parameters and reduce systemic inflammation, recent studies have shown that their use may negatively affect skin regeneration and accelerate skin aging. These agents act on receptors expressed in adipose-derived stem cells (ADSCs) and dermal fibroblasts, reducing the production of protective cytokines, increasing the generation of reactive oxygen species (ROS), inducing cellular apoptosis, and decreasing local production of dermal estrogens—factors that directly impact skin integrity and collagen synthesis. Furthermore, glucose uptake by ADSCs is impaired, which limits ATP production and compromises tissue repair processes.

The catabolic state induced by the combination of rapid weight loss, caloric restriction, and chronic use of GLP-1RAs can severely compromise the response to chemical injury caused by phenol. Therefore, patients using these medications, with a history of restrictive dieting or signs of nutritional frailty, should be carefully assessed, including laboratory tests, body composition analysis, and, when indicated, prior supplementation with amino acids, antioxidants, and micronutrients.

The decision to proceed with the intervention should be individualized, with postponement of the peeling procedure in cases where nutritional status poses a significant risk to tissue integrity or increases the likelihood of complications. Clinical judgment and transparent communication with the patient are essential to ensure safety, efficacy, and long-lasting aesthetic outcomes.

5.4.1.20 Skin Previously Compromised by Surgery or Specific Anatomical Conditions

Phenol-croton oil peel is contraindicated in areas of skin previously subjected to surgical procedures involving subcutaneous undermining, such as the flaps used in rhytidoplasty, due to the high risk of necrosis, poor wound healing, and unsatisfactory aesthetic outcomes. Vascular compromise in these regions, particularly due to disruption of the dermal and subdermal plexuses, leads to a permanent reduction in tissue nutrition and regenerative capacity, rendering the skin more susceptible to phenol-induced chemical injury and predisposing it to the development of areas of ischemia, necrosis, and irreversible dyschromia. Histological studies have demonstrated persistent structural changes in the vascular architecture of these areas, justifying the contraindication of deep caustic agents in such regions.

Furthermore, special attention should be paid to the eyelid and periorbital regions, particularly in patients with a history of previous blepharoplasty or recent ophthalmic surgery, such as ptosis correction, vitrectomy, or refractive surgery. In these situations, the tissue may exhibit scarring, underlying fibrosis, or anatomical fragility, increasing the risk of post-peel complications such as persistent edema, eyelid retraction, ectropion, and, in more severe cases, functional ocular impairment. A minimum interval of 6 months after blepharoplasty is recommended before the application of deep caustic agents to the treated area.

Highly myopic patients, especially those with a history of retinal detachment, also require careful assessment. Although there is no formal contraindication described in the literature, clinical observations by specialists suggest that the intense and prolonged edema occurring in the periorbital region after phenol-croton oil peel—particularly when applied to the full face including the eyelids—may transiently increase external pressure on the globe. In predisposed patients, this compression could theoretically trigger retinal detachment, especially in retinas already weakened by axial elongation or previous vitreous traction.

As a precaution, patients with high myopia (> −6.00 D), recent ocular surgery, or a history of retinal detachment should be evaluated by an ophthalmologist prior to the procedure. In such cases, it is recommended to avoid treatment of the eyelid region or to opt for segmental protocols with strict clinical monitoring in the postoperative period.

In summary, careful mapping of the facial and ocular surgical history, as well as identification of areas of anatomical fragility, is essential in the pre-peel assessment. This approach enables a safe, individualized, and technically appropriate indication for phenol-croton oil peel, respecting the biological and vascular limits of each patient.

5.4.1.21 Active Skin Neoplasia (Melanoma or Non-melanoma Skin Cancer)

The presence of active cutaneous neoplasia, whether melanoma or non-melanoma skin cancer (basal cell or squamous cell carcinoma), constitutes an absolute contraindication to the use of phenol-croton oil peel in the affected area. This is a matter of clinical and ethical prudence, based on oncological, immunological, and therapeutic principles.

Risk of Clinical Masking and Delayed Diagnosis

Deep peels induce necrosis of the epidermis and portions of the reticular dermis, followed by intense inflammation and remodeling. This process can conceal early lesions of cutaneous neoplasms, making subsequent visual detection more difficult. In particular, in cases of melanoma in situ or superficial forms of intraepidermal squamous cell carcinoma (Bowen's disease), the application of a deep caustic agent may mask tumor architecture, hinder histopathological diagnosis, and delay appropriate treatment, thereby compromising prognosis.

Stimulation of Pro-oncogenic Pathways

Although there is no direct evidence that phenol-croton oil peel induces malignant transformation, the dermal regeneration process is characterized by intense activation of cytokines, growth factors (TGF-β, PDGF, VEGF), and matrix metalloproteinases (MMPs), all of which play a dual role in regeneration and tumor progression. In experimental models, persistent activation of these pathways is associated with the promotion of tumor growth, tissue invasion, and angiogenesis in cutaneous carcinomas and melanomas. Therefore, the application of a deep peel to skin with active neoplasia may theoretically enhance disease progression, especially in tumors that have not been completely excised or identified.

Impairment of Local Immunological Surveillance

The acute inflammatory process induced by phenol-croton oil causes destruction of keratinocytes, sterile necrosis, and subsequent recruitment of neutrophils, macrophages, and fibroblasts. During this phase, there is modulation of local immunity and release of immunosuppressive mediators such as IL-10 and TGF-β. In tumor models, this environment favors tumor immune evasion, allowing proliferation of residual neoplastic cells. Thus, the post-peel inflammatory microenvironment may potentially permit the progression of subclinical or active cutaneous neoplasms.

Interference with Specific Therapeutic Strategies
Patients with active melanoma or NMSC frequently require surgical, immunotherapeutic, topical (imiquimod, 5-FU), or photodynamic approaches, the success of which depends on tissue integrity, histological accuracy, and the absence of external interference. Performing a deep peel compromises both the application and the response to these therapies. Furthermore, it may delay the surgical excision of suspicious lesions or interfere with the assessment of clinical and histological margins.

Distinction Between Field Cancerization and Active Neoplasia
It is important to distinguish cases of cutaneous field cancerization—for which phenol-croton oil peel is a valid and effective indication—from those with invasive tumors or proven proliferative activity. While field cancerization is characterized by multifocal, subclinical, and reversible dysplastic changes, active neoplasms require specific oncological treatment and targeted surgical or destructive intervention. Indiscriminate application of deep peeling to areas with untreated tumoral lesions may compromise oncological control and expose the patient to unnecessary risks.

In conclusion, the presence of active melanoma or NMSC is an absolute contraindication to phenol-croton oil peel, especially in the affected area. A comprehensive dermatological assessment, preferably with dermoscopy and, if necessary, biopsy, should precede any deep ablative procedure. In patients with a history of cutaneous cancer, careful selection of treatment areas and rigorous follow-up are mandatory to ensure safety, efficacy, and oncological integrity.

5.4.2 Relative Contraindications

Relative contraindications do not absolutely preclude the use of phenol-croton oil peel, but represent conditions that increase the risk of local or systemic complications. In such cases, it is necessary to carefully assess the patient's clinical profile, weigh risks and benefits, and consider the possibility of alternative treatments or modifications to the technique. The main relative contraindications are detailed below (Table 5.3):

5.4.2.1 Thick Skin, Enlarged Pores, and Phymatous Phenotypes

Patients with thick skin—characterized by dermal thickening, dilated pores, irregular texture, sebaceous hyperplasia, or phymatous phenotypes (as seen in early rhinophyma)—present additional technical challenges for the application of phenol-croton oil peel. In such cases, penetration of the caustic agent may be uneven and unpredictable, increasing the risk of undertreated areas (with insufficient therapeutic response) or overtreated areas (with necrosis and risk of scarring).

This skin profile may also delay the onset of frosting, making visual assessment of the clinical endpoint more difficult and increasing the risk of technical error. Furthermore, the presence of hypertrophic sebaceous glands may interfere with the homogeneous diffusion of phenol, resulting in areas of uneven absorption and raising the risk of dyschromia, scarring, and asymmetrical aesthetic outcomes.

Table 5.3 Relative contraindications to phenol-croton oil peel

Condition	Rationale/main risk	Objective criteria/ examples	Management
Thick skin/ enlarged pores/ phymatous phenotype	Irregular penetration of the solution; risk of unaesthetic result and abnormal scarring	Early rhinophyma, sebaceous and thick skin	Adjust formula/ concentration; procedure should be performed by experienced hands
Thin/atrophic/ fragile skin	Higher risk of overpenetration, necrosis, and dyspigmentation	Senile skin, chronic corticosteroid therapy, advanced photodamage	Assess risk/benefit; prefer segmental areas; close monitoring
Recent oral isotretinoin use	Altered dermal repair; increased risk of hypertrophic scarring	Treatment within the last 6–12 months	Postpone procedure until safe interval (≥6–12 months)
Recurrent herpes simplex	Risk of viral reactivation after peeling	Positive history of orolabial herpes simplex >6 episodes/year	Antiviral prophylaxis and follow-up
Controlled asthma/ bronchospasm	Possibility of exacerbation	Clinical history of asthma or bronchitis	Proceed with caution; keep bronchodilator available
Controlled cardiac arrhythmias	Vulnerability to cardiotoxic effects of phenol	Stable arrhythmias under treatment	Individual cardiological assessment; strict monitoring
Functional or cognitive dependence for self-care	Difficulty in following postoperative protocol	Frail elderly, patients with cognitive impairment	Proceed only with reliable caregiver support
Personality disorders/ unrealistic expectations	High risk of dissatisfaction and litigation	Body dysmorphic disorder, borderline disorder, unrealistic expectations	Assess psychological stability; contraindicate if adherence is not ensured
Pain intolerance	Low tolerance may compromise adherence	Previous history of abandoning painful procedures	Consider additional analgesia or alternative technique
Active inflammatory skin diseases	Risk of exacerbation and abnormal scarring	Psoriasis, lichen planus, active dermatitis	Postpone until disease control
Vitiligo	Risk of Koebner phenomenon	Clinical diagnosis of vitiligo	Avoid in active lesions; proceed only in stable areas
Systemic disease under investigation	Undefined risk; lack of clinical stability	Ongoing laboratory tests, unexplained symptoms	Postpone until diagnostic clarification
Use of drugs that prolong QT interval	Potentiation of phenol cardiotoxicity	Tricyclic antidepressants, antipsychotics, antiemetics, thiazide diuretics, antifungals, antihistamines	Assess need for suspension/ substitution; contraindicate if not feasible

Relative contraindications to phenol-croton oil peel. Clinical situations that do not represent an absolute contraindication, but require careful assessment, prior preparation, and close monitoring to reduce risks and ensure procedural safety. (*Source: Table prepared by the author (Dr Carolina Marçon)*)

To mitigate these risks, it is recommended to adjust both the formulation and the application technique. Adaptations may include:

- Use of more homogeneous and carefully measured concentrations, with strict control of the volume applied
- Application in thin, targeted passes, with intervals between them to assess frosting
- Pre-treatment with oral isotretinoin at a subclinical dose for 6–12 weeks, in selected cases, to reduce sebaceous hyperplasia and even out epidermal thickness
- Avoiding application in areas of active rhinophyma or advanced dermal fibrosis, which require alternative therapeutic approaches (such as surgery, ablative laser, or electrosurgery)

In all cases, careful clinical judgment, individualized protocol design, and rigorous monitoring of the cutaneous response during and after the procedure are essential. Although a thick skin phenotype does not constitute a formal contraindication, it demands technical skill, experience, and precise modulation to ensure safety and predictability of the final outcome.

5.4.2.2 Thin, Atrophic, or Fragile Skin

Skin thickness is a critical factor in determining the depth of action and safety of chemical peels. In thin skin—particularly in areas such as the eyelids, perioral region, forehead, and in individuals with a naturally atrophic or aged skin phenotype—there is a lower density of cutaneous appendages, a thin epidermal layer, and reduced thickness of the papillary and superficial reticular dermis. These anatomical features make the penetration of caustic agents faster and deeper, significantly increasing the risk of extensive dermal injury, dyschromia, atrophic scarring, and poor wound healing.

Histological studies show that the palpebral epidermis, for example, measures on average 0.04 mm (40 μm), while the dermis in this region is only 0.3–0.6 mm thick. In contrast, in the malar region, these layers combined may exceed 1.5 mm. This anatomical difference means that in thin skin, even a small amount of phenol may rapidly surpass the intended therapeutic zone and reach deeper dermal layers or even underlying vascular structures. Histological studies show that the palpebral epidermis, for example, measures on average 0.04 mm (40 μm), while the dermis in this region is only 0.3–0.6 mm thick. In contrast, in the malar region, these layers combined may exceed 1.5 mm. This anatomical difference means that, in thin skin, even a small amount of phenol can rapidly penetrate beyond the intended therapeutic zone and reach deeper layers of the dermis or even underlying vascular structures.

Furthermore, the low density of cutaneous appendages (pilosebaceous units, sweat glands) and reduced superficial vascularization in thin skin compromise rapid re-epithelialization and the dissipation of the chemical agent, favoring focal necrosis, prolonged ulceration, and increased risks of infection and persistent dyschromia.

Patients with extremely thin or atrophic skin due to chronological aging or severe photoaging also exhibit a reduced reserve of active fibroblasts, fragmented collagen, and a disorganized extracellular matrix. These factors impair the scarring response and dermal remodeling after peeling, increasing the likelihood of atrophic scars, post-inflammatory dyschromia, and permanent textural changes.

In addition to histological aspects, there is also greater functional susceptibility to ectropion (lower lip retraction), eyelid retraction (ectropion), and worsening of dynamic laxity in thin or very lax skin, especially if the peel is performed in conjunction with highly mobile regions or over areas with compromised ligamentous support.

Given these risks, prior assessment of skin thickness through thorough clinical examination, and when necessary, supported by imaging (such as high-frequency cutaneous ultrasound or optical profilometry), may be decisive in selecting the concentration, application time, and extent of the procedure. In cases of very thin skin, it is recommended to:

- Avoid deep phenol-croton oil peels in critical areas (such as the eyelids and nasolabial fold)
- Use diluted or segmented formulations
- Consider milder and progressive combination treatments
- Undertake preconditioning with topical bio-stimulatory and antioxidant agents that improve the structure of the superficial dermis

5.4.2.3 Recent Use of Oral Isotretinoin

For decades, recent use of oral isotretinoin was considered a contraindication for ablative dermatological procedures, especially those with the potential to reach deep dermal planes, such as phenol-croton oil peels. This precaution was based on theoretical premises and anecdotal reports suggesting a possible increased risk of scarring changes, such as exuberant dermal fibrosis, hypertrophic scars, and keloids. This recommendation, widely disseminated in the 1990s and 2000s, ultimately established an empirical clinical consensus that persists to this day, despite the lack of robust supporting evidence.

Over the past two decades, however, this paradigm has begun to be challenged by a growing body of scientific research. An extensive literature review conducted by Truax et al. encompassing publications in dermatology, plastic surgery, ophthalmology, otorhinolaryngology, orthopedics, and oral and maxillofacial surgery, demonstrated a lack of consistent data supporting the need to postpone elective surgeries in patients previously treated with isotretinoin. The analysis concluded that the practice of delaying procedures for 6–12 months after discontinuation of the medication lacks a solid scientific foundation and should be re-evaluated, particularly in light of contemporary data.

In the specific field of dermatology, Mysore et al. reinforced this shift in perspective by critically reviewing the available data on the safety of procedures such as peels, lasers, dermabrasion, and excisions in patients currently or recently treated with oral isotretinoin. The authors concluded that there is no absolute contraindication to performing these procedures, provided technical criteria are observed and an individual patient assessment is conducted. The incidence of complications such as hypertrophic scarring or wound dehiscence was considered very low and more closely related to the aggressiveness of the procedure than to the presence of systemic retinoid.

Additionally, a seminal study published by Spring et al. in JAMA Dermatology further supported this critical review by systematically compiling the available evidence on the association between oral isotretinoin and surgical risks. The analysis covered multiple categories of procedures—including fractional lasers, dermabrasion, and chemical peels—and concluded that most data do not support the need for a mandatory interval between isotretinoin use and the performance of dermatological interventions. Based on this review, the authors proposed consensus recommendations that relax the traditional approach, allowing many procedures to be performed safely even during or shortly after isotretinoin treatment, provided a careful individual risk-benefit assessment is conducted.

Recent experimental evidence also strengthens the hypothesis that isotretinoin may, under certain conditions, play a beneficial role in tissue regeneration. An innovative animal model study published by Maleki et al. evaluated the impact of different administration durations of isotretinoin (1 and 2 months) on the wound healing process in rats. The findings demonstrated that administration for 2 months significantly accelerated the proliferative phase of healing, with increased expression of key mediators such as VEGF, TGF-β1, IL-6, IL-10, IL-1α, IL-8, ICAM-1, and L-selectin. Histological analysis revealed greater recruitment of mast cells to the wounds, with no evidence of keloid formation. These data indicate that isotretinoin may positively modulate the inflammatory and angiogenic environment of healing, contradicting the traditional belief in its inhibitory potential.

From a pathophysiological perspective, oral retinoids modulate multiple immunological and cellular pathways relevant to tissue repair. Isotretinoin influences the differentiation of regulatory T cells, promotes IgA secretion, modulates macrophage activity, and stimulates the release of growth factors and pro-reparative cytokines. Its impact depends on factors such as cumulative dose, duration of use, nutritional status, and the type of procedure to be performed.

In light of this, it is recommended to abandon dogmatic approaches and adopt a clinical practice based on individual risk assessment. In patients with intact skin and no history of abnormal scarring, using standard doses of isotretinoin (<1 mg/kg/day) or having completed treatment several months prior, phenol-croton oil peel can be considered safe, provided that other clinical criteria are favorable. On the other hand, in individuals with multiple risk factors—such as a personal or family history of keloids, very thin or significantly atrophic skin, or previous procedures in adjacent areas—the decision should be more cautious, with the option of less aggressive treatments or postponing the procedure until complete tissue recovery.

In summary, the absolute contraindication to the use of deep peels in patients on isotretinoin is no longer supported by current literature. Management should be guided by careful clinical assessment, understanding of the mechanisms involved in healing, and individualized medical judgment, always aiming for safety, predictability, and excellence in therapeutic outcomes.

5.4.2.4 Frequently Recurrent Herpes Simplex

Frequent recurrence of herpes simplex is not an absolute contraindication to phenol-croton peel, but it does represent a significant risk factor for viral reactivation and infectious complications in the postoperative period. The risk of herpes simplex reactivation after deep chemical peels, such as phenol, is well documented and may result in extensive lesions and residual scarring, especially in the perioral region.

However, the literature shows that antiviral prophylaxis with agents such as acyclovir, initiated before the procedure and continued for several days afterward, significantly reduces the incidence and severity of herpetic recurrences even in patients with a history of frequent recurrences. Antiviral prophylactic strategies are considered standard for all patients undergoing facial resurfacing, regardless of herpes history, given the high prevalence of latent HSV-1 infection and the safety of antiviral use.

Therefore, patients with a history of recurrent herpes simplex may undergo phenol-croton oil peel provided they receive appropriate antiviral prophylaxis, with strict postoperative monitoring for early detection and management of potential infectious complications.

Bronchial asthma and a history of bronchospasm are considered relative contraindications to deep phenol-croton oil peels, particularly in procedures involving large areas or application in poorly ventilated environments. Although phenol is not a typical allergen, its volatility and direct irritant effect on the respiratory mucosa may trigger exacerbated inflammatory responses in the airways of patients with preexisting bronchial hyperreactivity.

5.4.2.5 Controlled Asthma or History of Bronchospasm

Phenol-induced respiratory toxicity occurs via two main mechanisms: direct caustic action and systemic absorption with secondary inflammatory response. Experimental studies have shown that inhalation of phenol vapors can cause lesions of the tracheobronchial mucosa, including epithelial erosion, focal hemorrhage, edema, and mixed inflammatory infiltration—changes consistent with an exacerbated Th2-type inflammatory response in asthmatic patients. This is due to the release of mediators such as histamine, leukotrienes, and prostaglandins, which promote bronchoconstriction, increased vascular permeability, and mucus production.

Furthermore, the literature reports cases of laryngeal edema and reflex laryngospasm following deep chemical peels with phenol, particularly in smokers, raising concerns about possible upper airway reactions in asthmatic patients as well. Although there are no clinical studies that formally contraindicate phenol-croton oil peels in patients with controlled asthma, the theoretical risk of acute bronchospasm induced by inhalation of irritant vapors, compounded by anxiety and the use of sedatives, should be considered with caution.

Therefore, patients with a history of moderate to severe asthma, bronchospasm induced by chemical irritants, or previous hospitalizations for respiratory exacerbations should be carefully evaluated before the procedure is indicated. When indicated, the peel should be performed in a well-ventilated environment, with continuous pulse oximetry, immediate medical support, and a preference for small, segmental applications. It is advisable that the patient's asthma is clinically stable, with no recent use of systemic corticosteroids, and that short-acting bronchodilators are used prophylactically prior to the procedure, as directed by the respiratory physician.

The decision should always consider the individual risk-benefit ratio, and may be postponed or replaced by alternative methods in cases of clinical instability. Communication between dermatologist and pulmonologist is essential to ensure patient safety.

5.4.2.6 Controlled Cardiac Arrhythmias

Patients with previously diagnosed cardiac arrhythmias under pharmacological control—such as atrial flutter, isolated extrasystoles, or first-degree atrioventricular block—should be considered at relatively increased risk for phenol-croton oil peel, even if stable or asymptomatic. Although the risk of serious events is lower than that observed in uncontrolled arrhythmias, systemic absorption of phenol may precipitate acute decompensation, especially when associated with factors such as severe pain, hyperventilation, anxiety, or electrolyte disturbances.

From a pathophysiological perspective, phenol exerts direct toxicity on the cardiovascular system, affecting myocardial contractility and electrical conduction. Experimental studies have demonstrated significant hemodynamic changes following phenol exposure, such as tachycardia, bradycardia, premature ventricular contractions, and, in extreme cases, sustained ventricular tachycardia and atrial fibrillation. These effects result from a combination of depressive action on cardiac ion channels, acid-base disturbances, and interference with autonomic homeostasis.

It should be noted that sex, age, previous cardiac history, and serum phenol levels have not proven to be consistent predictors of arrhythmia occurrence. Evidence reviewed in Chap. 3 (Systemic Toxicity) indicates that the main variable associated with cardiac risk is the body surface area treated within a short period, rather than the isolated concentration of the solution. Even slow applications may trigger changes, underscoring the need for strict precautions.

In light of this, it is recommended that patients with controlled cardiac arrhythmias:

- Undergo prior assessment by a cardiologist, with an up-to-date ECG and, if necessary, Holter monitoring
- Undergo only segmental procedures, with safety intervals between treated areas
- Receive continuous cardiac monitoring, with a trained team and advanced life support equipment
- Have any electrolyte disturbances corrected and the use of potentially arrhythmogenic drugs reviewed
- Undergo the procedure in a setting with adequate ventilation and immediate access to emergency care

Although this does not constitute an absolute contraindication, the risk of arrhythmic decompensation remains even in patients with controlled disease, and only a cautious, judicious, and closely monitored approach can mitigate this risk and allow the benefits of the procedure to outweigh its potential harms.

5.4.2.7 Functional or Cognitive Dependence for Self-Care

Patients with significant functional or cognitive impairment who have limitations in their ability to perform their own post-procedural care should be carefully assessed before being considered for phenol-croton oil peel. In such cases, this is regarded as a relative contraindication, as although there is no technical barrier to the procedure itself, the lack of adequate support during the recovery phase may compromise both outcomes and patient safety.

The phenol-croton oil peel is a deep procedure that requires strict adherence to the postoperative protocol, including appropriate use of dressings, application of ointments, pain management, rigorous photoprotection, home rest, monitoring for signs of infection, and attendance at follow-up appointments. Individuals with cognitive deficits (such as dementia, intellectual disability, or neurological sequelae) or with significant motor limitations (resulting from stroke, Parkinson's disease, muscular disorders, etc.) may be unable to understand or correctly follow these instructions, placing themselves at risk of secondary infections, abnormal crust formation, hypertrophic scarring, dyspigmentation, or even systemic complications.

Furthermore, institutionalized patients, those who are bedridden, or those under the care of untrained third parties often face environmental, emotional, and social barriers that hinder adequate follow-up, even when legal consent is in place. In these contexts, clinical autonomy must be assessed with ethical responsibility, ensuring that the patient (or their legal representative) is fully informed about the risks and requirements of the procedure, and that there is a concrete support structure for postoperative care.

The decision to perform the procedure in this group should be individualized, considering:

- Level of patient understanding regarding the treatment and its risks
- Presence of competent and committed caregivers to provide the required care
- Access to a hygienic and protected environment for recovery
- Ability to attend post-peel follow-up assessments
- Assessment of clinical, aesthetic, and emotional risks versus benefits

In the absence of minimum conditions to ensure a safe postoperative period, it is prudent to postpone or contraindicate the procedure, opting for less invasive alternatives or preparatory strategies aimed at improving the patient's support context.

5.4.2.8 Personality Disorders and Unrealistic Expectations

The presence of psychiatric disorders, particularly those involving disturbances in self-image perception, impulsivity, affective instability, and low frustration tolerance, constitutes a significant relative contraindication to phenol-croton oil peel. Although these patients may clinically meet the indications for the procedure, a lack of adequate emotional preparation or the presence of unrealistic expectations regarding outcomes can severely compromise the therapeutic result, both from an aesthetic and psychosocial perspective.

Individuals with body dysmorphic disorder (BDD) often exhibit a distorted and obsessive perception of minor or non-existent facial flaws, making them highly prone to chronic dissatisfaction, repeated interventions, and an increased risk of litigation. Similarly, patients with borderline, histrionic, or narcissistic personality disorders may present with emotional instability, intense reactivity to minor frustrations, unrealistic idealizations regarding outcomes, and difficulty adhering to self-care routines, thereby increasing the risk of clinical complications and therapeutic conflict.

Invasive, painful procedures or those with a prolonged recovery period, such as phenol-croton oil peel, require a high level of adherence, emotional maturity, and rational understanding of the risks, limitations, and expected course. Under these circumstances, any misalignment between expectation and reality may result in psychological distress, unfounded accusations, or premature discontinuation of post-procedural follow-up.

For these reasons, it is recommended:

- Careful psychological screening, especially in cases with a history of multiple cosmetic surgeries, obsessive verbalization of minimal defects, or reports of recurrent frustration with previous procedures
- Use of standardized screening tools, such as the Body Dysmorphic Disorder Questionnaire (BDDQ) or PRIME-MD
- Postponing or contraindicating the procedure in patients lacking emotional stability or with a distorted perception of aesthetic reality
- Providing detailed clarification of the risks, recovery time, progressive nature of the results, and the actual limitations of the procedure
- Careful documentation of the consent process, ensuring that the patient has understood and rationally accepted the terms

It is important to remember that phenol-croton oil peel acts on the skin structure but cannot correct deep-seated psychological distortions of self-image. Clinical prudence with this patient profile is essential to prevent emotional harm, legal complications, and therapeutic frustration for both parties.

5.4.2.9 Pain Intolerance

Pain intolerance constitutes a relative contraindication to phenol-croton oil peel, particularly in its traditional form, which is associated with severe pain both during and in the hours following the procedure. Despite advances in anesthetic techniques and multimodal analgesia protocols, this procedure remains among the most painful in aesthetic dermatology, requiring physical resilience, psychological preparation, and the patient's active cooperation.

From a physiological perspective, phenol acts as a local neurotoxic agent, inducing immediate protein coagulation and marked necrosis of the epidermis and superficial dermis, with activation of cutaneous nociceptors and release of inflammatory mediators (prostaglandins, bradykinin, and substance P) that intensify the pain response. Pain is most pronounced in the initial hours after application, often described as a deep, continuous, and diffuse burning sensation, and may persist for 24–48 h. Even with the use of regional anesthetic blocks, conscious sedation, and systemic agents such as ketorolac, clonidine, and opioids, many patients report significant post-procedural pain.

Patients with a low pain threshold, marked anxiety, a history of traumatic pain experiences, or functional hyperalgesia (as in fibromyalgia) may exhibit disproportionate responses, including agitation, tachycardia, hyperventilation, and even vasovagal or panic reactions, compromising both the safety of the procedure and the patient's experience. Furthermore, poorly controlled pain is a recognized trigger for cardiovascular events, arrhythmias, and hypertensive crises, particularly in patients with comorbidities.

From an emotional standpoint, severe pain is also associated with a poorer perception of the procedure and its outcomes, reduced overall satisfaction, risk of early discontinuation of follow-up, and catastrophic interpretation of the experience. Studies indicate that pain perception is closely linked to the patient's emotional state and prior preparation. Anxious, sensitive, or inadequately informed patients regarding the expected intensity of pain tend to react more negatively, with a higher risk of regret and strain in the therapeutic relationship.

Accordingly, it is recommended:

- Prior assessment of the patient's pain threshold and emotional profile, including a history of tolerance to previous medical procedures
- Use of combined anesthetic techniques, including regional blocks, supervised conscious sedation, and stepwise systemic analgesia
- Clear and objective explanation regarding the expected intensity and duration of pain, as well as the strategies that will be employed for relief
- Preference for segmental and gradual procedures in patients suspected of having low tolerance
- Consideration of less invasive alternatives in cases where the emotional profile is incompatible with the discomfort associated with phenol-croton oil

- Although this does not constitute an absolute contraindication, significant intolerance to pain may compromise the safe technical execution of the procedure, increase the risk of systemic complications, and deteriorate the patient's therapeutic experience. Therefore, it should always be carefully considered during the rigorous selection process of candidates for deep peeling.

5.4.2.10 Active Inflammatory Skin Diseases

The presence of active inflammatory skin diseases—especially those associated with the Koebner phenomenon—represents a significant relative contraindication to deep chemical peeling with phenol-croton oil. The main risk lies in the potential activation or dissemination of the underlying disease in areas subjected to chemical trauma, with important aesthetic, functional, and immunological repercussions.

The Koebner phenomenon (or Koebner isomorphism) refers to the ability of certain inflammatory dermatoses to manifest in previously unaffected areas following physical, chemical, or thermal trauma, even if mild. The phenomenon was first described in 1877 in patients with psoriasis, but is now recognized in a broader spectrum of diseases, including lichen planus, cutaneous lupus erythematosus, vitiligo, atopic dermatitis, lichen sclerosus, pemphigus vulgaris, and other autoimmune and immune-mediated conditions.

Phenol-croton oil peeling, by its nature, induces a deep chemical injury with necrosis of the epidermal and superficial dermal layers, activating local and systemic inflammatory cascades that may trigger the activation of autoreactive lymphocyte clones in genetically susceptible individuals. This can result in the recurrence of characteristic lesions of the underlying inflammatory disease precisely in the treated areas, worsening the clinical picture and compromising the aesthetic outcome.

Several studies and clinical reports have documented activation of lichen planus, psoriasis, and cutaneous lupus in traumatized areas, including surgery, tattoos, radiotherapy, laser, and chemical peels. In some cases, the Koebner phenomenon may occur weeks after the initial injury, making direct causal association difficult, but nonetheless compromising the clinical and scarring evolution of the procedure.

In addition to the risk of direct disease activation, these dermatoses often present with alterations of the skin barrier, increased dermal vascularization, and chronic inflammatory infiltration, which may affect the depth of phenol penetration, predispose to post-inflammatory dyschromia, atrophic or hypertrophic scarring, and delay physiological tissue repair.

It is therefore recommended:

- Avoid performing phenol-croton oil peel in patients with active inflammatory skin diseases, especially those known to be associated with the Koebner phenomenon.
- Carefully assess the clinical history, even in patients without apparent lesions at the time, seeking previous signs of chronic dermatoses.
- When the diagnosis is established and the disease is in sustained remission, the procedure may be considered with caution, provided that there is:
  - Absence of active lesions for at least 3–6 months.
  - Photographic and dermatological documentation of clinical stability.
  - Detailed informed consent regarding the risks of reactivation.
- Avoid application to areas previously affected by the inflammatory disease, even if currently inactive.
- Maintain strict monitoring in both the early and late postoperative periods, with prompt intervention in the event of signs of recurrence.
- In patients with a history of inflammatory dermatoses, the option of superficial peels or procedures with lower inflammatory potential should be considered as a safer alternative, especially when immunological factors are not yet well controlled.

5.4.2.11 Vitiligo

Phenol-croton oil peel is not recommended in areas affected by vitiligo, except in very specific contexts and with precise indication. The main risk is the induction of permanent depigmentation, worsening of achromic lesions, and the appearance of sharp demarcation lines between treated and untreated skin, especially in patients with higher phototypes. The risk of pigment loss is particularly high with higher concentrations of croton oil, potentially resulting in areas of irreversible depigmentation.

In the context of vitiligo, high-concentration phenol has been used as a depigmenting agent in cases of universal or extensive vitiligo, when the therapeutic goal is complete depigmentation of the remaining pigmented skin, aiming to achieve a uniform skin tone in patients with significant psychosocial impact and refractoriness to other therapies. In such cases, phenol may be applied in a controlled manner to promote depigmentation, but this use is restricted to specific indications, with informed consent and close monitoring, due to the potential for adverse effects and the possibility of exacerbating cutaneous autoimmunity.

Therefore, phenol-croton oil peel is contraindicated for conventional aesthetic purposes in areas of vitiligo, due to the high risk of further depigmentation and unsatisfactory cosmetic outcomes. Its application should only be considered in total depigmentation protocols, in selected cases of universal or extensive vitiligo, and always with careful assessment of risks and benefits. careful assessment of risks and benefits.

5.4.2.12 Systemic Disease Under Investigation or Without Definitive Diagnosis

The presence of clinical symptoms without an established cause, abnormal test results of indeterminate etiology, or systemic conditions still under investigation constitutes a significant relative contraindication to phenol-croton oil peel. Given the depth and complexity of the procedure, any latent or underdiagnosed pathology may unpredictably alter the inflammatory, scarring, or systemic response, exposing the patient to serious complications, unsatisfactory aesthetic outcomes, and even the risk of clinical deterioration.

Hidden autoimmune or systemic inflammatory diseases (such as systemic lupus erythematosus, dermatomyositis, vasculitis, or autoinflammatory syndromes) may be triggered or exacerbated by the inflammatory trauma induced by the peel, due to activation of the innate immune system and local release of DAMPs (damage-associated molecular patterns), with potential systemic recruitment of autoreactive T cells and release of inflammatory cytokines such as IL-6, TNF-α, and IFN-γ.

Primary or secondary immunodeficiencies, often subclinical, may present belatedly with bacterial, viral, or fungal infections after the procedure, particularly in the context of extensive and prolonged loss of the cutaneous barrier. The literature documents cases of disseminated herpes, severe impetiginization, and even necrotizing fasciitis following aesthetic procedures in previously undiagnosed immunocompromised patients.

Early hematological or hepatorenal disorders may directly interfere with wound healing, phenol metabolism, and clearance of toxic metabolites, increasing the risk of systemic toxicity. Phenol is metabolized predominantly by the liver (via conjugation with sulfate and glucuronide) and excreted by the kidneys. Hepatic or renal dysfunction, even if subclinical, may prolong the plasma half-life of phenol, predisposing to arrhythmias, central nervous system depression, hypotension, or respiratory failure.

Patients with subclinical cancer or undergoing oncological investigation (such as enlarged lymph nodes, uncharacterized masses, or unexplained hematological abnormalities) represent an additional risk group. Although there is no evidence that phenol has direct carcinogenic action at the doses used in peels, the local and systemic oxidative stress induced by chemical trauma and the potential activation of the inflammatory-immunological axis may theoretically worsen occult neoplastic diseases or interfere with the progression of immunosensitive cancers, such as lymphomas and cutaneous carcinomas. Moreover, undiagnosed oncology patients may present with hematological and immunological alterations that increase the risk of infection, prolonged necrosis, poor wound healing, or bleeding. bleeding.

Undiagnosed metabolic and endocrine disorders—such as early-stage diabetes mellitus, hypothyroidism, or mitochondrial disorders—also alter cellular metabolism, reduce tissue regeneration capacity, increase the risk of post-inflammatory hyperpigmentation, and may mask early signs of local complications such as infections or cutaneous dysbiosis.

Unrecognized drug interactions associated with clinical conditions under investigation represent another critical issue. Phenol may potentiate the toxicity of drugs with shared hepatic metabolism (e.g., benzodiazepines, antiarrhythmics, anticonvulsants). Furthermore, drugs that prolong the QT interval (such as certain antidepressants or antiemetics) may increase the risk of severe arrhythmias, especially when combined with phenol and intense pain, as described in the chapter on cardiac toxicity.

Phenol-croton oil peel is a medical procedure of high inflammatory, metabolic, and systemic complexity, the risk-benefit of which can only be properly assessed in a patient with a well-defined clinical profile, up-to-date investigations, and no outstanding diagnostic uncertainties. Procedures performed in patients with undiagnosed conditions may compromise both aesthetic and medical outcomes and pose ethical and legal risks.

Therefore, it is strongly recommended that:

- No patient with a systemic disease of uncertain etiology under investigation should undergo peeling.
- Any clinical complaints or laboratory abnormalities must be fully investigated and stabilized prior to indication.
- Symptoms such as persistent asthenia, lymphadenopathy, unintentional weight loss, fever of indeterminate origin, or changes in blood count, liver or renal function require diagnostic exclusion before the procedure.

- Clinical documentation must record that the patient has a complete diagnosis, up-to-date investigations, and no apparent medical contraindications, with validated informed consent.

Prudence in this context is a hallmark of good medical practice. In the event of diagnostic uncertainty, postponing the procedure is a responsible and safe clinical decision, protecting both patient and practitioner.

5.4.2.13 Use of Drugs That Prolong the QT Interval

Among the relative contraindications for phenol–croton oil peel, particular attention should be given to the use of medications that prolong the QT interval, such as certain tricyclic antidepressants, antipsychotics, antiemetics, thiazide diuretics, antifungals, and antihistamines. Phenol is well known to be associated with a risk of cardiac arrhythmias, including torsades de pointes (TdP), due to its systemic toxicity when absorbed over large areas or with sequential applications without adequate intervals. Patients taking these drugs are at a potentially increased risk of electrophysiological disturbances during the procedure, especially when undergoing extensive facial peels. Studies have shown that phenol–croton oil peel can cause transient prolongation of the QTc interval even in patients not using these medications, with minor arrhythmic events occurring in up to 80% of cases evaluated. Therefore, the use of QT-prolonging drugs should be considered a relative contraindication, requiring careful risk–benefit assessment, prior cardiological stratification, continuous electrocardiographic monitoring during the procedure, and, whenever possible, suspension or adjustment of these medications in collaboration with the attending physician. Cardiovascular safety should be maximized, particularly in extensive area peels or when performed at short intervals, situations in which the systemic phenol load tends to be higher.

5.5 Final Considerations

Careful patient selection is the cornerstone for the safe and effective performance of phenol–croton oil peel. Although the aesthetic outcomes can be remarkable, especially in well-established indications such as advanced photoaging, atrophic scars, dermal melasma, and field cancerization, it is essential that the indication is supported by thorough clinical assessment, proper documentation, and clear alignment of expectations. Likewise, contraindications—whether absolute or relative—must be strictly observed with technical rigor and ethical responsibility, considering the local, systemic, and psychosocial risks involved. Skin integrity, emotional stability, control of comorbidities, and the patient's ability to adhere to postoperative care are all decisive for therapeutic success (Table 5.4). Prudence in contraindication is as vital as precision in indication: the best outcome lies not only in flawless technical execution, but in the conscious decision of when, where, how, and for whom the procedure should be performed. Given its potential for systemic toxicity, risk of serious complications, and the need for refined clinical judgment, phenol–croton oil peel must

Table 5.4 Absolute and relative contraindications for phenol–croton oil peel

Absolute contraindications	Relative contraindications
Unstable/uncontrolled cardiovascular disease	Thick skin/enlarged pores/phyma-like phenotype
Uncontrolled arrhythmias or use of class I/III antiarrhythmics	Thin/atrophic/fragile skin
Uncontrolled arterial hypertension	Recent use of oral isotretinoin
Moderate/severe decompensated COPD or recent onset dyspnea	Recurrent herpes simplex
Severe or decompensated hepatic or renal disease	Controlled asthma/bronchospasm
Decompensated diabetes mellitus (HbA1c $\geq$7%)	Controlled cardiac arrhythmias
Severe immunosuppression or AIDS	Functional/cognitive dependence for self-care
Severe autoimmune diseases	Personality disorders/unrealistic expectations
History of extensive keloids/abnormal scarring	Pain intolerance
Frontal fibrosing alopecia	Active inflammatory skin diseases
Active cutaneous or systemic infection	Vitiligo
Pregnancy or breastfeeding	Systemic disease under investigation
Severe or decompensated psychiatric conditions	Use of drugs that prolong the QT interval
Malnutrition	
Skin previously compromised by surgery or specific anatomical conditions	
Smoking	
Active cutaneous neoplasia (melanoma or NMSC)	

Comparative summary of absolute contraindications, which preclude the procedure, and relative contraindications, which require individual assessment, technical adjustment, or postponement. (*Source: Table prepared by the author (Dr Carolina Marçon)*)

never, under any circumstances, be performed by individuals without medical training. This is a procedure that demands in-depth knowledge of pathophysiology, pharmacology, cutaneous anatomy, and the management of complications—competencies acquired only through medical education and practice. Clinical judgment, supported by scientific evidence and experience, is the tool that transforms a potentially hazardous procedure into a safe, ethical, and transformative intervention.

Sources

1. Wambier CG, Lee KC, Soon SL, Sterling JB, Rullan PP, Landau M, Brody HJ, International Peeling Society. Advanced chemical peels: phenol-croton oil peel. J Am Acad Dermatol. 2019;81(2):327–36.
2. Wambier CG, Lee KC, Bertolini TM, Rullan PP, Beltrame FL. Comment on "Anti-ageing effects of ingenol mebutate for patients with actinic keratosis" and phenol-croton oil peels. J Am Acad Dermatol. 2019;80(6):e185–6.
3. Larson DL. Phenol-croton oil peel: an update. Aesthet Surg J. 2005;25(2):197–200.
4. Vasconcelos KMS, Vasconcelos GSP, Rittes PG, Vasconcelos FRS, Vasconcelos JA. Phenol peel for facial rhytids: clinical comparison between Baker-Gordon and Hetter formulas. Surg Cosmet Dermatol. 2013;5(3):213–8.

5. Cardoso FAMES, Moura RD, Pilar EFS, Moura ICG, Miot HA, da Costa A. Phenol-croton oil peel increases type-1 and type-3 collagen by stimulating SIRT-6 and SIRT-7. Int J Dermatol. 2022;61(2):e71–4.
6. Gross BG, Maschek F. Phenol chemosurgery for removal of deep facial wrinkles. Int J Dermatol. 1980;19(3):159–64.
7. Mackee GM, Karp FL. The treatment of post-acne scars with phenol. Br J Dermatol. 1952;64(12):456–9.
8. Lee K, Rullan P. A combination approach to treating acne scars in all skin types: carbolic CROSS, blunt bi-level cannula subcision, and microneedling. Surg Cosmet Dermatol. 2019;11(2):145–47.
9. Leheta TM, Abdel Hay RM, El Garem YF. Deep peeling using phenol versus percutaneous collagen induction combined with 20% trichloroacetic acid in atrophic post-acne scars; a randomized controlled trial. J Dermatolog Treat. 2014;25(2):130–6.
10. Soon SL, Wambier CG, Rullan PR, Sterling JB, Brody HJ, Lee KC, Kreyden OP, Landau M, International Peeling Society. Phenol-croton oil chemical peeling induces durable improvement in constitutional periorbital dark circles. Dermatol Surg. 2023;49(4):368–73.
11. Platsidaki E, Stravodimou A, Kouris A, Markantoni V, Kontochristopoulos G. Efficacy and Safety of Phenol and Trichloroacetic Acid Combination Peel for the Management of Dark Circles. Actas Dermosifiliogr. 2022;113(10):988–90.
12. Lee KC, Wambier CG, Soon SL, Sterling JB, Landau M, Rullan P, Brody HJ; International Peeling Society. Basic chemical peeling: Superficial and medium-depth peels. J Am Acad Dermatol. 2019;81(2):313–24.
13. Paiva ML, Justo AS, Lemes BM, Capote ACMO, de Castro Maymone MB, Lipinski LC, Rullan PP, Beltrame FL, Miot HA, Wambier CG. Repigmentation of skin of colour following phenol-croton oil chemical peel. J Am Acad Dermatol. 2023;89(5):1068–70.
14. Sun HF, Lu HS, Sun LQ, Ping WD, Mao DS, Li D. Chemical Peeling with a Modified Phenol Formula for the Treatment of Facial Freckles on Asian Skin. Aesthetic Plast Surg. 2018;42(2):546–52.
15. Handog EB, Datuin MS, Singzon IA. Chemical peels for acne and acne scars in asians: evidence based review. J Cutan Aesthet Surg. 2012;5(4):239–46.
16. Park JH, Choi YD, Kim SW, Kim YC, Park SW. Effectiveness of modified phenol peel (Exoderm) on facial wrinkles, acne scars and other skin problems in Asian patients. J Dermatol. 2007;34(1):17–24.
17. Truax L, Hendrixson M, Naqvi J, Trevino J. Use of oral retinoids in the perioperative period by surgical specialty: a literature review. Arch Dermatol Res. 2025;317(1):174.
18. Mysore V, Omprakash HM, Khatri GN. Isotretinoin and dermatosurgical procedures. Indian J Dermatol Venereol Leprol. 2019;85(1):18–23.
19. Spring LK, Krakowski AC, Alam M, Bhatia A, Brauer J, Cohen J, Del Rosso JQ, Diaz L, Dover J, Eichenfield LF, Gurtner GC, Hanke CW, Jahnke MN, Kelly KM, Khetarpal S, Kinney MA, Levy ML, Leyden J, Longaker MT, Munavalli GS, Ozog DM, Prather H, Shumaker PR, Tanzi E, Torres A, Velez MW, Waldman AB, Yan AC, Zaenglein AL. Isotretinoin and timing of procedural interventions: a systematic review with consensus recommendations. JAMA Dermatol. 2017;153(8):802–9.
20. Maleki MH, Miladpour B, Mazhari SA, Far MH, Rajabi M, Alinejad M, Dehghanian A, Beigmohammadi F, Esmaeli N, Siri M, Aryanian Z. Investigating isotretinoin's unexpected acceleration of wound healing: a rat model study. Int Immunopharmacol. 2025;148:114145.
21. Marçon CR. Phenol in dermatology: updated evidence on efficacy and safety. An Bras Dermatol. 2025;100(5):501200.
22. Hetter GP. An examination of the phenol-croton oil peel: part IV. Face peel results with different concentrations of phenol and croton oil. Plast Reconstr Surg. 2000;105(3):1061–83; discussion 1084–1087.
23. Atiyeh B, Oneisi A, Ghieh F. Medium-depth trichloroacetic acid and deep phenol-croton oil chemical peeling for facial rejuvenation: an update. J Craniofac Surg. 2021;32(8):e745–50.

24. Justo AS, Lemes BM, Nunes B, Antunes KA, Capote ACMO, Lipinski LC, Campagnoli EB, Emiliano J, Meurer EC, Ezemma O, Miot HA, Beltrame FL, Wambier CG. Characterization of the activity of *croton tiglium* oil in Hetter's very heavy phenol-croton oil chemical peels. Dermatol Surg. 2021;47(7):944–6.
25. Stone PA, Lefer LG. Modified phenol chemical face peels: recognizing the role of application technique. Clin Plast Surg. 2001;28(1):13–36. Erratum in: Clin Plast Surg 2001 Jul;28(3):preceding xi.
26. Stone PA. The use of modified phenol for chemical facial peeling. Clin Plast Surg. 1998;25(1):21–44.
27. Ozturk CN, Huettner F, Ozturk C, Bartz-Kurycki MA, Zins JE. Evaluation of outcomes of combined facelift and perioral phenol-croton oil peel. Plast Reconstr Surg. 2013;132(5):743e–53e.
28. de Mendonça MCC, Segheto NN, Aarestrup FM, Aarestrup BJV. Punctuated 88% phenol peeling for the treatment of facial photoaging: a clinical and histopathological study. Dermatol Surg. 2018;44(2):241–7.
29. Garbers LEFM, Miola AC, de Souza V, de Castro Brommonschenkel C, Lima FO, Minicucci EM, Miot HA. Efficacy and tolerability of 1.6% phenol-croton peel vs. topical 5% imiquimod in the treatment of actinic cheilitis: a randomized controlled trial. Clin Exp Dermatol. 2025;50(4):826–35.
30. Kaminaka C, Yamamoto Y, Yonei N, Kishioka A, Kondo T, Furukawa F. Phenol peels as a novel therapeutic approach for actinic keratosis and Bowen disease: prospective pilot trial with assessment of clinical, histologic, and immunohistochemical correlations. J Am Acad Dermatol. 2009;60(4):615–25.
31. Langsdon PR, Milburn M, Yarber R. Comparison of laser and phenol chemical peel in facial skin resurfacing. Arch Otolaryngol Head Neck Surg. 2000;126(10):1195–9.
32. Hetter GP. An examination of the phenol-croton oil peel: part I. Dissecting the formula. Plast Reconstr Surg. 2000;105(1):227–39; discussion 249–251.
33. Brown AM, Kaplan LM, Brown ME. Phenol-induced histological skin changes: hazards, technique, and uses. Br J Plast Surg. 1960;13:158–69.
34. Han A, Chien AL, Kang S. Photoaging. Dermatol Clin. 2014;32(3):291–9.
35. Kligman AM, Zheng P, Lavker RM. The anatomy and pathogenesis of wrinkles. Br J Dermatol. 1985;113(1):37–42.
36. Fitzpatrick RE, Tope WD, Goldman MP, Satur NM. Pulsed carbon dioxide laser, trichloroacetic acid, Baker-Gordon phenol, and dermabrasion: a comparative clinical and histological study of cutaneous resurfacing in a porcine model. Arch Dermatol. 1996;132(4):469–71.
37. Rullan PP, Olson R, Lee KC. A combination approach to treating acne scars in all skin types: carbolic chemical reconstruction of skin scars, blunt bi-level cannula subcision, and microneedling—a case series. J Clin Aesthet Dermatol. 2020;13(5):19–23.
38. Platsidaki E, Stravodimou A, Kouris A, Markantoni V, Kontochristopoulos G. Efficacy and safety of phenol and trichloroacetic acid combination peel for the management of dark circles. Actas Dermosifiliogr. 2022;113(10):988–90.
39. Kaminaka C, Yamamoto Y, Yonei N, Furukawa F. Phenol application to angiosarcomas: implications and histological studies. Int J Dermatol. 2009;48:470–5.
40. Maymone MBC, Mirza FN, Steiner D, Ribeiro F, Landau M, Marçon C, Celidonio TC, Soon SL, Wambier CG, International Peeling Society. Comparative long-term efficacy of phenol-croton oil chemical peels for persistent melasma at varied *Croton tiglium* oil concentrations. J Am Acad Dermatol. 2024;91(2):336–8.
41. Rullan P, Karam AM. Chemical peels for darker skin types. Facial Plast Surg Clin North Am. 2010;18(1):111–31.
42. de Oliveira Ciaramicolo N, Bisson GB, Ferreira Júnior O. Adverse effects associated with the irresponsible use of phenol peeling: literature review. Oral Surg Oral Med Oral Pathol Oral Radiol. 2025;139(2):161–5.
43. Peters W. The chemical peel. Ann Plast Surg. 1991;26(6):564–71.
44. Gill JF, Yu SS, Neuhaus IM. Tobacco smoking and dermatologic surgery. J Am Acad Dermatol. 2013;68(1):167–72.

45. Coon D, Tuffaha S, Christensen J, Bonawitz SC. Plastic surgery and smoking: a prospective analysis of incidence, compliance, and complications. Plast Reconstr Surg. 2013;131(2):385–91.
46. Krueger JK, Rohrich RJ. Clearing the smoke: the scientific rationale for tobacco abstention with plastic surgery. Plast Reconstr Surg. 2001;108(4):1063–73; discussion 1074–1077.
47. Álvarez-Jiménez J, Córdoba-Fernández A. Influence of smoking on wound healing in patients undergoing nail matrix phenolisation: a prospective randomized clinical study. Adv Skin Wound Care. 2014;27(5):229–36; quiz 237–238.
48. Stechmiller JK. Understanding the role of nutrition and wound healing. Nutr Clin Pract. 2010;25(1):61–8.
49. Munoz N, Litchford M, Cereda E. Nutrition and wound care. Phys Med Rehabil Clin N Am. 2022;33(4):811–22.
50. Penny H, Flores R, Pennington E, Pedersen A, Tran S. The role of macronutrients and micronutrients in wound healing: a narrative review. J Wound Care. 2022;31(Suppl 5):S14–22.
51. Landau M, Tosti A, Kroumpouzos G, Eims E, Goldust M. Frontal fibrosing alopecia—a new absolute contraindication for deep chemical peels. Clin Dermatol. 2024;42(6):696–700.
52. Ding G, Wang C, Vinturache A, Zhao S, Pan R, Han W, Chen L, Wang W, Yuan T, Gao Y, Tian Y. Prenatal low-level phenol exposures and birth outcomes in China. Sci Total Environ. 2017;607–608:1400–7.
53. Becerro de Bengoa Vallejo R, Losa Iglesias ME, Jules KT, Trepal MJ. Renal excretion of phenol from physicians after nail matrix phenolisation: an observational prospective study. J Eur Acad Dermatol Venereol. 2012;26(3):344–7.
54. Losa Iglesias ME, Veiga de Cabo J, Tejedor Traspaderne J, Aguilar Franco J, Bernaola Alonso M, Becerro de Bengoa Vallejo R. Safety of phenol vapour inhalation during chemical matrixectomy for the treatment of ingrown toenails. Dermatol Surg. 2008;34(11):1515–9.
55. Joseph AW, Ishii L, Joseph SS, Smith JI, Su P, Bater K, Byrne P, Boahene K, Papel I, Kontis T, Douglas R, Nelson CC, Ishii M. Prevalence of body dysmorphic disorder and surgeon diagnostic accuracy in facial plastic and oculoplastic surgery clinics. JAMA Facial Plast Surg. 2017;19(4):269–74.
56. Gonser P, Kaestner S, Jaminet P, Kaye K. Histological case-control study of peeling induced skin changes by different peeling agents in surgically subcutaneous undermined skin flaps in facelift patients. J Plast Reconstr Aesthet Surg. 2017;70(11):1660–5.
57. Paschou IA, Sali E, Paschou SA, Tsamis KI, Peppa M, Psaltopoulou T, Nicolaidou E, Stratigos AJ. GLP-1RA and the possible skin aging. Endocrine. 2025;89(3):680–5.
58. Egorov VI, Sambulov VI, Magomedov MU, Mustafaev DM. Rhinophyma through the prism of time. Vestn Otorinolaringol. 2021;86(4):95–8.
59. Rosenbaum C, Whitworth M. Optimising wound healing and cosmesis of surgical closures on rhinophymas skin. JAAD Case Rep. 2024;46:18–22.
60. Paichitrojjana A, Paichitrojjana A. Oral isotretinoin and its uses in dermatology: review. Drug Des Devel Ther. 2023;17:2573–91.
61. Dias RPP, Rodrigues JLT, Jabour MSD, Albuquerque ROE, Friedrich HA, Westphalen MS, Caropreso CA. Isotretinoin in thick-skin rhinoplasty: a review. Int Arch Otorhinolaryngol. 2025;29(2):1–6.
62. Solovev I, Sergeeva A, Geraskina A, Shaposhnikov M, Vedunova M, Borysova O, Moskalev A. Ageing and physiological barriers: mechanisms of barrier integrity changes and implications for age-related diseases. Mol Biol Rep. 2024;51(1):917.
63. Rorteau J, Chevalier FP, Fromy B, Lamartine J. Ageing and skin integrity—from cutaneous biology to anti-ageing strategies. Med Sci (Paris). 2020;36(12):1155–62.
64. Yasui T, Yonetsu M, Tanaka R, Tanaka Y, Fukushima S, Yamashita T, Ogura Y, Hirao T, Murota H, Araki T. In vivo observation of age-related structural changes of dermal collagen in human facial skin using collagen-sensitive second harmonic generation microscopy equipped with a 1250-nm mode-locked Cr:Forsterite laser. J Biomed Opt. 2013;18(3):31108.
65. Pham TTQ, Kuo YC, Chang WL, Weng HJ, Huang YH. Double-sided niche regulation in skin stem cell and cancer: mechanisms and clinical applications. Mol Cancer. 2025;24(1):147.

66. Rezazadeh H, Nayebi AR, Garjani A, Sheikhulislami A, Babaei H. Evidence that iron overload plus croton oil induce skin tumors in mice. Hum Exp Toxicol. 2005;24(8):409–13.
67. Shubik P. Chemical and viral oncogenesis. J Dermatol Surg Oncol. 1983;9(8):604–7.
68. Diamond L, O'Brien TG, Baird WM. Tumor promoters and the mechanism of tumor promotion. Adv Cancer Res. 1980;32:1–74.
69. Ungarelli LF, Hetem CM, Farina Junior JA. Is it safe to operate on patients taking isotretinoin? Aesthet Plast Surg. 2016;40(1):139–48.
70. Perkins SW, Sklarew EC. Prevention of facial herpetic infections after chemical peel and dermabrasion: new treatment strategies in the prophylaxis of patients undergoing procedures of the perioral area. Plast Reconstr Surg. 1996;98(3):427–33; discussion 434–435.
71. Gilbert S. Improving the outcome of facial resurfacing—prevention of herpes simplex virus type 1 reactivation. J Antimicrob Chemother. 2001;47 Suppl T1:29–34.
72. Klein DR, Little JH. Laryngeal edema as a complication of chemical peel. Plast Reconstr Surg. 1983;71(3):419–20.
73. Marçon CR, Coppinger AJ, Salomão C, Alves Dos Reis V, Alves Dos Reis VN, de Menezes Gomes JL, Gianvecchio VAP, Medeiros de Aquino E, de Seixas Alves MT, Canzian M, Coelho Frenkelis Brandão SA, Fusel de Ue RR, Ribeiro F, Bageorgou F, Wambier CG, International Peeling Society (IPS) and São Paulo's Legal Medical Institute (IML-SP). Fatal phenol peel by an unlicensed social media practitioner: a forensic medical analysis. J Am Acad Dermatol. 2025;93(6):e211–3.
74. Piotrowski JK. Evaluation of exposure to phenol: absorption of phenol vapour in the lungs and through the skin and excretion of phenol in urine. Br J Ind Med. 1971;28(2):172–8.
75. Rullan P, Lin EM, Schaut E, Wambier CG. Cardiac safety in full-face phenol-croton oil peels: a 22-year retrospective study. J Am Acad Dermatol. 2024;91(4):762–3.
76. Litton C. Observations after chemosurgery of the face. Plast Reconstr Surg. 1963;32:554–6.
77. Stagnone GJ, Orgel MG, Stagnone JJ. Cardiovascular effects of topical 50% trichloroacetic acid and Baker's phenol solution. J Dermatol Surg Oncol. 1987;13:999–1002.
78. Truppman ES, Ellenby JD. Major electrocardiographic changes during chemical face peeling. Plast Reconstr Surg. 1979;63:44–8.
79. Gross BG. Cardiac arrhythmias during phenol face peeling. Plast Reconstr Surg. 1984;73:590–4.
80. Wexler MR, Halon DA, Teitelbaum A, Tadjer G, Peled IJ. Prevention of cardiac arrhythmias induced in an animal model by the topical application of a commonly used phenol preparation for facial peeling. Plast Reconstr Surg. 1984;73:595–8.
81. Beeson WH. The importance of cardiac monitoring in superficial and deep chemical peeling. J Dermatol Surg Oncol. 1987;13:949–50.
82. Landau M. Cardiac complications in deep chemical peels. Dermatol Surg. 2007;33:190–3.
83. Zheng P, Lyu Z. The impact of fear of pain on the temporal processing of emotional faces: modulation of attentional resources. Cogn Process. 2025;26(2):237–45.
84. Morton DL, Sandhu JS, Jones AK. Brain imaging of pain: state of the art. J Pain Res. 2016;9:613–24.
85. Gorczyca R, Filip R, Walczak E. Psychological aspects of pain. Ann Agric Environ Med. 2013;Suppl 1:23–7.
86. Brown JJ, Ollier WE, Thomson W, Bayat A. Positive association of HLA-DRB1*15 with keloid disease in Caucasians. Int J Immunogenet. 2008;35(4–5):303–7.
87. Ogawa R. The most current algorithms for the treatment and prevention of hypertrophic scars and keloids: a 2020 update of the algorithms published 10 years ago. Plast Reconstr Surg. 2022;149(1):79e–94e.
88. Marneros AG, Krieg T. Keloids—clinical diagnosis, pathogenesis, and treatment options. J Dtsch Dermatol Ges. 2004;2(11):905–13.
89. Boyd AS, Neldner KH. The isomorphic response of Koebner. Int J Dermatol. 1990;29(6):401–10.

90. Karampinis E, Georgopoulou KE, Goudouras G, Lianou V, Kampra E, Roussaki Schulze AV, Zafiriou E. Laser-induced koebner-related skin reactions: a clinical overview. Medicina (Kaunas). 2024;60(7):1177.
91. Sanchez DP, Sonthalia S. Koebner phenomenon [Updated 2022 Nov 14]. In: StatPearls. Treasure Island, FL: StatPearls Publishing; 2025 [cited 2026 Mar 14]. NCBI Bookshelf.
92. Weiss G, Shemer A, Trau H. The Koebner phenomenon: review of the literature. J Eur Acad Dermatol Venereol. 2002;16(3):241–8.
93. Haen P, Laversanne S, Graillon N, Foletti JM. Facial necrotizing fasciitis following rhytidectomy. Br J Oral Maxillofac Surg. 2019;57(7):685–7.
94. McGonagle D, McDermott MF. A proposed classification of the immunological diseases. PLoS Med. 2006;3(8):e297.
95. Mantovani A, Allavena P, Sica A, Balkwill F. Cancer-related inflammation. Nature. 2008;454(7203):436–44.
96. Grivennikov SI, Greten FR, Karin M. Immunity, inflammation, and cancer. Cell. 2010;140(6):883–99.
97. Nikalji N, Godse K, Sakhiya J, Patil S, Nadkarni N. Complications of medium depth and deep chemical peels. J Cutan Aesthet Surg. 2012;5(4):254–60.
98. Wambier CG, Wambier SPF, Pilatti LEP, Grabicoski JA, Wambier LF, Schmidt A. Prolongation of rate-corrected QT interval during phenol-croton oil peels. J Am Acad Dermatol. 2018;78(4):810–2.
99. Seneschal J, Boniface K, Ezzedine K, Taieb A. Accelerating bleaching in vitiligo: balancing benefits versus risks. Exp Dermatol. 2014;23(12):879–80.
100. El-Mofty M, Mostafa WZ, Esmat S, Zayed A, Mashaly H, Hussien MF, Ismail SI. Site-oriented depigmentation in vitiligo patients using Q-switched Nd:YAG laser (1,064/532 nm), cryotherapy and chemical peels: a comparative study. Dermatol Ther. 2019;32(5):e13052.

Patient Assessment and Selection

6

6.1 Introduction

The clinical success and safety of phenol-croton oil peel are intrinsically dependent on the careful selection of candidates for the procedure. This is a deep ablative intervention, recognized for its capacity to induce intense dermal remodeling, but also associated with potential systemic toxicity, local complications, and significant functional and aesthetic implications. Unlike less aggressive techniques, which have a broader safety margin and tolerate greater heterogeneity among patients, phenol-croton oil peel requires a selective process based on multiple clinical and contextual domains.

The assessment must synergistically integrate anatomical and cutaneous aspects, physiological and laboratory parameters, pharmacological profile, emotional state, social support network, logistical conditions, and, above all, alignment between expectations and therapeutic reality. Appropriate selection is not limited to the exclusion of absolute contraindications, discussed in the previous chapter, but also involves understanding the biological and psychosocial context in which the procedure will be performed.

This chapter proposes a systematic and evidence-based approach to selecting the ideal patient for phenol-croton oil peel, drawing on the best available scientific evidence, accumulated experience with the technique, and guidelines aimed at maximizing therapeutic benefits while minimizing associated risks.

6.2 Cutaneous and Morphofunctional Analysis

Cutaneous and morphofunctional analysis is a critical step in selecting patients for phenol-croton oil peel, being decisive for the safety, efficacy, and naturalness of the results. This involves a thorough clinical examination, integrating observation, palpation, photographic documentation, the use of auxiliary devices, and

C. Marçon, C. Wambier, *Phenol-Croton Oil Peel*,
https://doi.org/10.1007/978-3-032-25993-6_6

analysis of the patient's dermatological history. This assessment should encompass not only morphological but also functional aspects of the skin and its healing capacity.

Anatomical evaluation of candidates for phenol-croton oil peel should include a detailed analysis of facial characteristics, such as skin thickness, laxity, degree of elastosis, presence of telangiectasias, atrophies, presence and depth of rhytids, distribution of actinic lesions, previous scars, areas of surgical undermining, and local vascularization. The delicate thickness of the eyelid skin requires caution, especially in cases of ligamentous laxity, which may predispose to ectropion. Identifying areas at increased risk of complications, such as regions with reduced blood supply or a history of previous procedures, is essential for safe procedural planning. The presence of previous scars, rhinoplasties, rhytidectomies, or other procedures involving subdermal undermining alters phenol distribution and increases the risk of demarcation or necrosis.

The presence of solar elastosis, telangiectasias, enlarged pores, actinic keratoses, melanoses, and static wrinkles should be mapped in advance. These changes not only form part of the clinical picture of aging but also influence the absorption and distribution of phenol in the skin. The resulting frosting may vary according to the thickness and density of the stratum corneum and epidermis, requiring a trained eye for intraoperative interpretation.

The ideal candidate for phenol-croton oil peel is classically a patient with fair skin (typically Fitzpatrick phototypes I–II) , good dermal density, and moderate to deep facial rhytids, especially in areas such as the periorbital and perioral regions (Fig. 6.1). These patients have a lower risk of pigmentary complications, such as post-inflammatory hyperpigmentation and demarcation lines, which are more common in individuals with higher phototypes or thicker skin.

Patients with a history of good wound healing, no active cutaneous diseases, no tendency to hypertrophic scars or keloids, and without systemic contraindications to phenol are preferred candidates. Regarding age group, middle-aged to elderly adults are frequently selected, as they derive greater aesthetic benefit and have a lower risk of pigmentation-related complications.

6.2.1 Skin Thickness, Dermal Density, and Facial Topography

Skin thickness is one of the main determinants of the depth of action and safety of phenol-croton oil peel. Patients with thin, dry, aged skin with significant solar elastosis respond better to phenol than those with oily, thick, or very young skin. Very thin and atrophic skin tends to allow greater penetration of the caustic agent, increasing the risk of complications such as dyschromia, ulceration, and atrophic scarring. In contrast, thick skin with higher dermal density and a greater number of cutaneous appendages generally tolerates the chemical action better and shows a more predictable clinical response, with a lower risk of overpeeling.

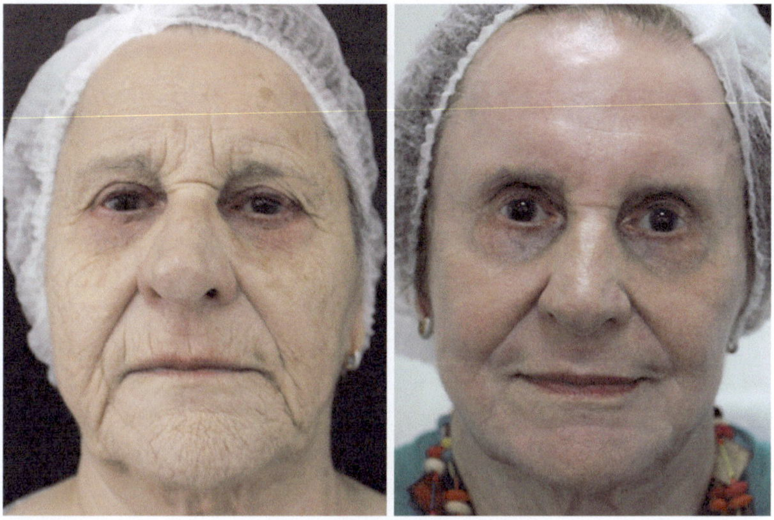

Fig. 6.1 Patient with fair skin (Fitzpatrick phototype II) , good dermal density, and moderate to deep facial rhytids, especially in the periorbital and perioral regions—classic characteristics of the ideal candidate for phenol-croton oil peel. These patients have a lower risk of pigmentary complications, such as post-inflammatory hyperpigmentation and demarcation lines, compared to individuals with higher phototypes. (*Source: Personal archive of Dr Carlos Wambier*)

This thickness varies significantly between different facial regions, directly influencing the uniformity of phenol penetration. Areas such as the lower eyelids, upper malar region, and preauricular area have thin skin and are particularly susceptible to excessive penetration, whereas regions such as the lower cheeks, nose, and chin have increased thickness, higher sebaceous density, and fibrous tissue, which may hinder the homogeneous absorption of the caustic agent.

The presence of solar elastosis, telangiectasia, dilated pores, actinic keratoses, melanosis, and static wrinkles should be mapped beforehand. These changes not only form part of the clinical picture of aging but also influence the absorption and distribution of phenol in the skin. The resulting frosting may vary according to the thickness and density of the stratum corneum and epidermis, requiring a trained eye for intraoperative interpretation (Fig. 6.2).

6.2.1.1 Assessment Methods

Assessment of skin thickness should be performed by clinical inspection, gentle digital palpation, and, when available, by objective methods such as high-frequency ultrasonography, cutometry, or digital optical analysis. This analysis allows precise mapping of high-risk zones—such as the eyelids, medial malar region, preauricular area, mandibular line, and areas of previous scarring—which require technical adaptations during peel application, such as adjustment of the number of layers, pressure, and formula composition.

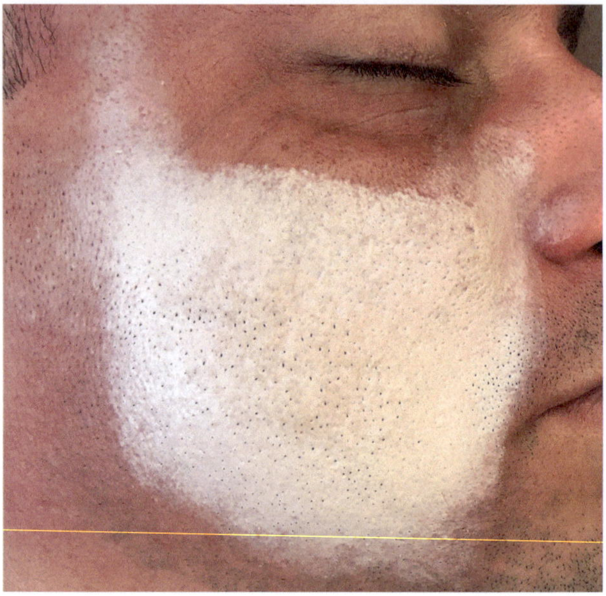

Fig. 6.2 Solid white frosting observed immediately after application of phenol–croton peel to the malar region. The intensity and pattern of frosting may vary according to the thickness and density of the stratum corneum and epidermis, requiring experience and a trained eye for correct intraoperative interpretation. (*Source: Personal archive of the author (Dr Carolina Marçon)*)

6.2.1.2 Areas Requiring Special Attention

Certain facial areas require extreme caution due to reduced thickness, terminal vascularization, or intense functional mobility:

Lower eyelids: high risk of ulceration, ectropion, and atrophic scarring. Assessment of ligamentous laxity and protrusion of fat pads is mandatory.

Perioral region: dynamic folds and high sebaceous density predispose to overcorrection, thick crusts, and visible scarring.

Glabella and nose: terminal vascularization with increased risk of necrosis. The application should be delicate, with fewer layers.

Chin and mandibular line: transition zones prone to demarcation and accumulation of agent. Require a feathering technique to ensure uniformity.

Detailed mapping of these areas in the preoperative period should guide technical adjustments and, in some cases, the exclusion of specific points from application (Table 6.1).

6.2.1.3 Thick Skin Phenotype: Technical Implications and Therapeutic Considerations

Patients with thick skin—characterized by dermal thickening, irregular texture, enlarged pores, sebaceous hyperplasia, or phymatous phenotypes (such as early rhinophyma)—present additional technical challenges. In these cases, penetration of the caustic agent may be irregular, making it difficult to achieve the clinical endpoint (frosting), with a risk of both undertreatment and localized necrosis.

Table 6.1 Areas of concern by facial region: thickness, risks, and technical adjustments

Facial region	Relative thickness	Main risks	Technical adjustments
Lower eyelids	Very thin	Ulceration, ectropion, atrophic scar	Fewer layers; drier applicator, minimal pressure; caution if *snap test* +
Zygomatic region	Thin	Overpenetration, dyschromia, scarring—area of bony projection	Lower pressure and fewer layers; segment the area
Pre-auricular	Thin	Demarcation, necrosis	Feathering at transitions; lower agent load
Glabella	Medium-thin	Necrosis due to terminal vascularization	Gentle application; reduce the number of layers
Nose	Thick	Irregular penetration, focal necrosis	Gradual layering; monitor frosting; caution in patients with previous rhinoplasty
Chin/perioral	Thick	Demarcation at transition, thick crust, dyschromia, scarring (area of high mobility), overcorrection	Feathering along the mandibular line; even passes, fractionated layers
Mandibular line	Medium	Agent accumulation, demarcation lines, scarring—bony projection	Broad feathering; reduce applied volume

Areas of concern by facial region in phenol–croton peeling, considering relative skin thickness, main associated risks, and recommended technical adjustments for greater safety and predictability of outcomes. Note: Feathering = blending at anatomical transition borders; "layers" refer to passes of the solution. (*Source: Table prepared by the author (Dr Carolina Marçon)*)

The presence of hypertrophic sebaceous glands may interfere with the homogeneous diffusion of phenol, resulting in areas of uneven absorption and increasing the likelihood of dyschromia, scarring, and aesthetic asymmetries. Furthermore, this skin profile tends to have a less predictable inflammatory and scarring response.

Although thick skin is not a formal contraindication, it requires greater technical skill, precise modulation, and strict intra- and post-procedural monitoring to ensure predictability and safety.

6.2.1.4 Thin Skin: Risk Factors and Technical Considerations

In contrast, thin skin—particularly in areas such as the eyelids, forehead, perioral region, or in patients with advanced ageing—has lower density of adnexal structures, a thin epidermis, and a reduced superficial dermis, which favors rapid and deep penetration of phenol, with possible involvement of vascular or deep ligamentous structures, significantly increasing the risk of poor healing, persistent dyschromia, and atrophic scarring.

In addition, the low density of glands and reduced vascularization compromise re-epithelialization and dissipation of the caustic agent, prolonging healing time and increasing the risk of infection or permanent changes in texture and color.

Patients with atrophic skin, whether due to intrinsic aging or severe photoaging, also tend to have fragmented collagen, disorganized extracellular matrix, and reduced fibroblast reserve, which impairs the expected dermal remodeling after peeling. In these cases, association with excessive facial mobility may favor adverse events such as ectropion, eclabium, or worsening of dynamic laxity.

6.2.2 Pigmentary Risk Stratification: Phototype, Ethnicity, and Melanocytic Reactivity

Proper classification of skin phototype is an essential step in pre-peeling assessment, especially in procedures with high inflammatory intensity, such as phenol-croton oil. Phototype directly influences the risk of post-inflammatory hyperpigmentation (PIH), formation of demarcation lines, and persistent dyschromia, even when using agents with depigmenting potential, such as phenol.

Although phenol exerts a strong caustic effect on epidermal melanocytes, the inflammation induced by the procedure may activate residual melanocytes in deeper layers or in adjacent untreated areas, triggering pigmentary processes that are difficult to resolve. In such cases, the risk is proportional to the melanocytic reactivity and the inflammatory capacity of the patient's skin.

6.2.2.1 Phototype Classification: Methods and Limitations

The Fitzpatrick system is the most widely used method for stratifying pigmentary risk. It is based on the skin's response to sun exposure, particularly the tendency to burn (*sunburn*) and to tan (*tanning*), and classifies individuals from I to VI. Assessment should include a targeted medical history, with questions regarding previous sunburns, ease of tanning, and observation of skin color in non-photoexposed areas.

- **Lower phototypes (I–III)**: lower risk of PIH, greater safety for deep peels.
- **Higher phototypes (IV–VI)**: increased risk of dyschromia, need for rigorous preconditioning and, in some cases, relative contraindication.

However, the Fitzpatrick system has significant limitations, especially in multi-ethnic populations. Asian, African-descendant, Hispanic, and mixed-race individuals do not always fit precisely into the original criteria, which were developed based on Caucasian populations. Terms such as "redness" or "tanning" often do not reflect the actual experience of these patients after sun exposure, compromising the accuracy of the classification. In such cases, it is necessary to adapt the medical history using more appropriate descriptors. Instead of asking only about sunburn or tanning, the clinician should enquire whether the skin darkens or develops marks after sun exposure, whether there is a history of burning, itching, or cutaneous sensitivity to sunlight, and whether the patient has noticed residual hyperpigmentation after wounds, previous procedures, insect bites, acne, or other inflammatory processes. These adaptations make the classification more faithful to the individual's physiology and cutaneous experience, especially in patients with increased melanocytic reactivity.

Furthermore, the tendency to classify all Black individuals as phototype VI is incorrect, as there is wide intra-ethnic variability—self-identified Black individuals may present with phototypes IV, V, or VI, which directly impacts the response to peeling.

6.2.2.2 Objective Methods for Pigmentary Assessment

In cases of diagnostic uncertainty or in highly mixed populations, objective methods may complement clinical assessment:

- **Colorimetry and spectrophotometry**: measuring melanin density in the skin with high precision.
- **Melanin index (MI)** and **individual typology angle (ITA)**: parameters derived from spectrophotometry, useful for determining functional phototype regardless of ethnicity.
- **Optical profilometry and high-resolution digital photography**: allowing comparative analysis of pigmentation in different anatomical areas.

These tools increase the accuracy of classification and assist in the individualized stratification of pigmentary risk.

6.2.2.3 Other Clinical Indicators of Risk for PIH

In addition to formal phototype, it is essential to identify clinical and historical signs indicating a propensity for post-inflammatory hyperpigmentation, even in patients with lower phototypes:

- Presence of residual PIH on physical examination, in previously inflamed, acne-prone, or manipulated areas.
- History of marks following insect bites, minor trauma, sunburn, or aesthetic procedures.
- Marked pigmentation of the palmar creases, reflecting increased melanocytic activity and higher melanin density in the basal layers of the epidermis (Fig. 6.3).
- History of post-traumatic pigmentation (such as scratches, cuts, or hair removal) with prolonged duration (Fig. 6.4).

These findings serve as phenotypic risk markers and should directly influence the choice of formulation, exposure time, and the extent of the treated area (Table 6.2).

6.2.2.4 Practical Recommendations

- In patients with higher phototypes or clinical signs of hyperpigmentation risk, prolonged topical preconditioning should be instituted, using depigmenting agents, antioxidants, and retinoids.
- Application should be performed carefully in transition zones and in areas of increased mobility, such as folds, perioral contour, and eyelids.
- The use of segmented techniques or diluted formulations may be considered in higher-risk areas.

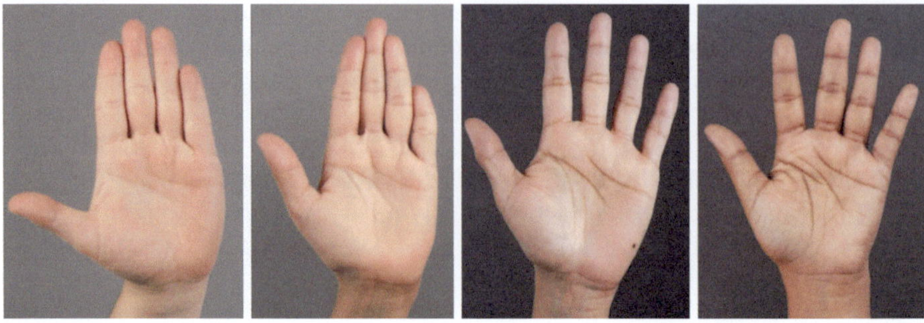

Fig. 6.3 Hyperpigmentation of the palmar creases, a clinical marker associated with increased risk of post-inflammatory hyperpigmentation (PIH) in patients undergoing deep ablative procedures. Assessment by pigmentation scale of the palmar creases (Palmar Crease Pigmentation—PCP). (*Source: Adapted from Khunger N, Kandhari R, Garg S. Predicting the risk of postinflammatory hyperpigmentation: The palmar crease pigmentation scale. J Cosmet Dermatol. 2021;20(2):584–590. doi:10.1111/jocd.14005. Reproduced with permission from the author/editor)*

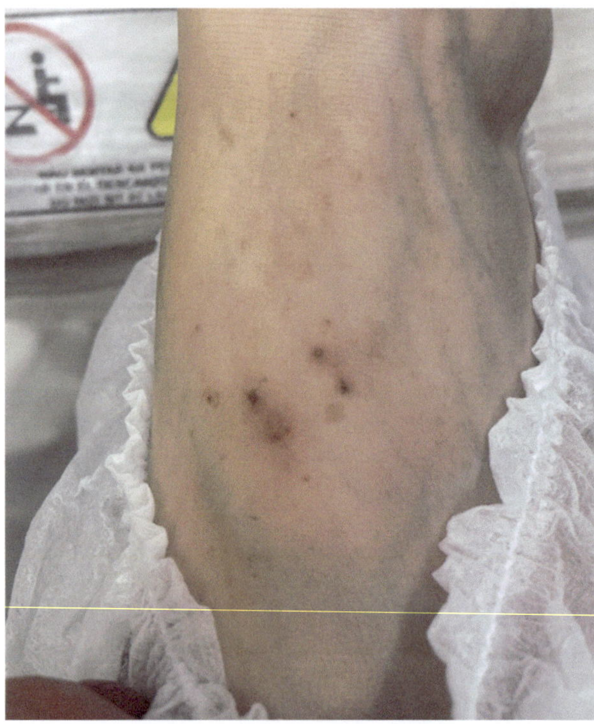

Fig. 6.4 Persistent hyperpigmentation following cutaneous trauma, indicating an individual predisposition to post-inflammatory hyperpigmentation (PIH). This clinical finding signals an increased risk for the development of dyschromia after deep ablative procedures, such as phenol–croton peel. (*Source: Author's personal archive (Dr Carolina Marçon)*)

- Individualized planning, considering not only phototype but also pigmentary history and clinical signs of PIH, is crucial for the safety and predictability of the procedure.

Table 6.2 Pigmentary risk stratification and preparation/follow-up protocols

Pigmentary risk	Profile (examples)	Clinical indicators	Pre-procedure preparation (4–8 weeks)	Intraoperative strategy	Follow-up
Low	Phototypes I–II; no previous PIH	Absence of post-inflammatory pigmentation	Mild retinoid + antioxidant; strict photoprotection	Standard technique; careful transitions	Review at 7–10 days; UV guidance
Moderate	Phototype III; history of mild PIH	PIH after previous acne/trauma	Depigmenting agent + retinoid; NIAC 4–5%	Dilution in critical zones; segment areas	Reviews at 1, 4, and 8 weeks; early PIH management
High	Phototypes IV–VI; mixed ancestry with easy PIH	Residual PIH, darkens after inflammation	Dual depigmenting agents + antioxidant + progressive retinoid; maximum photoprotection	More conservative formulation; avoid transition zones	Close follow-up; early initiation of depigmenting agents postoperatively

Pigmentary risk stratification in phenol–croton peel, with examples of clinical profiles, indicators of post-inflammatory hyperpigmentation, pre-procedure measures, intraoperative adjustments, and post-procedure follow-up recommendations. Note: “PIH” = post-inflammatory hyperpigmentation; NIAC = niacinamide. Adapt preparation to individual melanocytic reactivity, not just phototype. (*Source: Table prepared by the author (Dr Carolina Marçon)*)

6.2.3 History of Scarring, Cutaneous Reactivity, and Previous Surgeries

Prior assessment of the patient's scarring tendency is an essential step in the selection for phenol–croton peel. The presence of hypertrophic scars, keloids, or any history of Abnormal scarring, even in other areas of the body, should be considered a clinical marker of increased risk for an exacerbated inflammatory response, poor wound healing, or disorganized dermal fibrosis.

6.2.3.1 History of Pathological Scarring

Patients with a history of:

- Active or extensive keloids, especially in areas of trauma, surgery, inflamed acne, or vaccination.
- Hypertrophic scars or fibrotic contractures following previous procedures.
- Poor scar evolution after aesthetic, surgical, or traumatic procedures.

...should be carefully assessed, as they represent a high risk of developing post-peel complications such as unsightly scars, persistent dyschromia, and permanent deformities.

Personal and family predisposition to keloid formation should be investigated, with emphasis on the anatomical location of previous lesions and associated inflammatory or traumatic triggers. The presence of thickened scars in previously treated areas may require reassessment of the indication and restriction of the area to be exposed to the caustic agent.

6.2.3.2 Associated Ethnic and Genetic Factors

Individuals with phototypes IV–VI, especially those of African or Asian ancestry, are at greater risk of abnormal scarring. Studies show a keloid incidence of between 4.5% and 16% in people of African descent, compared to less than 1% in Caucasians. This risk is attributed to genetic variants in genes such as TGF-β1, SMAD3, and p53, as well as differences in inflammatory response and the biomechanical properties of the dermis.

Transition zones between aesthetic units—such as the nasolabial folds, mandibular line, and preauricular area—are particularly prone to unpredictable scarring responses, whether due to increased mechanical tension or heterogeneity in the penetration of the chemical agent (Figs. 6.5 and 6.6).

6.2.3.3 Management of Patients with Moderate Scarring Risk

In cases where the patient has a limited history of abnormal scarring, chemical peeling may be considered with caution, provided that:

- A prior test is performed on a restricted area (*test spot*).
- Critical anatomical zones are avoided.

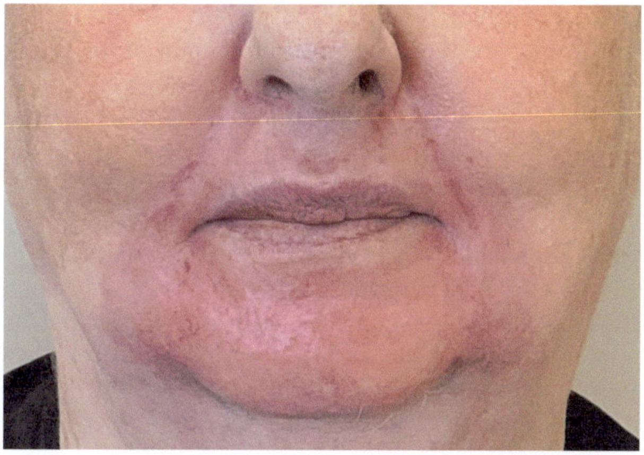

Fig. 6.5 Residual scars in the perioral region after segmental phenol–croton peel. Areas of high mobility, such as the labial and perioral regions, present an increased risk of scarring complications, especially when there is excessive penetration of the caustic solution or overlapping of layers. In these regions, local mechanical tension combined with greater tissue vulnerability may result in fibrotic contractures, irregularities, and functional aesthetic impairment. (Source: Author's personal archive (Dr Carolina Marçon))

Fig. 6.6 Marked inflammatory edema of the periorbital region following phenol–croton peel. Patients with high myopia (> −6.00 D), particularly those with a history of retinal detachment, require careful ophthalmological evaluation, as intense edema may transiently increase external pressure on the globe, representing a theoretical risk of vitreoretinal decompensation in anatomically predisposed individuals. (*Source: Author's personal archive (Dr Carolina Marçon)*)

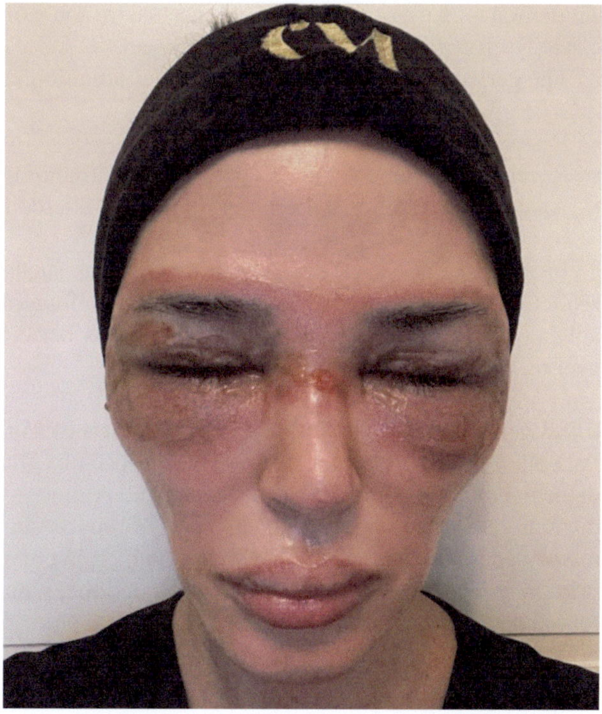

- The concentration of croton oil is reduced.
- Application is performed at a shallower depth with strict postoperative monitoring.

The decision should be individualized, based on a careful risk–benefit analysis, and formalized in a specific informed consent document.

6.2.3.4 Previous Facial Surgeries and Their Implications

Patients with a history of facial surgery—such as rhytidectomy, blepharoplasty, rhinoplasty, or lifting procedures—should be assessed using strict clinical criteria, considering the anatomical and physiological changes resulting from these interventions. Such procedures permanently alter vascular architecture, tissue elasticity, and dermal thickness, potentially resulting in areas of:

- Subcutaneous or dermal fibrosis.
- Relative tissue ischemia.
- Adhesions and changes in the regeneration pattern.

Phenol-croton oil peel is contraindicated in areas previously subjected to subcutaneous undermining, such as in rhytidoplasty flaps, due to the risk of necrosis, poor wound healing, and unpredictable aesthetic outcomes. Disruption of the dermal and subdermal plexuses reduces tissue perfusion and compromises the regenerative capacity of skin exposed to the caustic agent.

The periocular region requires particular attention, especially in patients with:

- History of blepharoplasty.
- Recent ophthalmic surgery (ptosis repair, vitrectomy, refractive surgery) .
- Anatomical fragility, underlying fibrosis, or altered local lymphatic drainage.

In these situations, the risk of complications such as persistent edema, eyelid retraction, ectropion, and even functional ocular impairment is increased. It is advisable to allow a minimum interval of 6 months between blepharoplasty and deep peeling in the same region.

6.2.3.5 Ophthalmological Considerations in Myopic Patients

Patients with high myopia (> −6.00 D), especially those with a history of retinal detachment, also require careful assessment. Although there is no formal contraindication described in the literature, clinical reports suggest that significant inflammatory edema in the periorbital region, which is common after phenol-croton oil peel, may increase external pressure on the globe, with a theoretical risk of vitreoretinal decompensation in eyes with anatomical predisposition (Fig. 6.6).

It is recommended to:

- Refer the patient for prior specialist ophthalmological assessment.

- Avoid application to the eyelids in patients with a high-risk ocular history.
- Opt for segmental protocols or exclude the eyelid region, always with close post-operative monitoring.

A detailed assessment of scarring and surgical history—including family predisposition, ethnic background, previous inflammatory responses, and any prior procedures on the face or eyes—is essential for a safe, individualized, and technically appropriate indication of phenol-croton oil peel. Respect for the biological, vascular, and structural limits of the skin is crucial for therapeutic success and for preventing permanent adverse events.

6.2.4 Laxity, Volume, and Facial Architecture

Morphofunctional changes related to skin laxity, volume loss, and imbalance of facial architecture decisively influence the indication, planning, and perception of outcomes in procedures using phenol-croton oil. Although deep peeling provides a secondary lifting effect—mediated by dermal contraction and stimulation of neocollagenesis—it does not address facial volumetry nor correct deep structures affected by ptosis or volume depletion.

Very thin faces, with marked lipodystrophy, loss of malar and temporal fat pads, or evident bone resorption, may show limited or even undesirable results, with accentuation of facial thinness and shadowing. In such cases, combination with deep volumizing strategies, such as structural fillers, autologous fat grafting, or biostimulators, is often necessary to restore facial contour and harmony.

Conversely, cases of severe tissue laxity, with advanced ptosis of the mid and lower thirds, detachment of supporting ligaments, and formation of platysmal bands, often exceed the lifting and support capacity provided by phenol-croton oil alone, and are better suited to surgical treatments such as cervicofacial lifting, sometimes combined with chemical peeling to optimize skin texture and pigmentation.

Three-dimensional facial assessment should be incorporated into the clinical analysis, including:

- Static and dynamic observation.
- Evaluation of bony support, depth of folds, and sagging of soft tissues.
- Presence of areas of volume loss and discontinuity in facial contour (such as nasolabial folds, jawline, and temples).

The distinction between dermal (cutaneous) laxity and structural ptosis is crucial to avoid unrealistic expectations. Phenol-croton oil is highly effective in improving skin quality, static wrinkles, and superficial texture, but has a limited effect on volumetric restoration and correction of deep anatomical changes.

Therefore, the ideal indication for peeling should consider the degree of residual anatomical support, the balance between the aesthetic units of the face, and the tissue remodeling potential in response to the induced inflammatory stimulus. Personalization of the therapeutic plan, potentially in combination with complementary techniques, is essential to achieve harmonious and functional results.

6.2.5 Screening for Pre-existing Dermatoses

Rigorous screening for pre-existing dermatoses is a fundamental step in selecting candidates for phenol-croton oil peeling. The presence of inflammatory or neoplastic skin diseases—whether active or of historical relevance—can significantly interfere with the tissue response to the caustic agent, increasing the risk of aesthetic, functional, and systemic complications.

6.2.5.1 Active Inflammatory Diseases

Active inflammatory dermatoses, such as nodulocystic acne, severe seborrheic dermatitis, facial psoriasis, perioral dermatitis, rosacea with prominent telangiectasia, and cutaneous lupus erythematosus, should be considered relative contraindications to the procedure. These conditions compromise the uniformity of the inflammatory response, increase the risk of post-inflammatory dyschromia, atrophic scarring, and disease reactivation, as well as favoring unpredictable scarring outcomes. Ideally, the procedure should be postponed until sustained clinical remission has been confirmed for at least 3–6 months.

Even in remission, these dermatoses often exhibit persistent alterations in the skin barrier, dermal vascularization, and chronic inflammatory infiltrate, which may affect the depth of phenol penetration and compromise both scarring response and physiological re-epithelialization. Clinical assessment should be thorough and, when necessary, supplemented by diagnostic biopsy, standardized photographic documentation, and inspection with a dermatoscopic magnifier.

6.2.5.2 Immune-Mediated Diseases and the Koebner Phenomenon

In immune-mediated dermatoses known to be associated with the Koebner phenomenon—such as psoriasis, lichen planus, vitiligo, cutaneous lupus, atopic dermatitis, lichen sclerosus, and pemphigus vulgaris—the risk of disease activation or spread in treated areas must be carefully considered. Induction of chemical trauma in predisposed skin may trigger exuberant clinical manifestations, with potentially severe aesthetic and functional consequences.

It is recommended to avoid deep phenol-croton oil peeling in patients with active inflammatory manifestations of these conditions. In cases of stable remission, the procedure may be considered under strict criteria, provided that:

- Absence of active lesions for a minimum period of 3–6 months.
- Clinical and photographic documentation of stability.
- Detailed informed consent, with explicit discussion of the risk of reactivation and potential complications.

Strict clinical follow-up is mandatory in both the immediate and late postoperative periods, with early intervention should any sign of recurrence arise.

6.2.5.3 Vitiligo

Vitiligo should be considered a relative contraindication to phenol-croton oil peeling, especially in active or unstable cases. The condition is frequently associated with the Koebner phenomenon, implying a high risk of new depigmented lesions developing in areas subjected to chemical trauma. Furthermore, the absence of functional melanocytes in affected regions renders the pigmentary response to the procedure unpredictable, with the possibility of pronounced dyschromia, irregular repigmentation, or undesirable lightening.

Although there are isolated and unsystematized clinical reports of partial repigmentation or homogenization of skin color following deep peeling in patients with stable vitiligo, such observations are not supported by controlled clinical studies, therapeutic guidelines, or systematic reviews of the medical literature. The currently available evidence on repigmentation in vitiligo focuses on topical immunomodulatory therapies, phototherapy, and surgical interventions based on cellular or grafting techniques, which have documented efficacy rates.

Phenol, on the other hand, has historically been used in contexts of definitive depigmentation, particularly in cases of universal or extensive vitiligo, aiming to achieve a uniform skin tone by residual elimination of melanocytes. Its known mechanisms of action do not promote melanocyte migration, proliferation, or repopulation—processes essential for repigmentation.

Thus, although vitiligo does not constitute an absolute contraindication to phenol-croton oil, its management requires rigorous clinical judgment, with individualized risk assessment and documentation of stability. Clinical remission for at least 6–12 months, absence of signs of activity, and specific informed consent. The decision must be supported by professional experience, and the procedure should be restricted to highly selected cases, with intensive postoperative monitoring.

6.2.5.4 Frontal Fibrosing Alopecia (FFA)

The presence of frontal fibrosing alopecia is an absolute contraindication to deep phenol-croton oil peels. This condition is characterized by progressive loss of pilosebaceous units and follicular stem cells in the frontotemporal region, which severely impairs the skin's regenerative capacity. The absence of these elements, essential for wound healing, increases the risk of skin necrosis, deep atrophy, and permanent unsightly scarring.

Recent reports have documented severe complications, such as extensive tissue loss and disfiguring scarring, following phenol-croton oil application in patients with FFA. This has led to the consolidation of an international clinical consensus regarding its absolute contraindication, regardless of the disease stage.

6.2.5.5 Infections

The presence of active infections—viral (such as herpes simplex), bacterial, or fungal—constitutes a formal contraindication to the procedure. The disruption of the epidermal barrier caused by the peel may facilitate the spread of infection, with an increased risk of necrosis, secondary infection, and sepsis. The procedure should be postponed until complete clinical and laboratory resolution of the infection.

6.2.5.6 Cutaneous Neoplasms

Performing deep peels on areas with active melanoma or non-melanoma skin cancer (NMSC)—such as basal cell carcinoma and squamous cell carcinoma—is absolutely contraindicated. Chemical manipulation of areas with neoplastic activity may mask lesions, hinder subsequent histopathological diagnosis, and interfere with appropriate oncological management. This approach is based on clinical, therapeutic, and ethical principles of dermatological oncology.

It is essential to distinguish between a field of cutaneous carcinogenesis—defined by multifocal, subclinical, and reversible dysplastic changes—and active invasive neoplasms. While the former is a valid and promising indication for phenol-croton oil peels, active tumors require specific surgical or destructive management. Indiscriminate application of the peel to malignant lesions may compromise oncological treatment and expose the patient to risks.

A comprehensive dermatological assessment should include a detailed clinical examination, dermoscopy, biopsy when indicated, and careful stratification of candidate areas for treatment. In patients with a history of skin cancer, it is mandatory to perform careful mapping of affected areas, with the exclusion of suspicious lesions and strict surveillance throughout the follow-up.

6.2.6 Functional Skin Support and Barrier Status

In addition to morphological and structural characteristics, skin function plays a central role in the response to phenol-croton oil peels, directly influencing the depth of penetration, intensity of inflammation, quality of healing, and uniformity of the final result. The skin should not be assessed merely as an anatomical surface, but as a dynamic functional organ with biochemical, immunological, and regenerative properties that determine its ability to tolerate and recover from controlled chemical injury.

6.2.6.1 Epidermal Barrier Integrity

The skin barrier, composed mainly of the stratum corneum and intercellular lipids (especially ceramides, cholesterol, and free fatty acids), plays a crucial role in protecting against transepidermal water loss (TEWL), entry of pathogens and irritants, and modulation of inflammation. An intact barrier attenuates phenol penetration, promoting a more controlled and predictable distribution. Conversely, a compromised barrier, common in sensitized, dry, or inflamed skin, may facilitate excessive absorption, resulting in areas of hypersensitivity, dyschromia, or delayed healing.

Clinical assessment of the barrier can be performed by observing desquamation, erythema, dryness, irregular oily sheen, fissures, and tenderness to touch. In specific situations, objective instrumentation may be used, such as:

- Corneometry (measurement of epidermal water content).
- TEWL measurement (assessment of transepidermal water loss).
- Sebometry (quantification of skin oiliness).
- Colorimetry (for the detection of subclinical erythema).

6.2.6.2 Hydration, Sebum Regulation, and Cutaneous Homeostasis

Skin with adequate hydration, balanced sebum production, and a functional microbiome demonstrates greater resilience to controlled injury. In contrast, skin in cases of dysbiosis, excessive or deficient sebum production, or pH alterations, tends to react unpredictably. Very oily skin, for example, may exhibit areas of uneven penetration, while extremely dry or delipidized skin may have low tolerance to the caustic agent, with a higher risk of focal necrosis, exacerbated inflammatory response, or premature epidermal detachment, compromising the uniformity and healing of the procedure.

Sebometry and cutaneous pH assessment are useful tools in specialized settings, but in clinical practice, careful inspection and palpation, combined with dermatological history, are sufficient for effective functional screening.

The presence of subjective sensations such as stinging, pruritus, burning, or tingling at rest or upon application of common cosmetics may indicate cutaneous hyper-reactivity, often associated with low-grade inflammation or a compromised barrier. Additionally, areas with persistent erythema, telangiectasia, chronic scaling, or irregular texture may signal subclinical inflammation, which predisposes to an exaggerated or unpredictable inflammatory response to phenol.

Conditions such as subclinical rosacea, mild seborrheic dermatitis, or sensitive skin syndrome should be carefully screened, even in the absence of typical lesions, and prior use of potentially irritating products should be investigated.

6.2.6.3 History of Medications and Topical Products

The recent pharmacological history of the skin significantly influences its defensive and regenerative functions. The following should be investigated:

- Previous use of oral isotretinoin, which may alter healing and dermal vascularization for months after discontinuation.
- Topical or systemic corticosteroid therapy, which may cause dermal atrophy, prolonged vasoconstriction, and local immunosuppression.
- Chronic use of acids, potent depigmenting agents, chemical exfoliants, or sensitizing products, which disrupt homeostasis and increase the risk of uncontrolled response to peeling.

Attention should also be paid to the cumulative effects of multiple recent aesthetic treatments (such as lasers, microneedling, previous peels), which may leave the skin previously inflamed or in a phase of subclinical repair.

6.2.7 Safe Interval Between Previous Aesthetic Procedures and Phenol-Croton Oil Peel

The correct indication for phenol-croton oil peel requires consideration of the recent history of ablative or chemical aesthetic procedures that may compromise the integrity of the skin barrier, dermal vascularization, or the skin's regenerative capacity. Overlapping aggressive treatments at insufficient intervals may result in excessive phenol penetration, tissue necrosis, persistent dyschromia, unsightly scarring, and unpredictable recovery (Table 6.3).

Procedures such as ablative CO_2 laser, medium-depth chemical peels, deep microneedling, ablative radiofrequency, and even mild procedures performed repeatedly can cause significant structural changes in the epidermis and papillary dermis, directly impacting the absorption and diffusion of caustic agents.

Table 6.3 Minimum safe intervals after previous procedures before phenol-croton oil peel

Previous procedure	Depth/ intensity	Minimum interval	Notes
CO_2 laser (ablative/ fractional)	High	6–12 months	Assess for residual erythema/ fibrosis/vascular changes; individualize parameters
Medium-depth peels (e.g. TCA 35%)	Medium	3–6 months	Only perform if skin is completely intact and stable, with no inflammatory signs or previous PIH
Deep microneedling/ ablative RF	Medium	3–6 months	Avoid recent overlap; pay attention to previously sensitized areas
IPL/non-ablative Nd:YAG/non-fractionated RF/superficial peels	Low	4–8 weeks	Ensure absence of subclinical inflammation or residual hypersensitivity
Repeated mild procedures (e.g., serial peels, superficial microneedling)	Variable	4–8 weeks	Cumulative sensitization risk and persistent low-grade inflammation
Phenol–croton peel (full face)	High	≥12 months (ideally 18–24 months in selected cases)	Dermal remodeling must be complete before a new session
Segmental phenol–croton peel (periorbital, lips, forehead, malar, etc.)	High	≥6 months	Only if healing is complete and there is no residual inflammation
Successive applications to different areas	Variable	6–8 weeks	Permitted if there is no overlap, with good tolerance and no adverse events

Minimum recommended intervals between different previous procedures and the performance of phenol–croton peel, according to the depth of the prior intervention. Individualization should consider additional factors such as phototype, history of post-inflammatory hyperpigmentation (PIH), recent isotretinoin use, residual inflammation, and previous complications. (*Source: Table prepared by the author (Dr Carolina Marçon)*)

6.2.7.1 CO_2 Laser (Ablative or Fractional)

Histological studies have shown that CO_2 causes deep thermal damage, with reorganization of collagen fibers, partial destruction of the superficial dermal plexus, and prolonged changes in vascularization and dermal thickness. These alterations may persist for up to 12 months after application, depending on the intensity of the protocol used and the individual biological response.

For this reason, a minimum interval of 6–12 months is recommended between CO_2 treatment and phenol–croton peel. This interval allows for reconstitution of the dermal matrix and vascular function, reducing the risk of irregular penetration or disorganized healing. The decision should be individualized, especially in areas where the laser was applied with multiple passes, at high density, or with residual signs of erythema or fibrosis.

6.2.7.2 Medium-Depth Chemical Peels

In the case of medium-depth chemical peels, such as 35% trichloroacetic acid (TCA), functional skin recovery is faster than with CO_2, but still significant. In general, a minimum interval of 3–6 months is recommended, especially if there is a history of post-inflammatory hyperpigmentation, prolonged desquamation, or repeated use of aggressive agents. The interval may be shortened in cases where the skin already appears intact, with adequate thickness and no inflammatory signs.

6.2.7.3 Less Aggressive Procedures

Procedures considered less invasive—such as superficial microneedling, non-ablative Nd:YAG laser, intense pulsed light (IPL), superficial peels, or non-fractional radiofrequency—require shorter intervals, generally between 4 and 8 weeks, provided that the barrier function has been restored and there are no signs of subclinical inflammation or residual hypersensitivity.

Even in cases of superficial procedures, sequential or cumulative performance of multiple treatments may lead to skin sensitization, cutaneous dysbiosis, and persistent low-grade inflammation, which hinder a controlled response to phenol and increase the risk of complications.

6.2.7.4 Assessment Criteria for Determining the Interval

The ideal interval should consider:

- Depth and type of previous procedure.
- Extent of the treated area.
- Observed scarring response.
- Presence of previous adverse effects (PIH, hyposensitivity, prolonged crusting).
- Functional status of the skin at the time of assessment, which may be inferred by: presence of residual erythema, desquamation, or abnormal sheen.

Instrumental tests (when available), such as corneometry, TEWL measurement, sebumetry, or high-frequency cutaneous ultrasound, assess dermal thickness and architectural recovery.

6.2.7.5 Safe Interval Between Phenol–Croton Peel Sessions

The interval between phenol–croton peel sessions should respect the principles of deep tissue regeneration, complete dermal remodeling, and functional recovery of the treated skin. Unlike superficial or medium-depth peels, phenol–croton acts on the mid or deep within the reticular dermis, inducing controlled necrosis, intense inflammation, and subsequent complex tissue regeneration.

This process involves not only epidermal re-epithelialization (usually completed within 10 days), but also collagen remodeling and reorganization of the extracellular matrix, which may extend over weeks to months depending on the depth reached, the area treated, the formula used, the patient's phototype, and the individual scarring response.

Minimum recommended interval:

- Between two full-face phenol-croton oil peels:
  - Minimum interval: 12 months.
  - In cases of severely aged skin, higher phototypes, or intense inflammatory response, the ideal interval may be 18–24 months.
  - This allows the collagen maturation phase and dermal remodeling to be completed before a new chemical insult.
- Between segmental sessions (periorbital, lips, forehead, malar region, etc.):
  - Minimum interval: 6 months, provided the area has fully healed and there are no sequelae or residual inflammation.
  - Repeating sessions before this interval increases the risk of disorganized dermal fibrosis, permanent dyschromia, dermal atrophy, or visible scarring.
- Between successive applications to different anatomical areas:

A sequential staging strategy may be adopted with minimum intervals of 6–8 weeks, provided that:

- The areas do not overlap.
- The patient tolerates the regeneration process well.
- There are no local or systemic adverse events.
- There is strict supervision and photographic documentation.

6.2.7.6 Factors That Prolong the Required Interval

- Higher phototypes (IV–VI).
- Presence of PIH or hypopigmentation following previous peel.
- Recent use of isotretinoin.

- Autoimmune diseases, chronic inflammatory conditions, or abnormal healing.
- History of recent surgery or laser in the same area.
- Previous complications, even if mild.

6.2.7.7 Physiological and Histological Considerations

The dermal remodeling process induced by phenol-croton oil involves destruction and subsequent reorganization of type I and III collagen, with influx of fibroblasts, release of growth factors, vascular reorganization, and activation of the dermal matrix. Histological studies show that collagen density continues to increase up to 6–9 months after the procedure, and that complete reorganization of the dermal matrix may take up to 12 months or more, depending on the area and the patient.

6.2.8 Importance of Prior Skin Conditioning

In the presence of any sign of functional skin alteration—such as compromised epidermal barrier, subclinical inflammation, cutaneous dysbiosis, or hyperreactivity—a prior skin conditioning protocol is recommended before performing the phenol-croton oil peel. The main objectives of this preparation are to restore the integrity of the epidermal barrier, reduce low-grade chronic inflammation, modulate the immune response to the caustic agent, and promote more uniform penetration of the chemical solution, ensuring safety and clinical predictability. The protocol should be individualized according to skin type and function, and may include the use of topical antioxidants, physiological moisturizers, ceramides, niacinamide, hyaluronic acid, and, in specific cases, retinoids or low-potency acids. Strict photoprotection is mandatory at all stages of preparation. In patients who have undergone previous aesthetic procedures, especially those with ablative or inflammatory potential, skin conditioning becomes even more relevant and should be maintained for at least 4 weeks prior to the peel, in order to ensure complete recovery of barrier function and optimize aesthetic and scarring outcomes.

The principles, objectives, and protocols of skin conditioning will be explored in greater depth in a dedicated chapter of this book.

6.3 Systemic, Laboratory, and Pharmacological Assessment

Given the toxic potential of phenol, which may affect the cardiovascular, hepatic, renal, neurological, and hematological systems, it is imperative that patient selection includes clinical criteria and biochemical objectives, focusing on the identification of risk factors for systemic toxicity, even if subclinical.

6.3.1 General Clinical Assessment

The general clinical assessment of the patient is essential for the safety of phenol-croton oil peel, considering the potential systemic impact of the substance and the prolonged recovery period. Decompensated chronic diseases, harmful habits, or silent pathophysiological alterations may compromise not only wound healing but also increase the risk of intra- and post-procedural clinical complications.

Medical history should specifically investigate cardiovascular, renal, hepatic, hematological, autoimmune, pulmonary, neurological, and psychiatric comorbidities, as well as the presence of drug allergies, recent surgical history, adverse events with anesthetics or volatile substances, and vasovagal reactions or syncope induced by aesthetic procedures. Assessment of nutritional status, lifestyle habits, smoking, physical activity level, and capacity to respond to inflammatory stress should also be documented.

Physical examination must be thorough and include measurement of blood pressure at rest and after standing, in order to assess hemodynamic stability and identify possible dysautonomia. Cardiac and pulmonary auscultation is essential for detecting arrhythmias, murmurs, crackles, or other signs indicating cardiovascular or respiratory compromise. The presence of edema, pallor, cutaneous lesions suggestive of peripheral vascular insufficiency, or cutaneous manifestations of liver disease should also be observed. Finally, assessment of the patient's mental state and anxiety level is indispensable, as emotional disturbances may negatively influence tolerance to the procedure and postoperative recovery (Table 6.4).

Table 6.4 Comorbidities and risks associated with phenol-croton oil peel and recommended management

Clinical condition	Main risk(s)	Recommended parameters/ management
Diabetes mellitus/ glycemic control	↑ infection and persistent inflammation; delayed healing; higher propensity to dyspigmentation; risk of superficial necrosis/thick crusts/ scars; endothelial dysfunction and impaired skin microcirculation	Assess HbA1c beforehand; target <7% prior to procedure. Postpone if fasting glucose >126 mg/dL or postprandial >180 mg/dL; optimize with attending physician
Asthma, COPD, chronic smoking or history of bronchospasm	Bronchospasm/bronchial hyperreactivity due to phenol vapors; respiratory exacerbations	Spirometry and/or pulmonology consultation. Plan intraoperative preventive measures (bronchodilators/prophylactic inhalation). Investigate and control wheezing, cough, nocturnal dyspnea, or recent inhaled corticosteroid use

(continued)

Table 6.4 (continued)

Clinical condition	Main risk(s)	Recommended parameters/ management
Active/unstable autoimmune diseases (lupus, dermatomyositis, vasculitis)	Risk of paradoxical eruptions; activation; delayed healing; cutaneous autoimmune complications	Individualized evaluation; prefer clinical stability; consider specialist consultation
Metabolic diseases (hypothyroidism, dyslipidemia, metabolic syndrome)	Interference in inflammatory process and dermal metabolism	Preoperative optimization; request laboratory tests as clinically indicated
Oncologic patients (remission/recent treatment)	Persistent immunosuppression; cumulative hepatotoxicity; tissue fragility	Evaluate with oncology; postpone until stability; attention to associated hepatopathy
Chronic use of immunosuppressants (corticosteroids, methotrexate, cyclosporine, biologics)	Impaired wound healing; risk of opportunistic infections	Review with attending specialist; may represent absolute contraindication
HIV/AIDS	↑ opportunistic infections; delayed healing; dysfunctional inflammatory response (dyspigmentation/scarring)	Proceed only with undetectable viral load and CD4 >500 cells/ mm^3
Chronic hepatitis B and C	Compromised hepatic metabolism of phenol (↑ toxicity); fibrosis/cirrhosis; hypoalbuminemia	Request complete liver profile (AST, ALT, GGT, bilirubin, albumin, PT/INR) and elastography when available. HBV: suppressed viral load under treatment. HCV: treatment with direct-acting antivirals completed and no inflammatory activity
Herpes simplex (HSV-1/ HSV-2)	Reactivation (especially perioral); risk of disseminated disease/extensive ulcerations with sequelae	Screen history of herpes. Prophylaxis with acyclovir/ valacyclovir initiated 1–2 days before and continued for 7–10 days after. Recent ophthalmic herpes: contraindication → ophthalmology consultation
Herpes zoster	Reactivation/complications in immunosuppressed patients	Exclude in cases of immunosuppression or recent infection; evaluate need for specialist consultation
Smoking	Persistent vasoconstriction; ↑ oxidative stress; ↓ collagen synthesis/angiogenesis; risk of hypertrophic scarring and dyspigmentation	Absolute abstinence for ≥4 weeks before and ≥4 weeks after the procedure
Alcohol (chronic use)	Impaired hepatic function and phenol metabolism; worsened immune response	Careful assessment of usage pattern; consider postponement/ optimization

(continued)

Table 6.4 (continued)

Clinical condition	Main risk(s)	Recommended parameters/ management
Recreational substances (cocaine, cannabis, ecstasy, unsupervised benzodiazepines)	Cardiovascular interference; hepatic metabolism; inflammatory response and pain perception; postoperative adherence	Targeted screening; complementary exams (extended liver function, toxicology panel) and psychiatric evaluation as indicated

Relevant clinical comorbidities for phenol-croton oil peel, associated risks, and recommended management. Careful patient selection is essential to reduce cardiovascular, infectious, metabolic, and scarring complications. Note. NSAIDs = non-steroidal anti-inflammatory drugs; COPD = chronic obstructive pulmonary disease; PT/INR = prothrombin time/international normalized ratio; HSV = herpes simplex virus. (Source: Table prepared by the author (Dr Carolina Marçon))

6.3.1.1 Glycemic Control and Diabetes Mellitus

Adequate glycemic control is essential for procedural success. Patients with diabetes mellitus, even in mild stages, present:

- Increased risk of infection and persistent inflammation.
- Delayed wound healing and greater propensity for dyspigmentation.
- Higher risk of superficial necrosis, thick crusts, and abnormal scarring.
- Alterations in endothelial function and cutaneous microcirculation.

Glycated hemoglobin (HbA1c) should be assessed in all patients with a history or suspicion of diabetes, with recommended levels <7% prior to clearance for the procedure. Fasting glucose >126 mg/dL or postprandial glucose >180 mg/dL should prompt postponement and medical management.

6.3.1.2 Respiratory Assessment: Pulmonary Risk and Asthma

Phenol, even when handled in controlled quantities, may release irritant vapors capable of triggering bronchospasm or bronchial reactivity, especially in patients with:

- History of bronchial asthma (current or past).
- Episodes of bronchospasm induced by NSAIDs, perfumes, or irritants.
- Chronic obstructive pulmonary disease (COPD) or chronic smoking.
- Severe anxiety associated with hyperventilation, which may precipitate respiratory crises.

In such cases, respiratory function assessment with spirometry and/or pulmonology consultation should be performed, in addition to planning intraoperative preventive measures (such as pre-procedure bronchodilators or prophylactic inhalation). The presence of wheezing, frequent cough, nocturnal dyspnea, or recent use of inhaled corticosteroids should be investigated and controlled beforehand.

6.3.1.3 Autoimmune, Metabolic, and Oncological Diseases

Phenol can induce an intense inflammatory response, the healing of which requires immunological competence, hormonal balance, and metabolic integrity. Therefore, patients with the following conditions require individualized assessment: Active or unstable autoimmune diseases (lupus, dermatomyositis, severe psoriasis, vasculitis): increased risk of paradoxical eruptions, delayed wound healing, and cutaneous autoimmune complications;

- Metabolic diseases (hypothyroidism, dyslipidemias, metabolic syndrome): interfere with the inflammatory process and dermal metabolism.
- Oncology patients in remission or recent treatment: risk of persistent immunosuppression, cumulative hepatic toxicity, and general tissue fragility.
- Chronic use of immunosuppressants (corticosteroids, methotrexate, ciclosporin, biologics): should be reviewed in conjunction with the attending specialist to weigh risks.

6.3.1.4 Chronic Infectious Diseases: HIV, Hepatitis, and Other Relevant Viral Conditions

Screening for chronic infectious diseases, such as HIV and hepatitis B and C, is an essential step in the pre-assessment for phenol-croton oil peeling. These conditions, even when controlled, can significantly impact the patient's immunocompetence, tissue healing, inflammatory response, and risk of postoperative infection.

HIV/AIDS

Patients living with HIV, even those on effective antiretroviral therapy, may present with residual immune alterations that can interfere with the response to tissue injury. This is particularly relevant in deep resurfacing procedures, such as phenol peeling, which induce extensive epidermal necrosis and acute dermal inflammation.

Associated risks include:

- Increased risk of cutaneous or systemic opportunistic infections during the re-epithelialization period.
- Delayed wound healing.
- Dysfunctional inflammatory response, predisposing to dyschromia and unaesthetic scarring.

The procedure should only be considered when:

- The viral load is undetectable.
- The CD4 lymphocyte count is above 500 cells/mm^3.
- There are no associated comorbidities, such as liver disease or coinfections.
- The patient demonstrates excellent adherence to treatment and regular medical follow-up.

In cases with CD4 counts between 350 and 500 cells/mm^3, the decision should be individualized, with input from an infectious disease specialist and strict postoperative monitoring. A CD4 count below 350 is a relative or absolute contraindication, depending on clinical stability.

Hepatitis B and C

Patients with chronic viral hepatitis may present with subclinical hepatic dysfunction, which directly affects phenol metabolism, whose main biotransformation pathway is hepatic (phase I—cytochrome P450 and phase II—conjugation with sulfate and glucuronide).

The systemic toxicity of phenol is increased in situations of:

- Reduced hepatic conjugation capacity.
- Presence of fibrosis or cirrhosis.
- Alterations in serum albumin (compromising phenol distribution and excretion).

In these cases, it is recommended to:

- Request a full hepatic profile (AST, ALT, GGT, bilirubins, albumin, PT/INR).
- Assess the degree of fibrosis (liver elastography, when available).
- Refer to a hepatologist in cases of laboratory abnormalities or a history of viral hepatitis.

Patients with chronic hepatitis B should have suppressed viral load through antiviral therapy, and those with hepatitis C should have completed treatment with direct-acting antivirals, with no evidence of hepatic inflammatory activity. Performing peeling in patients with compensated hepatic cirrhosis (Child-Pugh A) remains controversial and requires joint evaluation with a specialist.

Herpes Simplex and Herpes Zoster

Reactivation of herpes simplex virus (HSV-1 or HSV-2) is common after deep chemical peels, especially in the perioral region. Epidermal necrosis and intense dermal inflammation act as local triggers, potentially causing severe presentations such as disseminated herpes or extensive ulcerations, with risk of scarring sequelae.

Recommended measures:

- Prior screening for a history of labial, genital, or ocular herpes.
- Prophylactic use of acyclovir or valaciclovir initiated 1–2 days prior to the peel and maintained for 7–10 days afterward, even in patients without a positive history.
- Relative contraindication in cases of recent ophthalmic herpes, with recommendation for ophthalmological assessment.

Herpes zoster should be excluded in immunosuppressed patients, or those with a history of persistent neuralgia or recent infection.

6.3.1.5 Smoking, Alcohol, and Recreational Substances

Smoking is one of the most detrimental factors to tissue oxygenation and healing. Even with moderate exposure, it leads to:

- Persistent vasoconstriction.
- Increased free radicals and oxidative stress.
- Reduced collagen synthesis and angiogenesis.
- Higher risk of hypertrophic scarring and post-procedural hypo/hyperpigmentation.

Absolute abstinence is recommended for at least 4 weeks before and 4 weeks after the procedure.

Chronic alcohol use impairs liver function, interferes with phenol metabolism, and compromises immune response. It should be carefully assessed, especially in daily users or those with clinical signs of liver disease.

Recreational substances such as cocaine, cannabis, ecstasy, or unsupervised use of benzodiazepines may interfere with:

- Cardiovascular function.
- Hepatic drug metabolism.
- Inflammatory response and pain perception.
- Adherence to post-procedural care and general management.

Additional laboratory screening, such as extended liver function tests, toxicology panel, and psychiatric evaluation, may be indicated according to clinical suspicion (Fig. 6.7).

6.3.2 Cardiovascular Assessment

Cardiac toxicity of phenol is one of the most relevant and potentially serious aspects of the procedure. Phenol can cause alterations in cardiac electrical conduction, bradycardia, atrioventricular blocks, ventricular arrhythmias, and even cardiac arrest, especially in patients with cardiovascular predisposition, those taking medications affecting contractility, or with myocardial hypertrophy.

Patients with uncontrolled hypertension, arrhythmias, bundle branch blocks, history of myocardial infarction, heart failure, valvular disease, or known electrocardiographic abnormalities should be considered at increased risk. In such cases, the procedure should be contraindicated or postponed, depending on the severity and stability of the condition.

As a routine, baseline blood pressure should be measured on at least three separate occasions, including readings at rest and after mild stimulation, in order to detect labile or masked hypertension.

A 12-lead electrocardiogram should be requested for all patients considered for phenol-croton oil peel. The examination must include automatic calculation of the

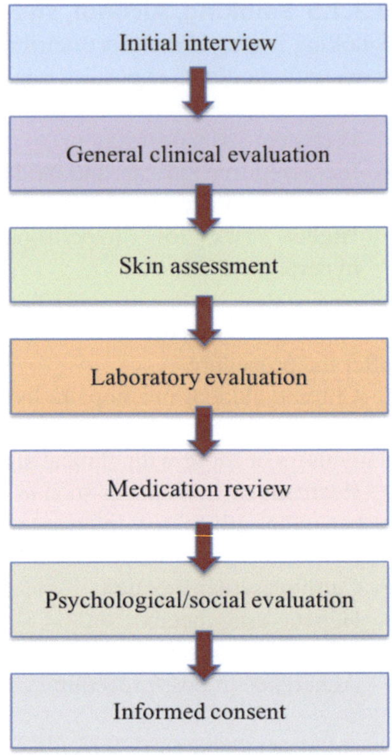

Fig. 6.7 Proposed flowchart for the clinical and laboratory assessment of candidates for phenol-croton oil peel, covering medical history, physical examination, complementary tests, medication review, psychological/social evaluation, and extended informed consent. (*Source: Figure prepared by the author (Dr Carolina Marçon)*)

corrected QT interval (QTc), preferably using Fridericia's formula ($QTc = QT/\sqrt[3]{RR}$), which is considered more accurate than Bazett's formula in cases of altered heart rate. The request should specify: "ECG with automatic QTc calculation, preferably using Fridericia's formula." QTc values above 475 ms represent an increased risk of severe ventricular arrhythmias and require specialist cardiology assessment before clearance for the procedure.

Although resting ECG is essential, it has low sensitivity for detecting intermittent arrhythmias or dysfunctions induced by physiological stress. For this reason, it is broadly recommended that a 24-h Holter monitor be performed for all patients considered for phenol-croton oil peel. Holter monitoring allows continuous assessment of cardiac rhythm, identifying extrasystoles, nocturnal bradycardia, pauses, and other changes that may go undetected in single-point examinations.

It is important to note, however, that Holter monitoring does not replace resting ECG for accurate QTc assessment, as physiological fluctuations over 24 h, artifacts, and heart rate variability hinder standardization and accuracy of measurement. Therefore, QTc measurement should be performed exclusively on resting ECG, under basal and controlled conditions.

Additionally, exercise testing (stress test) may be considered in the following situations:

- Sedentary individuals over 50 years of age.
- Patients with non-specific complaints, such as palpitations, exertional dyspnea, or atypical chest pain.
- Resting ECG or Holter monitoring with inconclusive findings.
- Personal or family history of coronary artery disease.

Exercise testing enables assessment of cardiovascular functional capacity, chronotropic and blood pressure response to physical stress, and detection of latent ischemia or exercise-induced arrhythmias, thereby increasing procedural safety.

Finally, any diagnostic uncertainty, conduction abnormality, presence of ectopy, history of heart disease, or borderline QTc should prompt referral to a cardiologist for comprehensive evaluation and formal clearance, ensuring an ethical, safe, and individualized approach for each patient (Fig. 6.8).

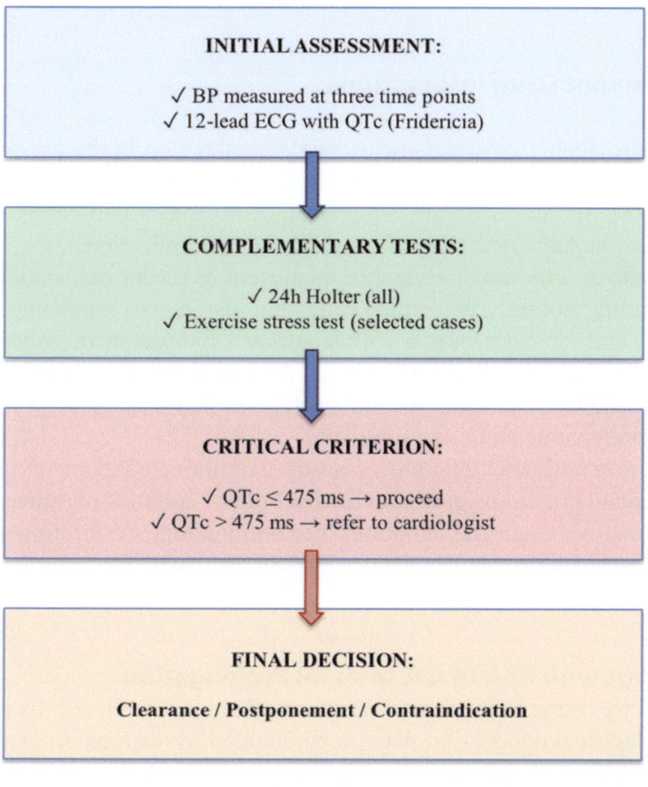

Fig. 6.8 Cardiovascular assessment and arrhythmia risk. Cardiovascular assessment flowchart for candidates for phenol-croton oil peel. Resting ECG with QTc calculation using Fridericia's formula is the central investigation, complemented by 24-h Holter monitoring and exercise testing in selected cases. QTc values above 475 ms indicate an increased risk of ventricular arrhythmias, requiring cardiology review prior to final decision. (*Source: Figure prepared by the author (Dr Carolina Marçon)*)

6.3.3 Hepatic and Renal Assessment

Phenol is primarily metabolized and eliminated via hepatic conjugation (glucuronidation and sulphation) followed by renal excretion. Alterations in these pathways increase the plasma half-life of phenol and its systemic bioavailability, raising the risk of acute toxicity.

Patients with a history of chronic liver disease (viral hepatitis, steatohepatitis, compensated cirrhosis), chronic alcohol use, cholestasis, unexplained jaundice, or abnormal transaminase levels should be screened with particular attention. Similarly, chronic kidney disease, mild to moderate nephropathies, persistent proteinuria, diabetes with microalbuminuria, or a history of acute renal failure should be considered risk factors.

Recommended laboratory investigations include:

- AST, ALT, GGT, bilirubin's, serum albumin.
- Urea, creatinine, estimated clearance (eGFR).
- Urinalysis + urine protein/creatinine ratio, when indicated.

6.3.4 Relevant Drug Interactions

Rigorous pharmacological assessment is an essential step in the pre-screening for phenol-croton oil peel, given the narrow therapeutic margin of phenol and its toxic potential across multiple systems. Drug interactions may significantly increase the risk of cardiac, hepatic, neurological, and scarring complications.

In this context, a thorough review of all current or recent medications is fundamental, including not only prescribed drugs but also herbal medicines, nutritional supplements, and topical products with significant transcutaneous absorption. The assessment should cover the potential for drug interactions, cumulative toxicity risks, and possible effects on wound healing, inflammatory response, and the patient's hemodynamic stability (Table 6.5).

Collaboration with attending physicians is essential in cases involving psychiatric, cardiological, immunosuppressive medications or complex regimens for chronic diseases. Decisions regarding temporary discontinuation, substitution or enhanced monitoring should be made on a multidisciplinary basis, focusing on safety and individualization of the therapeutic plan.

6.3.4.1 Drugs with Risk of QTc Interval Prolongation

Cardiac toxicity is one of the most feared complications of phenol. Its direct action on cardiac electrical conduction may be potentiated by various drugs that prolong the QTc interval, predisposing to malignant ventricular arrhythmias such as torsades de pointes. The main drugs with this effect include: antidepressants

Table 6.5 Relevant drug interactions in the context of phenol-croton oil peel

Class/examples	Risk/effect	Pre-procedure management
QTc-prolonging drugs: antidepressants (amitriptyline, citalopram, escitalopram), antipsychotics (haloperidol, ziprasidone), macrolides (azithromycin), fluoroquinolones (levofloxacin), azoles (fluconazole), antihistamines (astemizole, terfenadine), thiazide diuretics (HCTZ), antiarrhythmics (amiodarone), antiemetics (domperidone, ondansetron)	QTc prolongation; risk of ventricular arrhythmias (torsades de pointes)	Strict review; consider suspension or substitution when possible; check CredibleMeds® for risk classification (conditional/possible/known)
Sedation and analgesia: midazolam, propofol, ketamine, fentanyl	Potential QTc interference; cumulative risk in polypharmacy; cardiorespiratory depression	Prefer mild sedation; avoid polypharmacy; continuous cardiac rhythm monitoring; anesthesiologist present in high-risk cases
Beta-blockers (atenolol, propranolol)	Refractory bradycardia; masking of early signs of cardiovascular toxicity	Assess risk/benefit; consider adjustment/intraoperative monitoring
Calcium channel blockers (verapamil, diltiazem)	Hypotension; interference with chronotropic response	Evaluate adjustment and hemodynamic monitoring
Corticosteroids (systemic or potent topical)	Impaired healing and cutaneous immunosurveillance; ↓ collagen production; ↑ risk of infection	Minimize dose/duration when possible; evaluate real need
Anticoagulants/antiplatelets (warfarin, clopidogrel, rivaroxaban, ASA)	↑ risk of bleeding	Temporary suspension according to guidelines and prescribing physician evaluation; plan safe resumption
Oral isotretinoin (recent use)	Risk of abnormal scarring and post-inflammatory dyspigmentation	Recommend minimum interval of 6 months after last dose before deep peels
Hepatotoxic drugs (valproate, methotrexate, isoniazid, high-dose acetaminophen)	Hepatic overload; interference with phenol metabolism	Avoid when possible; monitor liver enzymes; evaluate alternatives
Systemic immunosuppressants (cyclosporine, methotrexate, biologics; corticosteroids in immunosuppressive doses)	↑ susceptibility to infections and delayed healing	Relative/absolute contraindication depending on case; multidisciplinary decision
Topical anesthetics and vasoconstrictors (lidocaine, prilocaine, topical adrenaline)	Potential myocardial toxicity and cumulative CNS effects	Avoid prior to procedure

(continued)

Table 6.5 (continued)

Class/examples	Risk/effect	Pre-procedure management
Herbal medicines/supplements (ginkgo biloba, vitamin E, omega-3, turmeric)	Antiplatelet/hemorrhagic effect; pharmacodynamic interaction	Suspend at least 10 days before
Photosensitizing antibiotics (e.g., doxycycline)	Cutaneous photosensitivity	Suspend at least 10 days before

Main drug interactions in the context of phenol-croton oil peel, including agents associated with QTc prolongation, bleeding risk, hepatotoxicity, and impaired wound healing. Systematic screening using specialized databases is mandatory. *Note. QTc = corrected QT interval; TdP = torsades de pointes; CNS = central nervous system; AAS = acetylsalicylic acid. For QTc risk screening, CredibleMeds®, Lexicomp® or Drugs.com Interactions Checker are recommended. (Source: Table prepared by the author (Dr Carolina Marçon))*

(amitriptyline, citalopram, escitalopram), antipsychotics (haloperidol, ziprasidone), macrolides (azithromycin), fluoroquinolones (levofloxacin), azole antifungals (fluconazole), antihistamines (astemizole, terfenadine), thiazide diuretics (such as hydrochlorothiazide), antiarrhythmics (amiodarone), and antiemetics (domperidone, ondansetron). Rigorous review of these medications should be performed prior to the procedure, and, whenever possible, temporary discontinuation or substitution should be considered. The use of the CredibleMeds® application is highly recommended as a screening tool, as it provides risk classification (conditional, possible, or known) for QT prolongation and risk of TdP.

6.3.4.2 Precautions with Sedation and QTc Prolongation

Drugs used for sedation and analgesia, such as midazolam, propofol, ketamine, and fentanyl, may also affect the QTc interval, especially when used concomitantly with other high-risk medications. In patients with borderline QTc or predisposing factors (advanced age, bradycardia, electrolyte disturbances), sedative polypharmacy should be avoided, and preference given to light sedation strategies, continuous cardiac rhythm monitoring, and individualized anesthetic supervision. Prior cardiological assessment with ECG and corrected QTc should be performed in all cases, and values above 475 ms require specialist investigation and may constitute a temporary contraindication.

6.3.4.3 Other Relevant Drug Interactions

- Beta-blockers (e.g., atenolol, propranolol): increase the risk of refractory bradycardia. Additionally, β-adrenergic blockade may mask early signs of phenol-induced cardiovascular toxicity, making it more difficult to identify episodes of hypotension or arrhythmias.
- Calcium channel blockers (verapamil, diltiazem): potentiate hypotensive episodes and may interfere with the chronotropic response during the procedure.
- Tricyclic antidepressants (amitriptyline) and selective serotonin reuptake inhibitors (citalopram, escitalopram): associated with QTc interval prolongation, increasing the risk of severe ventricular arrhythmias such as torsades de pointes, especially when combined with other drugs with the same effect.

- Systemic or potent topical corticosteroids: impair wound healing, immune response, and cutaneous immunosurveillance, increasing the risk of infection or abnormal scar formation.
- Anticoagulants and antiplatelet agents (e.g., warfarin, clopidogrel, rivaroxaban, acetylsalicylic acid): increase the risk of bleeding, including spontaneous bleeding, especially in delicate areas such as the eyelids. They should be temporarily discontinued according to risk-benefit assessment and clinical guidelines, in conjunction with the prescribing physician.
- Oral isotretinoin: recent use may interfere with the healing process, increasing the risk of hypertrophic or atrophic scarring, or post-inflammatory dyschromia. Although there is some controversy, a minimum interval of 6 months after the last dose is recommended before considering deep peeling, particularly in areas of thin skin or those prone to scar contracture.
- Hepatotoxic agents (valproate, methotrexate, isoniazid, high-dose paracetamol): increase the risk of hepatic overload and interfere with phenol metabolism, which already requires full hepatic capacity for proper elimination.
- Systemic immunosuppressants (e.g., ciclosporin, methotrexate, biologics, corticosteroids at immunosuppressive doses): represent a relative or absolute contraindication, as they impair healing and increase susceptibility to opportunistic infections.
- Topical anesthetics and vasoconstrictors (lidocaine, prilocaine, topical adrenaline): should be avoided prior to the procedure. Their combination with phenol may cause myocardial toxicity and cumulative effects on the central nervous system.

In view of these potential interactions, it is recommended that medication screening be active, systematic, and personalized, and that it decisively inform clinical decision-making. The presence of high-risk drugs may require prior therapeutic adjustments, multidisciplinary planning, or, in cases of high systemic risk, contraindicate the procedure.

6.3.4.4 Recommended Actions

Discontinuation should be advised, at least 10 days before the procedure, of:

- Non-steroidal anti-inflammatory drugs (NSAIDs).
- Photosensitizing antibiotics (e.g., doxycycline).
- Supplements containing ginkgo biloba, vitamin E, omega-3, turmeric, and natural anticoagulants.
- Irritant topical products not prescribed as part of the preparation (acids, retinoids, home-use peels).

All patients should have their medication list cross-checked with specialized databases (such as CredibleMeds®, Lexicomp®, or Drugs.com Interactions Checker), and the decision to continue or discontinue medications should be individualized. The opinion of the prescribing physician should be considered before any therapeutic modification.

6.3.5 Nutritional and Hydration Assessment

Adequate nutrition and systemic hydration are fundamental pillars for wound healing and for the success of phenol-croton oil peeling. States' deficiencies severely compromise the inflammatory response, dermal remodeling, and the skin's regenerative capacity, in addition to increasing the risk of infectious complications, dyschromia, atrophic or hypertrophic scarring, and delayed re-epithelialization.

6.3.5.1 Clinical Relevance

Phenol induces profound protein denaturation and requires tissue repair with high metabolic demand. This reparative response depends directly on:

- The integrity of the immune system.
- Adequate synthesis of collagen and extracellular matrix.
- Redox balance (antioxidant system).
- Sufficient protein, vitamins, and minerals.

Patients with mild to moderate malnutrition—often subclinical—exhibit reduced protein synthesis, altered inflammatory and immune responses, increased capillary fragility, and delayed wound healing. Deficiencies in micronutrients such as zinc, iron, selenium, vitamins A, C, D, E, and B complex have a direct impact on angiogenesis, re-epithelialization, immunocompetence, and dermal remodeling.

6.3.5.2 Clinical Signs of Nutritional Risk

During history taking and physical examination, signs suggestive of nutritional risk or dehydration should be investigated, such as:

- Recent weight loss (>5% in 3 months).
- Reduced muscle mass (temporal, scapular, thighs).
- Dry, scaly, or atrophic skin.
- Angular cheilitis, glossitis, diffuse hair loss.
- Fatigue, apathy, or persistent non-specific complaints.
- Previous hypoalbuminemia or episodes of slow wound healing.

6.3.5.3 Objective Nutritional Screening

Screening can be performed using simple, validated tools such as:

- Mini Nutritional Assessment (MNA).
- Subjective Global Assessment (SGA).
- MUST (Malnutrition Universal Screening Tool).

These instruments help identify patients at nutritional risk who should be referred for formal nutritional assessment prior to the procedure.

6.3.5.4 Recommended Laboratory Tests

Laboratory investigations may be guided by clinical suspicion and include:

- Full blood count: to detect anemia, leucopenia, or lymphopenia.
- Serum albumin and prealbumin: indirect markers of protein malnutrition.
- Ferritin, serum iron, and transferrin: assessment of iron metabolism.
- Plasma zinc and selenium: essential cofactors in tissue regeneration.
- 25-OH vitamin D: crucial for immunoregulation and cell proliferation
- Vitamin B12 and folate: associated with DNA and epithelial integrity.
- Fasting blood glucose and HbA1c: important for assessing wound healing response.
- Creatinine and urea: to assess renal function and hydration.
- Sodium and potassium: electrolyte disturbances that affect cellular homeostasis.

6.3.5.5 Hydration Status

Systemic hydration directly influences skin turgor, diffusion of substances within tissue, and inflammatory homeostasis. Patients with inadequate hydration may present with:

- Increased sensitivity to the caustic agent.
- Worsening of the inflammatory process.
- Impaired wound healing.
- Greater risk of post-peel complications.

6.3.5.6 Clinical Signs of Dehydration

- Reduced skin turgor.
- Dry mucous membranes.
- Mild orthostatic hypotension.
- Concentrated or scant urine.

6.3.5.7 Additional Assessment

- Plasma osmolality.
- Urine specific gravity.
- Elevated BUN/creatinine.

6.3.5.8 Recommended Management

- In patients with nutritional risk, malnutrition, or inadequate hydration, the procedure should be postponed until clinical optimization is achieved.
- Targeted supplementation with antioxidants, amino acids, vitamins, and minerals may be instituted, ideally under the guidance of a nutritionist or attending physician.
- Adequate fluid intake is recommended in the weeks preceding the procedure, based on individual parameters (weight, renal function, climate).

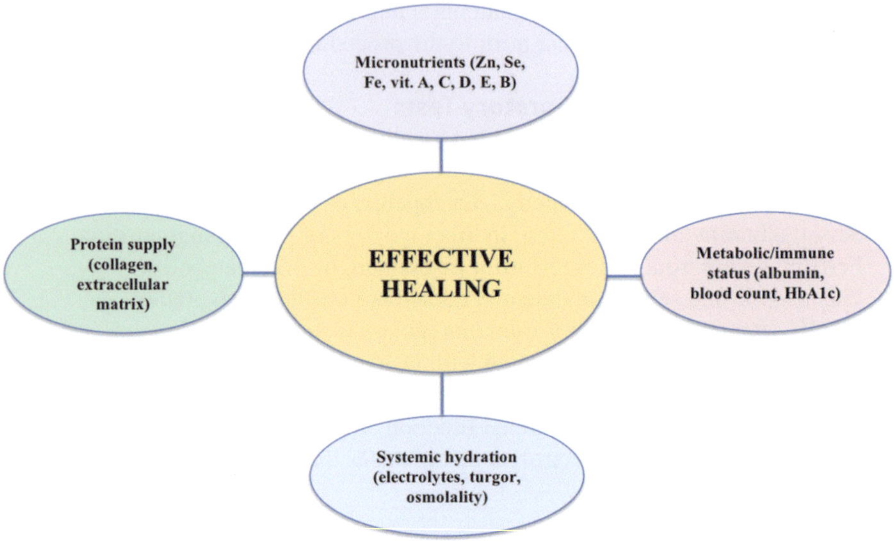

Fig. 6.9 Nutritional and hydration assessment. Proposed flowchart for the clinical and laboratory assessment of candidates for phenol-croton oil peel, encompassing medical history, physical examination, complementary tests, medication review, psychological/social evaluation, and extended informed consent. (*Source: Figure prepared by the author (Dr Carolina Marçon)*)

Nutritional assessment should be an integral part of the screening protocol for phenol-croton oil peel, especially in elderly patients, those with a history of weight loss, chronic diseases, prolonged use of medication, or restrictive diets. Prior attention to nutritional and hydration status is crucial for the safety, efficacy, and longevity of clinical outcomes (Fig. 6.9).

6.4 Psychological, Behavioral, and Social Assessment

Full adherence to preparation, social withdrawal, and post-procedure care is essential for the therapeutic success of phenol-croton oil peel. This is a demanding procedure, both clinically and emotionally, requiring a cooperative, emotionally stable patient who is aware of the initial phase of intense edema, prolonged erythema, pain, and temporary impairment of self-image.

The psychological profile of the candidate should be carefully evaluated, particularly regarding the presence of body dysmorphic disorders, severe depression, anxiety disorders, history of treatment abandonment, or low tolerance to discomfort. Such conditions may negatively impact the patient's experience, adequate recovery, and final perception of results.

It should be emphasized that unrealistic expectations and body image disorders must be considered exclusion criteria. Deep peels should not be indicated for patients seeking rapid, miraculous transformation or those with chronic body dissatisfaction. In these cases, the risk of frustration, litigation, or disproportionate emotional distress outweighs the potential clinical benefits of the intervention.

The absence of a home support network in the first 3–5 days postoperatively represents an additional risk, as the patient may require assistance with personal hygiene, nutrition, medication administration, and emotional support. It is strongly recommended that the patient has adequate home support and is prepared for complete withdrawal from usual activities for up to 14 days, considering the re-epithelialization period and possible complications. It should also be clarified that residual erythema may persist for several weeks or months after initial recovery, requiring emotional stability and a clear understanding of the healing process.

During the clinical interview, it is recommended to include:

- Assessment of expectations regarding outcomes and risks.
- Clear and realistic discussion of recovery time and possible complications (such as milia, dyschromia, scarring, ectropion, herpes activation, among others).
- Evaluation of commitment to pre-procedure preparation (including work and social withdrawal), post-procedure care, and follow-up appointments.

The patient should demonstrate:

- Emotional tolerance for the recovery process, which may be prolonged and temporarily impact body image.
- Realistic expectations regarding the effectiveness and limitations of the treatment.
- Commitment to prophylactic measures, strict photoprotection, and self-care regimen.
- Presence of a home support network in the initial days.

In cases of doubt regarding emotional stability, relevant psychiatric history, or difficulty understanding the therapeutic plan, a specialized psychological or psychiatric assessment is recommended before proceeding with the intervention.

6.5 Clinical and Laboratory Screening for Phenol-Croton Oil Peel: Practical Summary (Table 6.6)

Table 6.6 Practical clinical and laboratory screening by domain (operational summary)

Domain/system	Essential tests/ measurements	Key parameters/thresholds (where applicable)	Recommended action
Metabolic/ endocrine	Fasting blood glucose; HbA1c; lipid profile	Target HbA1c <7% prior to procedure. Postpone if fasting glucose >126 mg/dL or postprandial >180 mg/dL	Optimize glycemic control; endocrinology referral if required
Hepatic	AST, ALT, GGT, bilirubin's, albumin, PT/INR	Hepatic dysfunction, fibrosis/cirrhosis, and hypoalbuminemia increase the risk of phenol toxicity	Hepatology referral if abnormalities detected; HBV with suppressed viral load; HCV post-DAA without inflammatory activity

(continued)

Table 6.6 (continued)

Domain/system	Essential tests/ measurements	Key parameters/thresholds (where applicable)	Recommended action
Renal	Urea, creatinine, eGFR; urinalysis ± protein/ creatinine ratio	Proteinuria/ microalbuminuria and reduced eGFR indicate increased risk	Optimize renal function and hydration; consider contraindication or postpone until stabilized
Hematological/ immune	Full blood count; ferritin/B12/folate; CRP/ESR; serology (HIV, hepatitis, syphilis as indicated); coagulation profile	HIV: proceed only if undetectable viral load and CD4 >500; 350–500 = individualized decision; <350 = relative/ absolute contraindication depending on clinical context	Adjust management and involve infectious diseases/hepatology; plan HSV prophylaxis if indicated
Cardiovascular	BP at 3 time points (rest/stimulus/ standing); 12-lead ECG with QTc (Fridericia); 24-h Holter; exercise test (as per risk)	QTc > 475 ms = increased risk of ventricular arrhythmias; labile/masked hypertension	Refer to cardiologist in borderline/ abnormal cases; consider postponement/ contraindication/ optimization
Respiratory	Baseline and mild stimulus oxygen saturation (oximetry); spirometry in asthma/ bronchitis/COPD; respiratory specialist opinion	Bronchial reactivity/ bronchospasm increases risk	Prophylaxis with bronchodilators/ inhalation; disease control prior to procedure
Nutritional/ hydration	Albumin; electrolytes (Na, K, Mg); zinc and selenium (if available); BMI/body composition; clinical hydration assessment; plasma osmolality, urine specific gravity, urea/creatinine ratio (if necessary)	Weight loss >5% in 3 months; hypoalbuminemia; clinical signs of dehydration	Postpone until optimized; specific nutritional support; ensure adequate hydration in the weeks prior
Drug interactions	Systematic check (CredibleMeds®, Lexicomp®, Drugs.com); review NSAIDs, photosensitizing antibiotics, natural anticoagulants, etc.	Cumulative risk (e.g., QTc, bleeding, hepatotoxicity)	Discontinue ≥10 days prior if indicated; substitute/adjust; multidisciplinary decision

(continued)

Table 6.6 (continued)

Domain/system	Essential tests/ measurements	Key parameters/thresholds (where applicable)	Recommended action
Others (as suspected)	TSH/free T4; chest X-ray; psychiatric assessment; skin biopsy	–	Investigate and manage according to clinical findings

Practical clinical and laboratory screening by domain, summarizing essential tests and parameters for pre-assessment prior to phenol-croton oil peel. The standardized protocol assists in the standardization of the safety and efficacy of the procedure. *Note. Fridericia = preferred formula for QT correction ($QTc = QT/\sqrt[3]{RR}$). eGFR = estimated glomerular filtration rate; Ur = urea; Cr = creatinine; BP = blood pressure; COPD = chronic obstructive pulmonary disease. (Source: Table prepared by the author (Dr Carolina Marçon))*

6.5.1 Metabolic and Endocrine Assessment

- Fasting blood glucose.
- Glycated hemoglobin (HbA1c).

  Lipid profile (total cholesterol, HDL, LDL, triglycerides).

6.5.2 Hepatic and Renal Assessment

- ALT, AST, GGT, alkaline phosphatase.
- Total and fractionated bilirubin.
- Urea and creatinine.
- Albumin and total proteins.

6.5.3 Hematological and Immunological Assessment

- Full blood count.
- Ferritin, vitamin B12, folic acid.
- CRP or ESR (in cases of suspected inflammation).
- Serology (HIV, hepatitis, syphilis, if indicated).
- Coagulation profile (PT, aPTT, INR).

6.5.4 Cardiovascular Assessment

- Blood pressure measured on three separate occasions.
- ECG with QTc calculation (preferably using the Fridericia formula).
- 24-h Holter monitoring (for all patients).
- Exercise stress test (as indicated by risk).
- Cardiology assessment (if abnormalities or uncertainty).

6.5.5 Respiratory Assessment

- Spirometry in cases of asthma, bronchitis or COPD.
- Baseline and post-exertion oxygen saturation (oximetry).

6.5.6 Nutritional Assessment and Tissue Support

- Albumin.
- Electrolytes (sodium, potassium, magnesium).
- Zinc, selenium (if available).
- BMI and body composition assessment.
- Hydration status (clinical + laboratory tests).

6.5.7 Assessment of Drug Interactions

- QTc prolongation check (via CredibleMeds®).
- Discontinuation of NSAIDs, natural anticoagulants, photosensitizing antibiotics, etc.

6.5.8 Others (Specific Cases)

- Chest X-ray, spirometry, psychiatric assessment.
- C-reactive protein (CRP) and ESR, for screening of subclinical inflammation.
- Thyroid function tests (TSH, free T4), in cases with compatible symptoms.
- Skin biopsy in cases of diagnostic uncertainty in dermatology.

6.5.8.1 Clinical and Laboratory Assessment Flow

Initial interview: identification of motivations, clinical history, medication use, availability of time for recovery and home support.

Skin assessment: phototype, skin quality, presence of lesions, scars, laxity and tissue thickness.

Systemic and laboratory assessment: ECG with QTc, liver and renal function, electrolytes, full blood count, blood glucose, etc. (as above).

Medication review: identify relevant interactions and decide on discontinuation or substitution.

Psychological and behavioral assessment: identify emotional risk factors, adherence, and expectations.

Extended informed consent: clarify all potential risks, recovery time, possible complications, and contingency plan.

6.6 Final Considerations

Deep peels, such as phenol–croton oil peels, are highly effective therapeutic interventions for rejuvenation and the treatment of complex skin conditions. However, their potential for systemic impact requires that they be approached with seriousness, responsibility, and scientific rigor. Unlike purely cosmetic procedures, phenol–croton oil peels carry significant clinical risks and demand technical expertise from the practitioner, as well as informed engagement from the patient.

Appropriate candidate selection is a critical and multifactorial step. It involves not only the analysis of the skin and aesthetic indication, but also a comprehensive assessment of the overall clinical, functional, psychological, pharmacological, and laboratory status. Early identification of risk factors—cardiovascular, hepatic, infectious, psychiatric, nutritional, or social—is essential to prevent complications and ensure predictable and safe outcomes (Fig. 6.10).

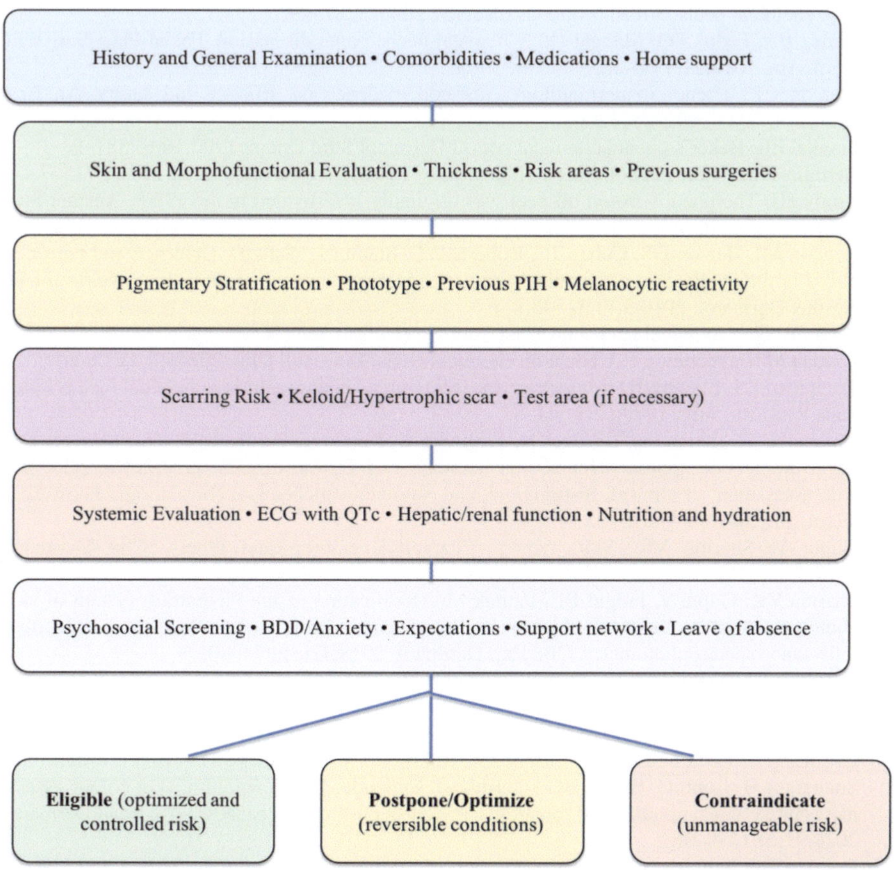

Fig. 6.10 Algorithm for selecting candidates for phenol–croton oil peel, encompassing general clinical assessment, pigment stratification, scarring risk analysis, review of systemic comorbidities, and psychosocial screening. The flowchart provides a practical synthesis of the criteria guiding indication, postponement for prior optimization, or formal contraindication of the procedure. (*Source: Figure prepared by the author (Dr Carolina Marçon)*)

Therapeutic success with phenol–croton oil peel is directly related to the accuracy of screening and specialized medical management. It is through this structured and rigorous process that superior clinical outcomes can be achieved with minimized risk. Thus, it is emphasized that deep peels should be performed exclusively by qualified physicians, in a controlled environment, with well-defined protocols and strict monitoring.

Excellence of outcome depends not only on the technique applied, but on the sum of all preceding precautions.

Sources

1. Wambier CG, Lee KC, Soon SL, Sterling JB, Rullan PP, Landau M, Brody HJ, International Peeling Society. Advanced chemical peels: phenol-croton oil peel. J Am Acad Dermatol. 2019;81(2):327–36.
2. Bensimon RH. Phenol-croton oil peels. In: Obagi S, editor. Procedures in cosmetic dermatology: chemical peels. 3rd ed. London: Elsevier; 2020. p. 81–99.
3. Cortez EA, Fedok FG, Mangat DS. Chemical peels: panel discussion. Facial Plast Surg Clin North Am. 2014;22(1):1–23.
4. Marçon CR. Phenol in dermatology: updated evidence on efficacy and safety. An Bras Dermatol. 2025;100(5):501200.
5. Frankel EB. Baker's phenol chemical peel. J Dermatol Surg Oncol. 1990;16(6):581–2.
6. Bertolini TM. Is the phenol-croton oil peel safe? Plast Reconstr Surg. 2002;110(2):715–7.
7. Brody HJ. The phenol-croton oil peel was originally investigated in the 1980s. Aesthet Surg J. 2009;29(5):446.
8. Rendon MI, Berson DS, Cohen JL, Roberts WE, Starker I, Wang B. Evidence and considerations in the application of chemical peels in skin disorders and aesthetic resurfacing. J Clin Aesthet Dermatol. 2010;3(7):32–43.
9. Peters W. The chemical peel. Ann Plast Surg. 1991;26(6):564–71.
10. Landau M, Bageorgeou F. Update on chemical peels. Dermatol Clin. 2024;42(1):13–20.
11. Truppman ES, Ellenby JD. Major electrocardiographic changes during chemical face peeling. Plast Reconstr Surg. 1979;63(1):44–8.
12. Kaminaka C, Yamamoto Y, Yonei N, Kishioka A, Kondo T, Furukawa F. Phenol peels as a novel therapeutic approach for actinic keratosis and Bowen disease: prospective pilot trial with assessment of clinical, histological, and immunohistochemical correlations. J Am Acad Dermatol. 2009;60(4):615–25.
13. Gupta V, Sharma VK. Skin typing: Fitzpatrick grading and others. Clin Dermatol. 2019;37(5):430–6.
14. Sharma VK, Gupta V, Jangid BL, Pathak M. Modification of the Fitzpatrick system of skin phototype classification for the Indian population, and its correlation with narrowband diffuse reflectance spectrophotometry. Clin Exp Dermatol. 2018;43(3):274–80.
15. Coleman W, Mariwalla K, Grimes P. Updating the Fitzpatrick classification: the skin colour and ethnicity scale. Dermatol Surg. 2023;49(8):725–31.
16. Harvey VM, Alexis A, Okeke CAV, McKinley-Grant L, Taylor SC, Desai SR, Jaleel T, Heath CR, Kang S, Vashi N, Lester J, Vasquez R, Rodrigues M, Elbuluk N, Hamzavi I, Kwatra SG, Sundaram H, Cobb C, Brown SG III, Kohli I, Callender VD. Integrating skin colour assessments into clinical practice and research: a review of current approaches. J Am Acad Dermatol. 2024;91(6):1189–98.
17. Roberts WE. Skin type classification systems old and new. Dermatol Clin. 2009;27(4):529–33.
18. Reserva J, Champlain A, Soon SL, Tung R. Chemical peels: indications and special considerations for the male patient. Dermatol Surg. 2017;43(Suppl 2):S163–73.

19. Seneschal J, Boniface K, Ezzedine K, Taieb A. Accelerating bleaching in vitiligo: balancing benefits versus risks. Exp Dermatol. 2014;23(12):879–80.
20. El-Mofty M, Mostafa WZ, Esmat S, Zayed A, Mashaly H, Hussien MF, Ismail SI. Site-oriented depigmentation in vitiligo patients using Q-switched Nd:YAG laser (1,064/532 nm), cryotherapy and chemical peels: a comparative study. Dermatol Ther. 2019;32(5):e13052.
21. de Mendonça MCC, Segheto NN, Aarestrup FM, Aarestrup BJV. Punctuated 88% phenol peeling for the treatment of facial photoaging: a clinical and histopathological study. Dermatol Surg. 2018;44(2):241–7.
22. Kligman AM, Zheng P, Lavker RM. The anatomy and pathogenesis of wrinkles. Br J Dermatol. 1985;113(1):37–42.
23. Sun HF, Lu HS, Sun LQ, Ping WD, Mao DS, Li D. Chemical peeling with a modified phenol formula for the treatment of facial freckles on Asian skin. Aesthet Plast Surg. 2018;42(2):546–52.
24. Larson DL. Phenol-croton oil peel: an update. Aesthet Surg J. 2005;25(2):197–200.
25. Platsidaki E, Stravodimou A, Kouris A, Markantoni V, Kontochristopoulos G. Efficacy and safety of phenol and trichloroacetic acid combination peel for the management of dark circles. Actas Dermosifiliogr. 2022;113(10):988–90.
26. Paiva ML, Justo AS, Lemes BM, Capote ACMO, de Castro Maymone MB, Lipinski LC, Rullan PP, Beltrame FL, Miot HA, Wambier CG. Skin of colour repigmentation after phenol-croton oil chemical peel. J Am Acad Dermatol. 2023;89(5):1068–70.
27. Rullan P, Karam AM. Chemical peels for darker skin types. Facial Plast Surg Clin North Am. 2010;18(1):111–31.
28. Gill JF, Yu SS, Neuhaus IM. Tobacco smoking and dermatologic surgery. J Am Acad Dermatol. 2013;68(1):167–72.
29. Stechmiller JK. Understanding the role of nutrition and wound healing. Nutr Clin Pract. 2010;25(1):61–8.
30. Munoz N, Litchford M, Cereda E. Nutrition and wound care. Phys Med Rehabil Clin N Am. 2022;33(4):811–22.
31. Penny H, Flores R, Pennington E, Pedersen A, Tran S. The role of macronutrients and micronutrients in wound healing: a narrative review. J Wound Care. 2022;31(Suppl5):S14–22.
32. Landau M, Tosti A, Kroumpouzos G, Eims E, Goldust M. Frontal fibrosing alopecia—a new absolute contraindication for deep chemical peels. Clin Dermatol. 2024;42(6):696–700.
33. Gonser P, Kaestner S, Jaminet P, Kaye K. Histological case-control study of peeling-induced skin changes by different peeling agents in surgically subcutaneous undermined skin flaps in facelift patients. J Plast Reconstr Aesthet Surg. 2017;70(11):1660–5.
34. Yan C, Wen R, Chen N, Fan Y, Li J, Peng Y, Li X, Xu X, Jia C, Wang Y. Psychological disorders are a non-negligible factor in medical aesthetic disputes. Aesthet Plast Surg. 2026;50(1):435–46.
35. Rosenbaum C, Whitworth M. Optimizing wound healing and cosmesis of surgical closures on rhinophymas skin. JAAD Case Rep. 2024;46:18–22.
36. Paichitrojjana A, Paichitrojjana A. Oral isotretinoin and its uses in dermatology: a review. Drug Des Devel Ther. 2023;17:2573–91.
37. Mysore V, Omprakash HM, Khatri GN. Isotretinoin and dermatosurgical procedures. Indian J Dermatol Venereol Leprol. 2019;85(1):18–23.
38. Perkins SW, Sklarew EC. Prevention of facial herpetic infections after chemical peel and dermabrasion: new treatment strategies in the prophylaxis of patients undergoing procedures of the perioral area. Plast Reconstr Surg. 1996;98(3):427–33.
39. Klein DR, Little JH. Laryngeal edema as a complication of chemical peel. Plast Reconstr Surg. 1983;71(3):419–20.
40. Piotrowski JK. Evaluation of exposure to phenol: absorption of phenol vapour in the lungs and through the skin and excretion of phenol in urine. Br J Ind Med. 1971;28(2):172–8.
41. Gross BG. Cardiac arrhythmias during phenol face peeling. Plast Reconstr Surg. 1984;73:590–4.
42. Wexler MR, Halon DA, Teitelbaum A, Tadjer G, Peled IJ. The prevention of cardiac arrhythmias produced in an animal model by the topical application of a phenol preparation in common use for face peeling. Plast Reconstr Surg. 1984;73:595–8.

43. Gorczyca R, Filip R, Walczak E. Psychological aspects of pain. Ann Agric Environ Med. 2013;Suppl 1:23–7.
44. Brown JJ, Ollier WE, Thomson W, Bayat A. Positive association of HLA-DRB1*15 with keloid disease in Caucasians. Int J Immunogenet. 2008;35(4–5):303–7.
45. Boyd AS, Neldner KH. The isomorphic response of Koebner. Int J Dermatol. 1990;29(6): 401–10.
46. Karampinis E, Georgopoulou KE, Goudouras G, Lianou V, Kampra E, Roussaki Schulze AV, Zafiriou E. Laser-induced Koebner-related skin reactions: a clinical overview. Medicina (Kaunas). 2024;60(7):1177.
47. Haen P, Laversanne S, Graillon N, Foletti JM. Facial necrotizing fasciitis following rhytidectomy. Br J Oral Maxillofac Surg. 2019;57(7):685–7.
48. Nikalji N, Godse K, Sakhiya J, Patil S, Nadkarni N. Complications of medium depth and deep chemical peels. J Cutan Aesthet Surg. 2012;5(4):254–60.
49. Wambier CG, Wambier SPF, Pilatti LEP, Grabicoski JA, Wambier LF, Schmidt JB. Prolongation of rate-corrected QT interval during phenol-croton oil peels. J Am Acad Dermatol. 2018;78(4):810–2.
50. Leal-Silva H. Predicting the risk of postinflammatory hyperpigmentation: the palmar creases pigmentation scale. J Cosmet Dermatol. 2021;20(4):1263–70.

7 Histology

7.1 Introduction

A detailed histological understanding of the effects of phenol-croton oil peel is essential to provide scientific support for its indications and outcomes, enabling an objective comprehension of the biological mechanisms of skin regeneration and remodeling triggered by this procedure. Through a controlled and deep chemical injury, phenol-croton oil peel induces necrosis of the epidermis and upper dermal layers, resulting in intense tissue regeneration characterized by reorganization of collagen and elastic fibers, increased dermal mucin, neovascularization, apoptosis of damaged cells, fibroblast activation, and, as more recently discovered, release of neutrophil extracellular traps (NETs) and activation of epigenetic pathways such as sirtuins.

Over the past 50 years, numerous histological, clinical, and immunohistochemical studies have been conducted in humans and animal models to assess the effects of phenol and its combinations, particularly with croton oil. The techniques employed have ranged from serial biopsies at different time points after the peel to analysis by light microscopy, electron microscopy and immunohistochemical methods using specific markers such as PCNA, p53, cyclin A, TUNEL, among others. The following section presents a critical and integrated analysis of the main histological studies available on phenol peeling, as well as comparisons with other agents such as trichloroacetic acid (TCA) and glycolic acid.

C. Marçon, C. Wambier, *Phenol-Croton Oil Peel*,
https://doi.org/10.1007/978-3-032-25993-6_7

7.2 Fundamental Concepts of Tissue Remodeling

Cutaneous regeneration following deep chemical peels involves epidermal re-epithelialization through proliferation of viable keratinocytes remaining in the pilosebaceous units and eccrine ducts, followed by intense dermal remodeling. This remodeling includes degradation of aged collagen fibers (mainly fragmented type I collagen), deposition of new type I and III collagen, reorganization of elastic fibers, and increased content of glycosaminoglycans and acidic mucopolysaccharides (mucin). In addition, there is stimulation of angiogenesis and sustained fibroblast activation. More recently, mechanisms such as NETs release, activation of protein kinases (PKC), TGF-β production, and epigenetic activation of sirtuins (SIRT-6 and SIRT-7) have been described as part of the complex rejuvenation process promoted by phenol-croton oil peel (Fig. 7.1).

The repair time and histological changes evolve over time, and studies show marked differences between the initial periods (days to weeks) and late effects (months). The main studies will be presented and analyzed in depth below (Fig. 7.2).

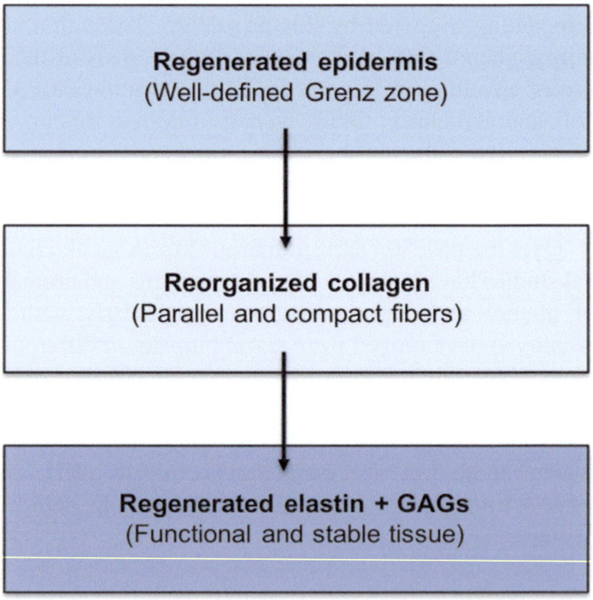

Fig. 7.1 Dermal remodeling after phenol–croton peel. Schematic representation of epidermal regeneration and dermal remodeling induced by phenol–croton peel, highlighting the formation of a new collagen-elastin band (Grenz zone), with collagen organized parallel to the surface and regenerated elastin. Figure created by the author. *Source: Figure created by the author (Dr Carolina Marçon)*

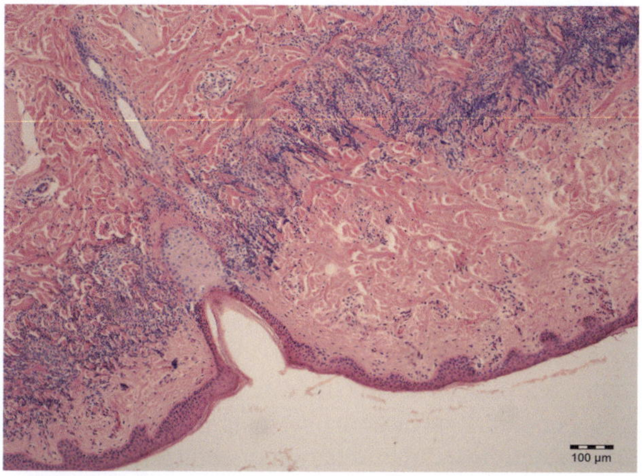

Fig. 7.2 Photomicrograph in HE, 24 h after phenol–croton peel (Hetter formula 1.6%). Extensive coagulative necrosis is observed extending to the reticular dermis, accompanied by a thick band of deep neutrophilic inflammation with a characteristic "ant-like" pattern, consistent with NETosis. The delimitation of dermal necrosis by the NETs band surrounding the coagulation area is also noted. Magnification 400×. *Source: Courtesy of Dr Flavio Beltrame and Dr Carlos Wambier*

7.3 Histological Evidence in Humans

The scientific understanding of the histological and clinical effects induced by phenol peeling—either alone or combined with croton oil—has been built over more than six decades of clinical and experimental research. From the pioneering studies of Brown (1960), through in-depth histological analyses by Baker (1974), Stegman (1982), Kligman (1985), and Hetter (2000), to recent studies employing immunohistochemical and epigenetic approaches, such as those by Kaminaka et al. (2009) and Cardoso et al. (2021), a robust body of evidence has been established regarding the mechanisms of action, durability of effects, and safety of deep phenol peeling.

The classic study by Brown et al. (1960), published in the *British Journal of Plastic Surgery*, was a pioneer in the systematic clinical and histological analysis of these effects. The authors applied phenol solutions at concentrations ranging from 60% to 95%, often combined with cresol and vegetable oils (such as olive or sesame) to modulate penetration. Although Brown did not explicitly mention croton oil in his articles and even omitted its presence from the registered patent, it is known that the substance was part of his formulations, being a key component in enhancing the dermal action of phenol. The protocol involved dividing the face into five regions treated sequentially, the use of occlusion (plastic film, adhesive tape, or latex mask) to intensify the effect, and rigorous clinical monitoring, including vital signs, urinary phenol, and serum urea. Serial biopsies were performed at different time points, including more than 15 years after the procedure.

Histologically, normal epidermis presents as uniform stratified squamous epithelium, with a thin and loosely adherent stratum corneum, and dermis with a spongy network of connective tissue and abundant dilated vascular and lymphatic channels. After phenol application, there is orderly hyperplasia of the squamous epithelium, thickening, and mild acanthotic ridges. In the dermis, fibro-hyaline transformation is observed, with collagen reorganized into laminated and compacted fibers, oriented parallel to the epidermal surface, associated with a significant reduction in solar elastosis. Dermal vascularization remains preserved, with occasional perivascular lymphocytes.

These changes are permanent and irreversible, histologically documented by Brown and colleagues up to 15 years after application. This dermal remodeling is considered the main factor responsible for skin tightening and the long-lasting smoothing of wrinkles, as the dermis, being 20–30 times thicker than the epidermis, is where the most relevant structural modifications occur. Although epidermal renewal produces a smoother surface, the most significant impact occurs in the dermis, with tissue compaction and reorientation of collagen fibers.

From a histochemical perspective, phenol denatures keratin proteins by breaking sulfur bonds and promoting protein coagulation. Brown et al. hypothesized that this denaturation produces a protective eschar that reduces dermal penetration and systemic absorption. Penetration also depends on the surface tension of the solution, which can be increased by surfactants (such as soap or bentonite) or reduced by oils. Absorption may occur through damaged epidermis as well as via cutaneous appendages, the latter being the preferential route according to Schwartz and Peck (1946).

Clinically, these histological changes manifest as tissue contraction, improved texture, wrinkle reduction, and overall rejuvenation, with greater durability than methods such as dermabrasion or surgical lifting. However, the authors also reported significant risks when the procedure was performed improperly, especially by non-medical personnel. Cases of hypertrophic scarring, ectropion, and even deaths due to pneumonia or pericarditis were associated with large-area applications without technical control, underscoring that the safety of phenol depends on medical expertise.

In 1974, Baker et al. published a landmark study that systematically and longitudinally evaluated the histological changes in human skin treated with phenol-croton oil peel (49%/2.1%—Baker's Formula). Biopsies were obtained from patients who had previously undergone the procedure and subsequently underwent rhytidectomy, with intervals ranging from 6 months to 13 years. Sampling was performed at the junction between treated and untreated areas, allowing intra-individual comparisons and precise anatomical control. The samples were processed with specific stains (hematoxylin-eosin, Fontana-Masson, Verhoeff, and Masson's trichrome) to assess the epidermis, melanin, elastic fibers, and collagen.

The main objective was to determine the durability of microscopic changes and correlate them with observed clinical effects. The results demonstrated homogenization and compaction of dermal collagen, with reorganization of the extracellular matrix and significant reduction of solar elastosis. The collagen architecture became reorganized parallel to the epidermal surface, resulting in denser and more uniform connective tissue. There was also an accumulation of fibers staining as elastic (elastotic tissue), interpreted by the authors as an adaptive rather than degenerative change, possibly functioning as a barrier against further chemical penetration or UV radiation.

In the epidermis, a persistent reduction in melanin granules and decreased melanocyte density in the basal layer were identified, findings present even more than a decade after the procedure. This alteration explains the long-lasting clinical skin lightening effect (bleaching effect). The regenerated epidermis appeared smoother and more regular, without the typical irregularities of photoaging.

Temporal analysis showed that the changes observed early, up to 2 years after the procedure, remained virtually unchanged at longer intervals (up to 13 years), indicating that the histological effects of phenol-croton oil are, in practice, irreversible. No clinical or histological evidence of late deleterious effects was identified. The structural basis for sustained clinical improvement lies in deep dermal remodeling, with collagen reorganization, reduction of elastosis, and modification of the epidermal pigmentation pattern, supporting the long-term rejuvenating effects of phenol peel.

In 1982, Stegman published a pioneering and carefully controlled comparative study to assess, in human skin, the histological changes induced by different escharotic agents—trichloroacetic acid (TCA) 60%, phenol 100%, Baker's formula, and dermabrasion—applied to both normal and photoaged skin. The study was conducted in a 55-year-old Caucasian patient with cutis rhomboidalis nuchae in the posterior cervical region. The surface was divided into 16 quadrants of 1 cm^2, including areas of normal and photoaged skin. The quadrants were randomized to receive each treatment, with and without 24-h occlusion, allowing assessment of regenerative dynamics under different conditions. Biopsies were obtained at 3, 60, and 120 days post-procedure, with hematoxylin-eosin, Verhoeff (elastic fibers), and colloidal iron (glycosaminoglycans) staining.

In the acute phase (day 3), TCA 60% produced the most superficial lesion, with partial epidermal necrosis, mild dermal edema, and homogenization limited to the papillary dermis, only superficially affecting the reticular dermis. In photoaged skin, penetration was slightly greater but still limited, with partial preservation of the elastotic band. Phenol 100% induced complete epidermal necrosis and injury to the papillary dermis and upper third of the reticular dermis, traversing the entire solar elastosis in photoaged skin. Baker's formula caused extensive necrosis of the epidermis, papillary dermis, and up to half of the reticular dermis, an effect accentuated by occlusion, which significantly increased penetration and destruction of the elastotic matrix. Dermabrasion produced a pattern similar to occluded Baker's formula, with equivalent depth but slightly less intense edema and collagen disorganization.

In the subacute and regenerative phase (60–120 days), TCA 60% showed a restored epidermis and regular architecture at 60 days, but with a thin Grenz zone and mild dermal remodeling, only partially replacing solar elastosis in photoaged skin. The "dermal scar" was barely evident, suggesting a limited rejuvenating effect. Phenol 100% and Baker's formula resulted in a restored and well-organized epidermis, with a thick Grenz zone composed of collagen and elastic fibers of normal appearance, and a well-defined "dermal scar" in the mid-dermis, replacing a significant portion of solar elastosis. Baker's formula, especially under occlusion, promoted the most intense remodeling and the more complete replacement of the elastotic matrix by organized connective tissue. Dermabrasion produced results comparable to those of the occluded Baker formula in terms of depth and replacement of elastosis, but with slightly less homogeneous collagen organization.

The histological changes were equivalent between normal and photoaged skin, refuting the notion that photodamage impairs the dermal regenerative capacity. Stegman concluded that the formation of a functional Grenz zone and a "dermal scar" rich in mature collagen, regenerated elastic fibers, and glycosaminoglycans constitutes the histological basis for the prolonged rejuvenation achieved with deep peels. Among the methods studied, 60% TCA induced the least structural remodeling, while the Baker formula and dermabrasion stood out for the intensity and durability of their results, with 100% phenol occupying an intermediate position.

In 1985, Kligman, Baker, and Gordon further advanced the understanding of the long-term effects of phenol-croton oil peels by publishing a seminal study that meticulously analyzed the long-term histological changes produced by deep peeling with the Baker formula—phenol at approximately 50%, croton oil 2.1%, water, and liquid soap (Septisol®)—in patients with severe actinic damage. The aim was to document, in histological sections obtained from 1.5 to 20 years after the procedure, the dermal and epidermal modifications responsible for the prolonged clinical effects of the treatment (Fig. 7.3).

The sample included 11 women, aged between 34 and 58 years, all with advanced photodamage characterized by marked solar elastosis, actinic keratoses, solar lentigines, and irregular hyperpigmentation. Material was obtained during rhytidectomies, using strips of skin 4–5 cm wide encompassing the sharp transition between treated and untreated areas. This strategy allowed direct intra-individual comparison, eliminating anatomical and environmental variables. Samples were fixed in formalin, cut in semi-serial sections, and stained with specific techniques for collagen, elastin, mucopolysaccharides, basement membrane, and melanin (H&E, PAS, Fontana-Masson, Verhoeff, Mowry, van Gieson, and others).

In untreated skin, findings were consistent with chronic actinic damage: pronounced solar elastosis, with thick, dense, disorganized, and often degenerated elastic fibers forming amorphous masses; fragmented collagen with irregular architecture; presence of telangiectasia and chronic perivascular inflammatory infiltrate (heliodermatitis). The epidermis showed irregular thickening, loss of polarity, keratinocytes of varying sizes, and cytological disarray. Microscopic actinic keratoses were common, and in one case, early lentigo maligna was observed. Melanin distribution was heterogeneous, with hyperpigmented areas adjacent to regions of scant pigment, and melanocytes were often increased and clustered. Solar lentigines and irregular pigment patterns were frequent findings.

In skin treated with phenol-croton oil, the findings were markedly different and explained the sustained clinical rejuvenation. The most characteristic finding was the formation of a new dermal band 2–3 mm thick, located immediately beneath the epidermis and sharply separated from the old elastotic dermis by an abrupt demarcation line. This band was composed of fine, dense collagen bundles arranged

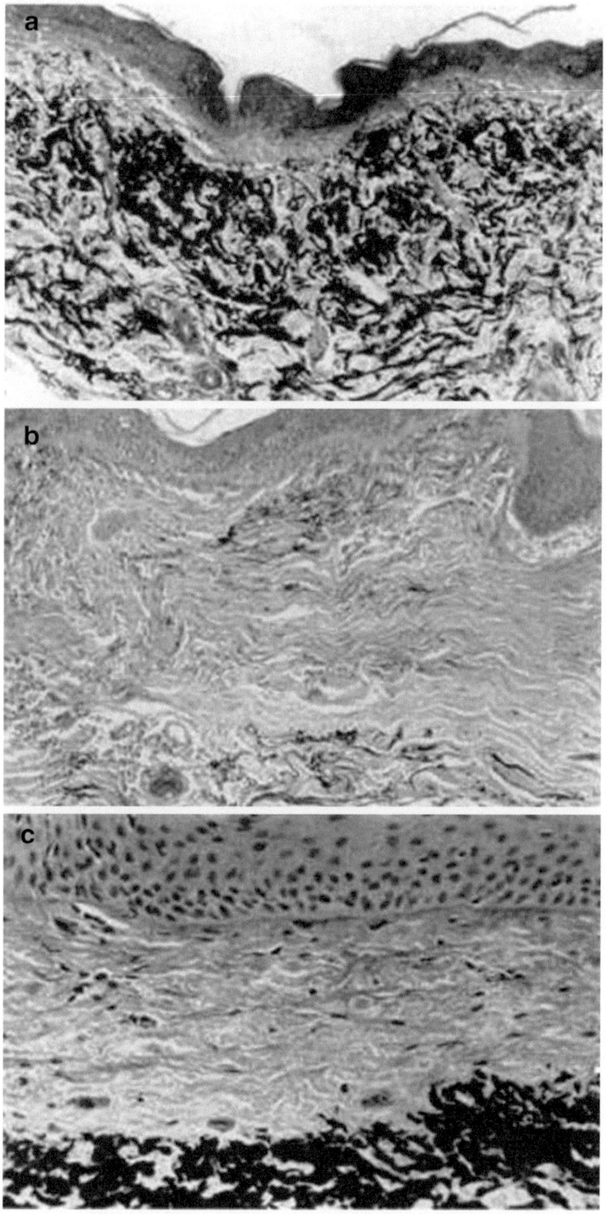

Fig. 7.3 Long-term dermal remodeling after phenol-croton oil peel. Long-term histological findings following phenol-croton oil peel. (**a**) Untreated skin, showing marked solar elastosis, with disorganized collagen bundles and degenerated elastic fibers. (**b**) Specimen 14 years post-peel, demonstrating a broad dermal band of homogeneous collagen and fine elastic fibers oriented parallel to the epidermal surface. (**c**) Specimen 4 years post-peel, showing a clear demarcation between the new collagen-elastic band and the residual elastotic dermis. Luna stain, original magnifications 382–406×. *Source: Kligman AM, Baker TJ, Gordon HL. Long-term histologic follow-up of phenol face peels. Plast Reconstr Surg. 1985;75* (5)*:652–659. Reproduced with permission from the publisher*

parallel to the surface, with an ordered and stable architecture even after two decades. Among the collagen bundles, numerous fine, regenerated elastic fibers were observed, often following the orientation of the collagen. The quality and density of these regenerated elastic fibers were sufficient to partially restore the biomechanical function of the skin, contributing to its firmness and ability to return after deformation. The ground substance showed increased glycosaminoglycans, as evidenced by special stains, enhancing tissue hydration and elasticity.

In the new dermal band, vessels were normal, with no telangiectasia or abnormal wall thickening. No skin appendages—hair follicles or sweat glands—were present in the reconstructed area, confirming that dermal regeneration results from organized but functionally adapted scar tissue, rather than pathological scarring. Cases of hypertrophic scarring were observed only in samples from patients treated by non-medical personnel using inadequate technique, which differed markedly from the regeneration pattern achieved by the standardized medical method.

The overlying epidermis exhibited normalized architecture: a basal layer with a continuous row of columnar cells, regular organization, absence of atypia, and complete elimination of actinic keratoses. The basement membrane was uniform and well defined, and the melanocytic population was preserved but distributed more homogeneously. Melanogenesis remained active, but the even distribution of melanin granules within the keratinocytes explained the long-lasting lightening effect—characterized by relative hypopigmentation rather than true depigmentation.

These changes were stable over time: even after 15–20 years, the regenerated collagen-elastic band remained intact, with an orderly arrangement of fibers and no signs of recurrence of solar elastosis in the treated area. In addition to the aesthetic benefit, the authors highlighted the preventive oncological potential of phenol-croton oil peel, given the complete destruction of precancerous lesions and the likely impact on reducing the risk of cutaneous carcinomas.

In summary, the study demonstrated that phenol-croton oil peel, when properly performed, promotes deep, permanent, and functional dermal reconstruction, normalizes epidermal architecture, evens out pigmentation, and eliminates preneoplastic lesions. These structural changes underpin the rejuvenating clinical effect that can last for decades, establishing the technique as one of the most durable aesthetic procedures with a significant impact on skin histology.

In 2000, Gregory Hetter published the fourth part of his series of studies on phenol–croton peel, presenting one of the most comprehensive and iconoclastic critical reviews ever conducted on the procedure. Based on clinical and experimental observations accumulated over the years, Hetter not only refined the technique and understanding of its histological effects but also broke with several dogmas perpetuated since the inception of the method.

The first and most striking of these dogmas was the belief that phenol was the main agent responsible for the depth and efficacy of the peel. Hetter demonstrated that isolated phenol, even at high concentrations (up to 49%), did not produce significant dermal necrosis when applied without croton oil—except when combined with prolonged occlusion. In practice, phenol acted more as a vehicle for the true cytotoxic agent: croton oil resin. This finding shifted the focus from phenol to croton oil as the determinant of the depth of dermal injury and the intensity of tissue remodeling.

Another historical dogma, originating from Brown's observations, held that the more diluted the phenol, the greater its penetration. The reasoning was that, at high concentrations, phenol would cause intense keratocoagulation in the epidermis, rapidly forming a barrier that would limit its diffusion to deeper layers; whereas more diluted solutions, with less initial keratocoagulation, would penetrate further. Hetter's systematic studies refuted this premise, showing that, in practice, the higher the concentration of phenol, the greater its penetration. And, in the context of phenol-croton oil peel, the depth is even more decisively determined by the concentration of croton oil and the method of application.

The second dogma challenged was the notion that the effect of the peel would be uniform across the entire face. Hetter demonstrated that facial skin exhibits great heterogeneity in thickness, density of adnexal structures, and tolerance, and that the use of standardized concentrations across the whole face is not only unnecessary but potentially harmful. He therefore proposed facial mapping by zones, varying the concentration of croton oil between 0.2% and 1.6%: higher values for areas of thick skin (perioral and nasal dorsum), intermediate for cheeks and forehead, and ultra-low for eyelids and neck.

Hetter also showed that depth depends not only on concentration, but also on the number of layers applied with the same solution—each successive layer increases penetration, corroborating previous findings by Stegman. Experiments in pigs showed no difference in the depth of necrosis and neutrophilic infiltrate between occlusion with adhesive tape or ointment. Epithelialization was faster with ointment than with tape, and slower in non-occluded skin.

Hetter further questioned the unit of measurement "drop," used since Baker, noting that the variation in volume between different droppers compromised reproducibility. He proposed standardizing the volume to 0.04 ml per drop, creating a universal and precise metric for calculating concentrations.

From a clinical-histological perspective, he demonstrated that concentrations above 1% croton oil significantly increase the risk of permanent hypopigmentation, and above 2% this risk is virtually inevitable outside areas of thick skin. On the other hand, in cases of severe photodamage, the strategic use of higher concentrations in specific zones (such as perioral and nasal) resulted in rejuvenation superior to any other available single-session method, with near-complete replacement of deep rhytids and intense dermal reorganization.

In his final considerations, Hetter speculated on the physics and chemistry of the phenol–water–croton oil system, suggesting that the affinity of croton resin for phenol could explain differences in penetration observed with different proportions. And, in a gesture that encapsulates the paradigm shift promoted by his work, he proposed that the term "croton peel" might be more accurate in reflecting the true active mechanism than "phenol peel."

In 2009, Kaminaka et al. published a prospective study evaluating the efficacy and the histological and immunohistochemical correlations of phenol peel in the treatment of actinic keratoses (AK) and Bowen's disease (BD) in Japanese patients. In total, 46 patients (32 with AK and 14 with BD), aged between 31 and 91 years (mean age 75.1 years), were treated with 100% pure phenol applied monthly, for up to eight sessions. The application was preceded by cleaning with acetone and gentle curettage of the superficial crust, and clinical and dermatoscopic follow-up was performed monthly. Four-millimeter biopsies were collected before and after treatment for histological and immunohistochemical evaluation.

The study demonstrated that 39 patients (84.8%) achieved complete response (CR), with BD requiring a greater number of sessions than AK (mean of 5.5 versus 2.9, $p = 0.005$). The one-year recurrence rate was only 4.3%. Patients with a previous history of skin cancer showed a lower response rate and required more sessions ($p = 0.0004$).

Histologically, clinical efficacy correlated with pre-treatment tumor thickness, but not with the thickness of the stratum corneum. Lesions with tumor thickness >400 μm had a lower probability of response. In cases with complete response in 1–2 sessions, the mean tumor thickness was 164 μm, increasing progressively in lesions that required more sessions or showed progressive disease (PD), in which the mean reached 570 μm.

Immunohistochemical analysis revealed that cyclin A expression, a marker of cellular proliferation, correlated directly with the number of sessions required for complete remission, and was considered a useful predictive marker. Low values (<11%) were associated with rapid response, while higher values (>25%) were found in resistant lesions. PCNA showed increased expression in PD lesions, but without statistical significance. p53 expression was variable and showed no consistent correlation with clinical response, while TUNEL staining, which indicates apoptosis, was elevated in both CR and PD groups, raising the hypothesis that high levels may reflect lesions with early malignant transformation, but was not directly associated with response to the peel.

Microscopically, after successful treatment, complete epidermal necrosis was observed with destruction of atypical cells and re-epithelialization by normal keratinocytes. In the papillary dermis, initial inflammation was followed by reorganization of collagen fibers and reduction of dilated vessels.

The authors concluded that phenol peel is highly effective for superficial AK and BD, especially in lesions with thickness ≤400 μm and low cyclin A index, and that these parameters, together with the patient's oncological history, may serve as predictive tools for response and safety. Furthermore, they emphasized that the method does not induce tumorigenesis in cured lesions, unlike reports with low-concentration TCA, and that hypopigmentation is a frequent and dose-dependent adverse effect.

More recently, Cardoso et al. (2021) investigated the clinical and histological effects of phenol–croton peel in perioral rejuvenation, with emphasis on dermal collagen remodeling and activation of epigenetic markers involved in cellular longevity. The sample comprised 30 patients with a mean age of 64.8 years and phototypes II to IV, all presenting with marked perioral aging.

The intervention consisted of application of the phenol–croton peel, with clinical assessment using the Glogau, Baker and Cohen scales before the procedure (D0) and after 90 days (D90 ± 2). The clinical results were highly significant: two-thirds of patients showed improvement of at least two grades on the Glogau and Baker scales, and more than half progressed from moderate/severe to mild or absence of wrinkles according to the Cohen scale. These clinical findings were supported by histochemical and immunohistochemical analyses performed on biopsies from the treated area.

Herovici and Picrosirius Red staining demonstrated a marked increase in type I and III collagen in the papillary and reticular dermis. Polarized light microscopy analysis revealed a statistically significant increase in the proportion of mature collagen fibers (COL1)—from 52.93% to 62.14%—and immature fibers (COL3)—from 54.71% to 64.77%, indicating intense neocollagenesis. This process was accompanied by increased density and organization of dermal fibers, indicative of profound and sustained structural remodeling.

Notably, immunohistochemical analysis revealed a significant increase in the expression of sirtuins SIRT-6 and SIRT-7 after treatment. SIRT-6, involved in DNA repair and regulation of genomic homeostasis, increased from 1.6 to 2.9, while SIRT-7, associated with collagen synthesis and cellular senescence, rose from 5.4 to 7.47 (both $p < 0.05$). These findings indicate that, in addition to the traditional escharotic action attributed to phenol and croton oil, there is activation of epigenetic pathways involved in cellular longevity and tissue repair, which may explain the clinical durability of the results observed with the procedure.

This study represents the first evidence in humans that phenol–croton peeling not only induces dermal regeneration and collagen synthesis, but also modulates the expression of genes related to the biology of aging and skin repair. The selective activation of SIRT-6 and SIRT-7 suggests a novel molecular mechanism of action for deep chemical peels, with clinical implications that extend beyond aesthetic remodeling, potentially involving genomic protection, improved tissue quality, and delay of senescent processes.

In 2024, a retrospective study published in the *Journal of the American Academy of Dermatology* investigated the histopathological effects of phenol–croton peeling in patients with recalcitrant melasma. In 12% of the cases evaluated, biopsies were performed before and after the procedure, revealing preservation of the melanocyte population in the regenerated epidermis, associated with a reduction in melanocyte density and a decrease in both the number and size of melanin granules. A more homogeneous redistribution of melanin among keratinocytes was also observed, with no evidence of total melanocyte destruction. This pigmentary reorganization corroborates the histological basis of the *bleaching effect* described in classical studies, but here documented specifically in skin with chronic hypermelanosis. The pigment uniformity achieved was consistent with sustained clinical improvement, even in higher phototypes, reinforcing that the observed lightening does not result from depigmentation, but from structural and functional modulation of melanocytes and melanin transfer.

The convergence of historical and modern findings reaffirms that phenol–croton peeling is one of the most effective, consistent, and scientifically substantiated methods for deep rejuvenation of human skin. It is a procedure capable of promoting complete restructuring of the papillary dermis, orderly epidermal regeneration, replacement of solar elastosis with a youthful matrix and mature collagen, sustained skin lightening, and possible prevention of early cutaneous neoplasms. (Table 7.1, Figs. 7.4 and 7.5).

However, the safety and predictability of outcomes are intrinsically linked to the medical qualifications of the practitioner, pharmacological knowledge, technical proficiency, and strict control of application parameters. The history of complications arising from lack of expertise underscores the necessity for phenol-croton oil peels to be performed exclusively by trained physicians in an appropriate setting.

Table 7.1 Histological evidence in humans after phenol–croton peeling

Author/ year	Sample/ population	Solution and parameters	Follow-up period	Epidermal findings	Dermal findings	Pigmentary changes	Clinical contribution/ duration
Brown, 1960	Treated patients, biopsies up to 15 years	Phenol 60–95% (+ cresol, oils); plastic/latex occlusion	Up to 15 years	Ordered hyperplasia, mild acanthosis	Collagen reorganized in compact lamellae; reduction of elastosis	Melanocyte preservation	Stable dermal remodeling; tissue contraction; results >15 years
Baker, 1974	Patients undergoing peeling and rhytidectomy (6 m–13y)	Baker's formula (phenol 49%, croton 2.1%); occlusion variation	6 months to 13 years	Smooth, homogeneous epidermis	Homogeneous collagen, reduction of solar elastosis	Persistent reduction of basal melanin	Long-lasting lightening; irreversible changes up to 13 years
Stegman, 1982	55-year-old patient, normal and photoaged skin	TCA 60%, phenol 100%, baker's formula, dermabrasion; with/without occlusion	3, 60, 120 days	Complete epidermal necrosis with phenol/ baker; faster regeneration with TCA	Thick Grenz zone, dermal scar; replacement of elastosis	Reduction of elastosis, structural reorganization	Showed that deep remodeling (Grenz zone) is the basis of rejuvenation
Kligman, 1985	11 women, aged 34–58 years, severe photodamage; biopsies 1.5–20 years	Baker's formula (~50% phenol, 2.1% croton oil, Septisol®)	Up to 20 years	Normalized epidermis, no atypia; elimination of keratoses	New dermal band 2–3 mm; organized collagen/elastin; ↑ GAGs	Homogeneous melanin distribution; relative bleaching	Permanent remodeling; oncological prevention; stable for up to 20 years
Hetter, 2000	Clinical and experimental observations	Phenol up to 49% + croton oil 0.2–1.6%; clinical and animal study	Long-term	Variable according to concentration/zone	Remodeling determined by croton oil; dose/ layer-dependent effect	Increased risk of hypopigmentation if croton oil >1% (>2% almost inevitable)	Challenged dogmas; highlighted the role of croton oil

Kaminaka, 2009	46 patients (32 AK, 14 BD), mean age 75 years	100% pure phenol; up to 8 sessions	Up to 1 year	Complete epidermal necrosis; re-epithelialization by normal keratinocytes	Collagen reorganization; vascular reduction	Frequent, dose-dependent hypopigmentation	High efficacy in superficial AK and BD; predictors: Tumor thickness and cyclin A
Cardoso, 2021	30 patients, mean age 64.8 years, phototypes II–IV; perioral rejuvenation	Phenol–croton oil, clinical assessment + biopsies	90 days	Normal re-epithelialization; regular epidermis	↑ collagen I and III; mature, organized fibers; ↑ SIRT-6 and SIRT-7	Homogeneous redistribution of melanin	First epigenetic evidence (sirtuins); significant clinical outcomes
Maymone et al., 2024	Patients with recalcitrant melasma (12% with biopsy)	Phenol–croton oil	Post-treatment	Regenerated epidermis; preserved melanocytes	Deep dermal remodeling	Reduced melanocyte density and melanin redistribution	Sustained lightening in higher phototypes; confirmed bleaching effect

Main histological studies in humans evaluating the effects of phenol and phenol–croton peels. The table summarizes study design, sample characteristics, solutions used, follow-up duration, histological findings, and documented clinical contribution. Notes. AK: actinic keratosis; BD: Bowen's disease; GAGs: glycosaminoglycans; PCNA: proliferating cell nuclear antigen; Cyclin A: cell proliferation marker; SIRT-6 and SIRT-7: sirtuins involved in DNA repair, collagen synthesis, and epigenetic regulation; Grenz zone: homogeneous dermal band of newly organized collagen/elastin, typical of deep peels; Dermal scar: compact dermal remodeling band replacing solar elastosis. *Source: Table prepared by the author (Dr Carolina Marçon)*

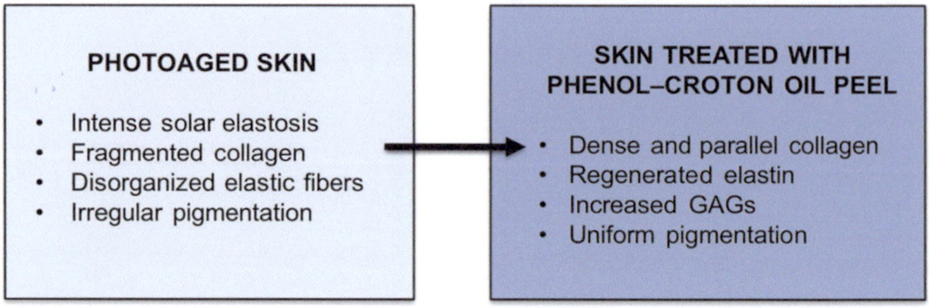

Fig. 7.4 Photoaged skin vs. treated skin. Comparative diagram between photoaged skin, characterized by solar elastosis, fragmented collagen, and irregular pigmentation, and skin treated with phenol–croton oil, showing homogeneous collagen, fine elastic fibers, increased glycosaminoglycans, and uniform pigmentation. *Source: Figure prepared by the author (Dr Carolina Marçon)*

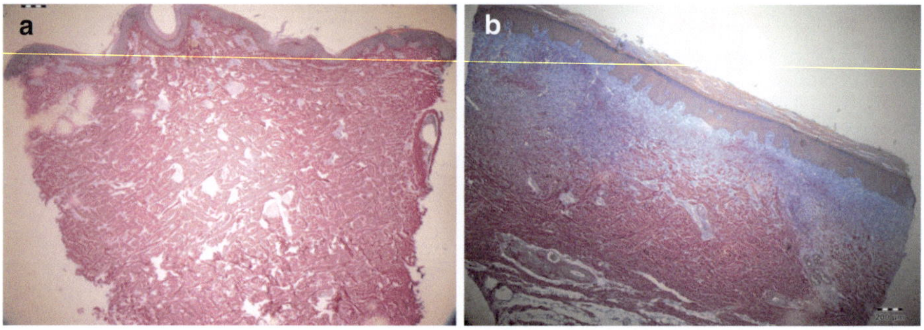

Fig. 7.5 Assessment of neocollagenesis in punch biopsies obtained on day 21 post-peel in a porcine model. (**a**) Negative control (emulsifier agent 5% in distilled water), showing predominance of mature collagen (type I, in red) throughout the dermal thickness. (**b**) Hetter's "very heavy" formula (phenol 35% + croton oil 1.6% + emulsifier agent 5% in distilled water), positive control, showing a dense band of 400–1000 μm of newly formed collagen (type III, in blue) immediately beneath the epidermis, associated with epidermal thickening. Herovici stain, original magnification 320×. *Source: Wambier CG* et al*; International Peeling Society. Advanced chemical peels: Phenol-croton oil peel. J Am Acad Dermatol. 2019;81 (2):327–336. doi:10.1016/j.jaad.2018.11.060. Reproduced with permission from the publisher*

When properly conducted, this is a regenerative and potentially preventive procedure, with lasting clinical and histological benefits supported by over six decades of robust scientific evidence.

7.4 Histological Evidence in Animal Models

Studies in animal models have played a fundamental role in understanding the tissue effects of phenol and phenol combined with croton oil, allowing for controlled analysis of the sequence of histological events and the influence of variables such as concentration, vehicle, occlusion, and number of layers. Before the establishment of clinical protocols, experiments conducted mainly in rabbits and pigs provided crucial information on the depth of injury, the dynamics of epidermal and dermal regeneration, and the durability of structural changes. These studies also helped elucidate the mechanisms of collagen-elastic remodeling, establishing the scientific basis for the safe and effective application of deep peels in humans.

The first controlled experiments to understand the effects of phenol on the skin were conducted by Brown et al. in 1960, using rabbits as the experimental model and correlating the findings with human biopsies. The aim was to systematically analyze the sequence of histological changes induced by different phenolic and cresolic formulations over a follow-up period of up to 98 days, as well as to assess the durability of changes in human skin, including a case with more than 15 years of post-peel evolution. Although Brown's publications made no mention of croton oil use—information also omitted from the patent—it is known that the substance was already part of his formulations, playing an important role in the intensity of the observed responses.

In the animal model, ten rabbits had the inner surface of one ear treated with phenol or cresol solutions at concentrations ranging from 50% to 100%, dissolved in different vehicles—oil, glycerin, ether, and saponified solutions—also varying the purity of the phenol. The contralateral ear and the untreated portion of the same ear served as controls. The areas underwent serial biopsies on days 7, 15, 60, and 98, and were analyzed with routine (H&E) and special stains (Masson's trichrome, Verhoeff, reticulin and elastin stains), allowing sequential observation of the injury and repair process.

In animals treated with more concentrated solutions and with vehicles that facilitated penetration, day 7 showed replacement of the epidermis by a thick, edematous necrotic crust, superficial collagen with a "smudgy" and narrow caliber appearance, vascular congestion, endothelial proliferation, and active fibroblasts depositing immature collagen in lamellae parallel to the surface. By day 15, there was complete epithelialization, with squamous hyperplasia and acanthosis, more fibrillar and organized collagen, persistent dilated vessels, and active fibroblasts. At 60 days, the epidermis displayed almost normal architecture, while the dermis exhibited dense, homogeneous, parallel bundles of mature collagen, with regenerating skin appendages. By day 98, the dermal pattern was stabilized, with persistent thickening due to the deposition of compact lamellar collagen arranged parallel to the epidermis—an alteration considered permanent.

Less concentrated solutions, especially those in oil vehicles, produced more superficial and reversible changes, confirming that penetration and injury intensity are directly related to concentration and vehicle.

The human biopsies analyzed included a case 36 hours after application of pure phenol, showing coagulative degeneration of the epidermis, nuclear vacuolization, and dermal edema; another at 7 days, with almost complete epidermal loss, dermal edema, and degeneration of appendages; and, notably, a case 15 years after a full facial peel, revealing a regular epidermis with slight hyperplasia, dermis with lamination and stratification of collagen and elastin parallel to the surface, and hyperplastic sebaceous glands.

These findings supported the notion that the most significant and lasting effect of phenol occurs in the dermis, with permanent remodeling of collagen and elastin, while the epidermis regenerates thin and orderly. The study also warned that inadequate dilution of phenol, in an attempt to increase safety, may paradoxically favor greater penetration and systemic absorption, increasing the risk of toxicity and scarring, thus reinforcing the need for strict technical control and individual assessment before clinical use.

In 1993, Zukowski et al. published a pilot study using the Yucatan minipig as an experimental model to investigate the impact of different methods of phenol application and occlusive dressings on lesion depth, re-epithelialization rate, and repigmentation. The choice of species was based on the fact that its skin exhibits epidermal thickness, dermoepidermal junction structure, and melanocyte distribution very similar to those of human skin.

A matrix of 35 squares (2.1 cm each) was drawn on both flanks, each treated differently. The application of Baker's solution in "wet" and "moist" forms was compared—where in the "moist" application, excess solution was removed by blotting before contact with the skin—as well as occlusion with impermeable adhesive tape, Xeroform gauze, or bacitracin ointment, maintained for 48 or 96 h. Other areas were subjected to dermabrasion and chemoabrasion (chemical peel immediately followed by dermabrasion) for comparison. Xeroform gauze, used as one of the occlusion methods, consists of cotton gauze impregnated with petrolatum and 3% bismuth tribromophenate, a combination that provides an occlusive effect, maintains local moisture, and exerts mild antimicrobial action. As it is non-adherent, it is widely used for burns, graft donor sites, and superficial wounds, protecting healing tissue and facilitating atraumatic dressing changes.

Histologically, on day 2, all phenol groups showed intact epidermis and dermis but with nuclear pyknosis, indicating cellular non-viability, associated with a dense inflammatory zone rich in neutrophils extending into the reticular dermis. The mean lesion depth ranged from 0.54 to 0.74 mm, with no statistically significant differences between "wet" and "moist" applications or between the different forms of occlusion and absence thereof. On day 4, epithelialization began from viable dermal appendages at the base of the inflammatory zone; it was more frequent and mature in groups kept occluded for 96 h, regardless of the material used. By day 8, all areas were completely re-epithelialized, with a gradual reduction of inflammation and formation of granulation tissue, followed by restoration of epidermal ridges and dermal papillae over the first month.

Repigmentation began around day 12, originating from hair follicles, and by day 29 there was almost complete recovery of melanocytes in both non-occluded and occluded "moist" groups, with marked pigment deposition in the upper layers of the epidermis. Repigmentation was less intense after dermabrasion, chemoabrasion, and non-occluded "wet" peeling.

Regarding microbiology, Staphylococcus epidermidis was the predominant microorganism in all groups, with a significant increase in bacterial counts between

48 and 96 h, but no statistical difference between occluded and non-occluded areas, and no association with greater lesion depth. Bacitracin ointment did not show any antibacterial advantage.

Comparatively, dermabrasion caused a more superficial and less inflammatory lesion than chemical peeling; chemoabrasion, in turn, produced a more intense inflammatory reaction and possibly more prolonged effects, although without immediate advantages in healing.

As a result of this study, the authors recommended that phenol solutions be applied in the moist form and that the treated skin remain occluded for at least 4 days. Occlusion with ointments proved as effective as with adhesive tape or gauze, with no advantage to using tape, which is more laborious to apply, painful to remove, and offers no additional benefit. Bacitracin ointment did not demonstrate antibacterial effect, is more expensive than petroleum jelly, and may cause allergic contact dermatitis in some cases. The "moist" application also prevents iatrogenic injury from phenol dripping, and for the same concentration, occlusion accelerates re-epithelialization and repigmentation. Based on these findings, the authors' preference shifted to intraoperative application of Xeroform gauze over the treated area, kept moist by the patient with sterile petroleum jelly twice daily. This method is easy to apply, usually allows the gauze to detach spontaneously between the fourth and sixth day with minimal discomfort, and, as an added benefit, conceals the unsightly crust during the healing process. Nevertheless, they conclude that, ultimately, the type of occlusive medium used does not alter the final outcome, provided it is properly maintained.

In 1980, Samuel J. Stegman developed an experimental model in Hartley strain guinea pigs (albino guinea pig) to systematically compare the histology of lesions induced by dermabrasion and by different agents used in chemical peels. The study assessed the impact of acid concentration, presence or absence of croton oil, use of occlusion, and number of passes on lesion depth, regeneration pattern, and healing time.

The dorsal skin was previously depilated and divided into distinct areas for treatment application: dermabrasion with a 5 mm diamond fraise; phenol alone in different doses; TCA at 40% and 60%; combination of TCA and phenol; and Baker's formula applied with and without croton oil, with and without occlusion. Occlusion was performed with multiple layers of adhesive tape (Holister Ace Adherent®, paper, and Blenderm®) and maintained for 24 h. Serial biopsies (3 mm) were collected at different time points and analyzed by H&E and immunofluorescence.

During the first 3 days, dermabrasion resulted in complete loss of the epidermis and deep dermal damage, with fragmented collagen, edema and changes in fiber staining. The Baker formula produced necrosis, yet intact epidermis and massive edema throughout the dermis; under occlusion, necrosis and cellular infiltration extended into deeper layers of the reticular dermis.

By day 6, all groups showed re-epithelialization, but the dermis still exhibited marked edema and disorganization in areas treated with occluded Baker, followed by non-occluded Baker and dermabrasion. Eschar separation in the Baker groups was slower with occlusion.

On day 12, skin treated with non-occluded Baker was already approaching histological normality, whereas occluded skin still showed diffuse edema and necrotic debris beneath the new epithelium. Dermabrasion maintained acanthosis, dermal edema, and deep collagen disorganization.

At 32 days, epidermal maturation remained incomplete in the dermabrasion and occluded Baker groups, with a less developed stratum corneum than in the non-occluded Baker group. In all groups, the dermis still contained newly formed, loosely organized, and mildly eosinophilic collagen fibers.

Comparing agents, Stegman observed that lesion depth increased progressively according to the agent: TCA 40% < TCA 60% < Baker formula. The number of passes also directly influenced depth, and the presence of croton oil resulted in a deeper and more intense lesion.

The author concluded that the Baker formula under occlusion induces a deeper and more extensive dermal injury than TCA and pure phenol, being particularly effective for treating deep wrinkles associated with severe actinic damage. It was also demonstrated that dermabrasion, although classically considered superficial, produces significant dermal injury requiring collagen regeneration, and that there is a dose-dependent response to phenol, without an "all or nothing" effect. The author further emphasized that, although results in guinea pigs cannot be fully extrapolated to humans, the data reinforce the importance of variables such as concentration, number of applications, occlusion, and the presence of croton oil in controlling depth and final outcome.

In 1995, Vagotis and Brundage published an experimental study to assess the impact of pre-treatment with topical tretinoin (Retin-A 0.1%) on skin regeneration after dermabrasion and chemical peeling, also using an albino Hartley guinea pig animal model, whose skin architecture resembles that of human skin. The aim was to determine, both histologically and clinically, whether tretinoin could accelerate re-epithelialization and promote dermal regeneration following these procedures.

The study included 12 guinea pigs, equally divided into a control group and a pre-treated group, the latter receiving daily topical tretinoin for 30 days. After the pre-treatment period, the dorsal skin of all animals was divided into two halves: one treated with dermabrasion and the other with 50% phenol chemical peel. Biopsies were performed before the start of the study, after pre-treatment, and at intervals over 6 weeks following the procedures.

Clinically, after 1 month of tretinoin, the treated group exhibited superficial irritant dermatitis, consistent with the expected effect of the medication, while the control group's skin remained unchanged. In the first 24 h and on the third day post-procedure, both groups showed similar clinical progression. However, from day 7 onwards, wounds in the pre-treated group displayed visibly faster re-epithelialization. Within 2 weeks, all areas in the treated group were fully epithelialized, compared to approximately 75% in the control group. After 6 weeks, both groups were healed.

Histologically, after 1 month of tretinoin, the treated group showed epidermal hyperplasia with 7–8 cell layers, in contrast to 4–5 layers in the control group. One week after the procedures, the treated group exhibited 1.5 times more epidermal regeneration than the control; at 14 days, this difference doubled, accompanied by dermal neovascularization observed only in the treated group. At 42 days, epidermal regeneration had stabilized but remained thicker in the treated group (8–9 layers) than in the control (4–5 layers). Greater collagen renewal was also observed in the treated group, although this finding was not quantified in a statistically robust manner.

The authors concluded that pre-treatment with tretinoin promotes faster and more intense epidermal regeneration, stimulates neovascularization, and possibly accelerates collagen turnover after dermabrasion or phenol chemical peel. They suggested that these effects are due to prior activation of epidermal regeneration mechanisms by tretinoin before chemical or mechanical injury, and recommended its clinical use prior to these procedures to enhance healing.

Butler et al. (2001) conducted a quantitative and qualitative study to assess the effects of chemical peeling on photoaged skin, using the Skh:HR-1 animal model (hairless mouse). One hundred animals were subjected to photoaging induced by chronic UVB radiation for 14 weeks and then divided into five groups: control, glycolic acid 50%, trichloroacetic acid (TCA) 30%, TCA 50%, and phenol (Baker-Gordon formula). The agents were applied to the dorsal skin of the animals and evaluated by biopsies at multiple time points (days 3, 7, 14, 28, and 60) for histological and biochemical analyses, including quantification of collagen and glycosaminoglycans (GAGs).

The control group exhibited the classic changes of photoaging: reduction in dermal thickness, loss of birefringence of collagen fibers under polarized light, presence of amorphous elastic masses, and disorganization of the elastic fiber network. In the groups subjected to peeling, especially with 50% TCA and phenol, there was significant dermal thickening on day 60 (mean: phenol 192 μm; 50% TCA 171 μm versus control 70 μm; $p < 0.02$), collagen reorganization with restoration of birefringence, and reorientation of elastic fibers in a finer and more horizontal pattern, in contrast to the thick and disorganized pattern seen in controls. These effects were more pronounced with deep (50% TCA and phenol) and medium-depth peels than with superficial peels (glycolic acid and 30% TCA).

Biochemically, collagen content per unit volume increased in all treated groups during the first 3 days, peaking at day 28 and returning to baseline by day 60, except for glycolic acid, where the increase was not significant. GAG content increased significantly only in the deep and medium-depth peel groups (50% TCA and phenol), peaking at day 14 and remaining elevated until day 28, returning to control levels by day 60. The increase in GAGs is associated with greater dermal hydration and may contribute to the temporary disappearance of wrinkles.

Dermal reorganization included replacement of pathological elastic masses with finer, more orderly fibers, reconstitution of the collagen network, and increased dermal volume, partially reversing the histological changes of photoaging. These findings indicate that the clinical benefit of deep peeling derives from two main mechanisms: structural reorganization of the extracellular matrix and increased dermal volume. The study also demonstrated that, even in an animal model, phenol and 50% TCA promote more intense and long-lasting tissue remodeling than shallower agents.

In 2009, Larson, Karmo, and Hetter developed an experimental model in pigs to validate, in a controlled manner, Hetter's clinical observations regarding the role of croton oil in phenol peeling. The aim was to analyze the individual contribution of each component of the classic formula—phenol, croton oil, Septisol, and water—as well as the impact of their concentrations and application technique on lesion depth and subsequent inflammatory response.

Forty different solutions were tested, organized into eight main groups: phenol diluted in water (20–80%); phenol in water with added Septisol; phenol in water with 0.2% croton oil; phenol in water with 2% croton oil; phenol in water with 0.2% croton oil and Septisol; phenol in water with 2% croton oil and Septisol; phenol in ethanol with 2% croton oil; and phenol in ethanol with 2% croton oil and Septisol. The solutions were applied to 2 × 2 cm grids on the animals' flanks using standardized gauze sponges, with 20 passes per cell. To assess the effect of the number of layers, two of these solutions were reapplied with 5, 20, and 45 passes.

Biopsies were collected on days 1, 8, and 22, assessed by a blinded dermatopathologist, with specific stains for elastin (orcein) and collagen (van Gieson). The results showed that, in the case of phenol alone, lesion depth increased proportionally with concentration, refuting the historical dogma proposed by Brown that higher dilutions would penetrate more deeply. The addition of Septisol intensified the inflammatory response and depth of penetration, an effect attributed to reduced surface tension of the solution, facilitating its diffusion. Croton oil proved to be the most impactful element: even at minimal concentration (0.2%), it significantly increased the depth of dermal necrosis, surpassing even high-concentration phenol-only formulations. Increasing croton oil concentration to 2% further potentiated the lesion, especially when combined with high-concentration phenol and Septisol.

Another relevant finding was the effect of ethanol as a solvent: when water was replaced by ethanol, the depth achieved was less, although application produced a more immediate "frost," indicating more rapid superficial protein precipitation but reduced intradermal diffusion. The number of passes was also a determining factor: additional layers progressively increased penetration, so that 45 passes of a solution considered weak (20% phenol +0.2% croton) produced a lesion equivalent to that obtained with 5 passes of a strong solution (50% phenol +2% croton).

Detailed histological analysis confirmed that:

- Formula A (0.4% croton oil): penetration to the deep papillary dermis.
- Formula B (1.2% croton oil): necrosis reaching the superficial reticular dermis, with visibly altered collagen.
- Formula C (2.1% croton oil): extensive necrosis extending to the mid and deep reticular dermis, with significant fibrillar damage.

The temporal progression of damage showed that, at 24 h, there was evident epidermal necrosis, dermal edema, and onset of inflammatory infiltrate; at 48 h, necrosis was more extensive and continuous, with crust formation and dense inflammatory infiltrate; and at 7 days, there was partial re-epithelialization of the superficial layers, persistence of dermal infiltrate, and ongoing remodeling. The epidermis was completely removed in all the formulations, and regeneration began at the edges of the hair follicles and sweat glands, indicating that these structures are key sources of regeneration. Areas treated with higher concentrations of croton oil exhibited greater edema, inflammation, and a tendency to form thick crusts.

Histologically, areas treated with croton oil and Septisol showed a dermis with compact collagen bundles arranged parallel to the surface, replacing the elastotic matrix present in the control areas, without loss of epidermal polarity. By day 22, all areas were re-epithelialized, with no signs of infection or scar contracture, although some dorsal regions still retained residual dry crusts.

This study confirmed, in an animal model, that the depth of peeling increases according to: (1) phenol concentration; (2) presence and increased concentration of croton oil; (3) use of Septisol; and (4) number of layers applied. It also demonstrated that replacing water with alcohol reduces penetration, and reinforced the concept that croton oil is the true cytotoxic agent responsible for the deep action of the procedure, objectively corroborating the clinical and histological conclusions previously presented by Hetter.

As a relevant historical note, in 2009, Harold J. Brody published a letter to the editor in the *Aesthetic Surgery Journal* in response to the study by Larson, Karmo, and Hetter on the porcine model in phenol-croton oil peeling. While acknowledging the quality and relevance of the work, Brody pointed out that the use of the minipig as an experimental model for studying the effects of phenol and croton oil had already been established decades earlier by Samuel Stegman, who published two pioneering articles on the subject: A study of dermabrasion and chemical peels in an animal model (J Dermatol Surg Oncol, 1980) and A comparative histologic study of the effects of three peeling agents and dermabrasion on normal and sun damaged skin (Aesthetic Plast Surg, 1982).

Stegman's work had already documented, in a controlled manner, fundamental aspects that would also be explored by Hetter: the dose-dependent response to phenol, the increase in lesion depth with the addition of croton oil, the effect of occlusion in intensifying penetration, and the comparison of findings in animal models with results obtained in humans. Brody emphasized that, although the study by Larson, Karmo, and Hetter expanded and detailed the analysis, Stegman's articles remain fundamental references for the scientific understanding of deep chemical peeling and deserve citation as historical milestones.

In 2022, Lemes et al. investigated, using a porcine model, the possibility of replacing phenol as a vehicle in phenol-croton oil peeling with non-cardiotoxic agents, while maintaining the ability to induce deep dermal remodeling. The study compared formulations containing 35% glycolic acid (GA), 35% trichloroacetic acid (TCA), and phenol as main agents, all combined with 1.6% croton oil, 5% Septisol, and distilled water as the vehicle. The choice of acids aimed to assess whether a highly water-soluble agent (GA) or a traditional coagulating agent (TCA) could produce histological effects similar to phenol when combined with croton oil.

The experiment was conducted on four domestic pigs (two males and two females, 5 months old, weighing between 30 and 35 kg), selected for their skin pattern similar to humans in terms of thickness and dermal structure. In each animal,

4 cm^2 areas were shaved and degreased with acetone. The solutions were applied with saturated cotton swabs, under uniform pressure, performing 30 circular movements per area.

Biopsies were collected on days 1, 7, and 21 after the procedure. On days 1 and 7, samples were stained with hematoxylin-eosin for general morphological analysis; on day 21, picrosirius red under polarized light was used to identify and quantify the deposition of type I collagen (mature) and type III collagen (immature, associated with active remodeling).

From a chemical perspective, the TCA solution had the lowest pH (1.97), followed by GA (2.55) and phenol (5.2). Phenol and TCA produced immediate white frosting after application, indicating superficial protein coagulation, whereas GA did not produce this visible effect.

On day 1, phenol induced epidermal necrosis associated with deep dermal necrosis, accompanied by a subcoagulative band of neutrophils. TCA also induced epidermal necrosis but it was limited to the superficial dermis. GA, in turn, caused only mild epidermal edema, with no evident necrosis.

On day 7, skin treated with phenol showed intense proliferation of fibroblasts in the deep dermis and marked neovascularization. GA showed more discrete dermal proliferation, accompanied by moderate neovascularization, while TCA exhibited proliferation limited to the superficial dermis, with restricted vascularization.

On day 21, phenol induced a deep and dense band of type III collagen in the dermis, overlaid by type I collagen in more superficial regions, a typical pattern of active remodeling following deep injury. GA promoted more superficial collagen deposition, but with a higher density of type I collagen than phenol and TCA, suggesting faster matrix maturation. TCA showed only a thin superficial band of type III collagen, with minimal type I collagen deposition, indicating limited remodeling.

Quantification confirmed that phenol, in combination with croton oil, induced deeper and more intense remodeling, characterized by predominance of type III collagen in the mid and deep layers of the dermis, whereas GA resulted in a greater relative amount of type I collagen, but more superficially. TCA showed the most modest results in terms of depth and density of collagen fibers.

The analysis of the results was complemented by an assessment of the physicochemical properties of the agents. Phenol, with a logP of 1.46, is more lipophilic, favoring the diffusion of phorbol esters from croton oil into the dermal matrix. TCA, although moderately lipophilic (logP 1.33), induces rapid superficial protein coagulation, creating a physical barrier that limits deeper penetration. GA, which is highly hydrophilic (logP -1.11), penetrates more diffusely but with lower affinity for cutaneous lipids, resulting in minimal necrosis, although still capable of stimulating superficial collagen remodeling.

The authors concluded that, at the tested concentration, neither GA nor TCA reproduced the pattern of deep dermal necrosis and robust remodeling achieved with phenol combined with croton oil. However, they observed that GA, as it does not cause epidermal necrosis or induce hypopigmentation, may have potential for safe use in darker skin types, justifying further investigation as a less aggressive alternative in skin rejuvenation protocols.

Additionally, it should be considered that the type of soap used in the experimental formulation may have interfered with the results, as its emulsifying capacity is influenced by pH, amphoteric characteristics, and the physicochemical properties of the substances present. Thus, further studies employing different emulsifiers are necessary to more accurately assess the contribution of each component. Another relevant aspect is that the combination of croton oil with TCA may enhance the penetration of this substance, deepening its action in the skin. Unlike phenol—whose penetration is more predictable and limited by rapid protein coagulation—TCA, upon reaching deeper dermal layers, maintains its caustic activity for a longer period, increasing the risk of necrosis and, consequently, scar formation. This greater depth may also favor more intense systemic absorption, which could compromise the safety of the procedure. Therefore, further investigations into the possible systemic effects of TCA, especially when combined with croton oil, are essential before such a combination can be considered safe for use in humans. This underscores the need for extreme caution and rigorous scientific validation of this practice, which has been widely promoted, including by non-medical individuals, without proper evidence of efficacy and safety.

In summary, studies in animal models have provided valuable information on the isolated and combined histological and biochemical effects of phenol, croton oil, and other caustic agents, allowing partial elucidation of their mechanisms of penetration, intensity of inflammatory response, and tissue remodeling potential (Table 7.2). However, these findings should be interpreted with caution, as anatomical, physiological, and cutaneous metabolic differences between animal and human skin may limit the direct extrapolation of results. Furthermore, methodological variables—such as the type of emulsifier, formulation pH, and application conditions—can significantly influence the observed outcomes, reinforcing the need for experimental standardization and validation in controlled clinical trials. These considerations are fundamental for understanding the biological basis and safety limits of chemical peels, and lay the groundwork for a more in-depth analysis of the cellular and molecular mechanisms responsible for dermal and epidermal remodeling, which will be addressed in the next section.

Table 7.2 Histological evidence in animal models

Author/year	Experimental model	Agent/concentration	Occlusion/no. of passes	Evaluation times	Main findings	Observations
Brown, 1960	10 rabbits (ears); correlation with human biopsies	Phenol/cresol 50–100% in oil, glycerin, ether or saponified solutions	None	Days 7, 15, 60, 98; human up to 15 years	Necrotic epidermis → complete re-epithelialization in 15 days; compact, persistent lamellar collagen; permanent remodeling	Vehicle influences depth; inadequate dilutions may ↑ systemic absorption
Stegman, 1980/82	Hartley albino Guinea pigs; dorsal skin	Isolated phenol, TCA 40–60%, baker's formula (± croton oil), dermabrasion	24 h occlusion (tapes); multiple passes ↑ depth	Days 3, 6, 12, 32	Phenol/baker → deep dermal necrosis; well-defined Grenz zone and dermal scar; dermabrasion also deep	Depth is dose-dependent; croton oil ↑ intensity; photodamage does not limit regeneration
Zukowski, 1993	Yucatan minipig; 35 areas of 2.1 cm	Baker's formula (wet vs moist)	Occlusion: Tape, Xeroform, ointment; 48–96 h	Days 2, 4, 8, 29	Mean depth 0.54–0.74 mm; complete re-epithelialization by D8; repigmentation from follicles	Ointment = tape in efficacy; moist application +4-day occlusion recommended
Vagotis & Brundage, 1995	Hartley albino Guinea pigs	Phenol 50% ± pre-treatment with tretinoin 0.1%	None	Up to 42 days	Pre-treatment → thicker epidermis; accelerated re-epithelialization; ↑ dermal neovascularization	Tretinoin enhances epidermal and collagen regeneration
Butler, 2001	Skh:HR-1 mouse, UVB photoaged	GA 50%, TCA 30–50%, baker's formula	None	Days 3, 7, 14, 28, 60	Phenol/TCA 50% → ↑ dermal thickness, reorganized collagen, fine elastic fibers; ↑ GAGs	Deep peels > medium > superficial in remodeling
Larson, Karmo & Hetter, 2009	Pig; 40 formulations	Phenol 20–80% ± croton oil 0.2–2% ± Septisol ± alcohol	5, 20, 45 passes	Days 1, 8, 22	Depth ↑ with phenol, croton oil, Septisol concentration and layers; alcohol ↓ penetration	Confirmed croton oil as main cytotoxic agent
Lemes, 2022	Domestic pig; 4 animals	GA 35%, TCA 35%, phenol; all + croton oil 1.6% + Septisol 5%	30 circular movements	Days 1, 7, 21	Phenol-croton oil → epidermal + deep dermal necrosis; GA → superficial type I collagen; TCA → superficial dermal necrosis	Phenol-croton oil is deeper; GA may be a safe alternative for darker skin phototypes

Main histological studies in animal models evaluating the effects of phenol, croton oil and alternative agents, according to concentration, vehicle, occlusion and number of layers. Notes: GA: glycolic acid; TCA/ATA: trichloroacetic acid; GAGs: glycosaminoglycans; HR-1: hairless mouse strain; Septisol®: anionic detergent used as surfactant; AK: actinic keratosis; BD: Bowen's disease. *Source: Table prepared by the author (Dr Carolina Marçon)*

7.5 Mechanisms of Dermal and Epidermal Remodeling

Cutaneous remodeling induced by phenol-croton oil peel results from a deep, controlled chemical injury, followed by a coordinated process of tissue regeneration. The initial phase is marked by immediate protein coagulation in the epidermis and papillary dermis, accompanied by keratinocyte necrosis and destruction of the extracellular matrix altered by photoaging. This injury triggers an intense acute inflammatory response, with recruitment of neutrophils and formation of neutrophil extracellular traps (NETs), which release enzymes and mediators capable of degrading damaged tissue and stimulating fibroblasts and endothelial cells.

During the proliferative phase, there is abundant deposition of type III collagen—fine, flexible fibers associated with a young matrix—in the mid and deep dermis, upon which type I collagen, thicker and more resistant and predominant in the superficial layers, is progressively organized. Unlike what is observed in fibrotic scars, phenol-croton oil preserves a significant proportion of type III collagen in the long term, contributing to the elasticity tecidual and for the natural appearance of rejuvenated skin. This balanced combination of types I and III, together with the reorganization of elastic fibers and the elimination of solar elastosis, results in a dense, orderly, and functionally adapted dermal matrix.

Another significant finding is the temporary increase in dermal mucin, which contributes to tissue hydration and flexibility during the initial phases of regeneration. Neovascularization, stimulated by inflammatory mediators and growth factors, ensures the metabolic supply necessary for extracellular matrix synthesis and maintenance of the newly formed tissue.

In the epidermal compartment, the procedure promotes orderly basal hyperplasia, restoration of the rete ridges, and reorganization of skin pigmentation. Histologically, there is preservation of the melanocyte population, but with a reduction in melanocyte density and a decrease in the number and size of melanin granules, which become more homogeneously distributed among keratinocytes. This structural and functional reorganization explains the long-lasting bleaching effect, resulting in sustained lightening and a more even skin tone.

The most striking histological observation is the formation of a dense zone of dermal neocollagenesis, which intensifies up to around 16 weeks, associated with the replacement of elastosis by organized elastic fibers. This reorganization remains evident for decades, with dense, compact collagen interposed between the regenerated epidermis and the underlying dermis, replacing previously disorganized structures of photoaged skin. Croton oil enhances the inflammatory response and neocollagenesis, deepening and improving the quality of remodeling.

The final result is skin with renewed dermal architecture, restructured collagen and elastic fibers, and sustained clinical improvement in wrinkles, texture, and tone—a unique regenerative effect, unmatched by other resurfacing methods.

7.6 Cellular Activation and Molecular Markers

The regenerative effects of *Croton tiglium* oil in phenol-croton oil peeling are largely due to the presence of phorbol esters, potent activators of protein kinase C (PKC). This family of serine/threonine-dependent kinases is involved in key processes such as cell proliferation, extracellular matrix remodeling, inflammation, and tissue differentiation. PKC activation mimics signals mediated by diacylglycerol (DAG), promoting the translocation of isoforms to the plasma membrane and, subsequently, phosphorylation of intracellular substrates that modulate gene transcription.

This activation triggers cascades such as MAPK/ERK and leads to the expression of inflammatory mediators (IL-1β, IL-6, TNF-α), activation of the NF-κB pathway, increased expression of TGF-β, and stimulation of type I and III collagen synthesis by dermal fibroblasts. TGF-β plays a central role, regulating fibroblast differentiation and activity, promoting collagen and elastin deposition, and modulating the expression of metalloproteinases (MMP-1, MMP-3) and their inhibitors (TIMPs), allowing selective degradation of the aged matrix. VEGF, induced in the early phases, promotes angiogenesis, while inflammatory cytokines modulate tissue remodeling and are subsequently regulated to prevent chronic inflammation.

Another relevant mechanism is the induction of NETosis—programmed cell death of neutrophils with the release of extracellular traps (NETs)—histologically visible as subcoagulative neutrophilic bands. This response contributes to the removal of damaged skin structures, such as solar elastosis, creating a microenvironment conducive to intense regeneration. In the epidermal compartment, there is sustained proliferation of basal keratinocytes, evidenced by increased PCNA and Cyclin A, until complete re-epithelialization.

At the epigenetic level, phenol-croton oil induces increased expression of sirtuins, especially SIRT-6 and SIRT-7. SIRT-6 is linked to the maintenance of chromosomal stability, DNA repair, and regulation of collagen synthesis, protecting against cellular aging. SIRT-7 regulates the transcription of genes involved in extracellular matrix production and the balance between type I and III collagen. This activation ensures that the resulting regeneration is not only structural but also functional and potentially more stable in the long term.

Experimental models demonstrate that croton oil rapidly increases dermal inflammatory markers, such as myeloperoxidase (MPO) and MMP-8/MMP-9, promoting controlled matrix degradation and facilitating subsequent remodeling. Direct comparisons between formulas with and without croton oil confirm its essential role: while phenol alone induces superficial necrosis and limited regeneration, the addition of the oil promotes deeper necrosis, intense inflammation, abundant type III collagen deposition, and increased vascularization.

The phenol–croton oil interaction is synergistic. Phenol induces controlled necrosis, vasoconstriction, and increased permeability, facilitating the penetration of phorbol esters, which initiate and sustain targeted inflammation and deep dermal remodeling. Systemic absorption of the esters is limited by phenol-induced vasoconstriction, but local effects are intense and long-lasting.

These combined mechanisms ensure that phenol-croton oil peeling promotes functional and genetic reprogramming of the skin tissue, resulting in skin that is more resilient, elastic, with even pigmentation and potentially more stable in the face of degenerative processes or recurrence of pigmentary and pre-neoplastic lesions. (Table 7.3 and Fig. 7.6)

Table 7.3 Histochemical, immunohistochemical, and epigenetic markers associated with phenol–croton peel

Marker	What it measures/ function	Observed change	Clinical/histological interpretation
PCNA	Basal keratinocyte proliferation	↑ in the initial phases, sustained until re-epithelialization	Indicates intense epidermal regeneration
Cyclin A	Proliferative activity and cell cycle	↑ sustained in basal keratinocytes	Correlates with the need for multiple sessions; predictor of clinical response
MPO	Neutrophil activity	↑ in the initial phases	Marker of acute inflammatory infiltration
MMP-8/ MMP-9	Neutrophil metalloproteinases	↑ induced by croton oil	Selective degradation of aged matrix
TGF-β	Regulation of fibroblasts, collagen, and elastin	↑ after PKC activation	Stimulates neocollagenesis and dermal remodeling
VEGF	Angiogenesis	↑ in the initial phases	Formation of new vessels; regenerative support
NF-κB, IL-1β, IL-6, TNF-α	Inflammatory mediators	↑ initially, then regulated	Targeted, non-chronic inflammation
NETs (NETosis)	Neutrophil extracellular traps	Subcoagulative bands visible histologically	Removal of solar elastosis, pro-regenerative microenvironment
SIRT-6	DNA repair, collagen synthesis	↑ after peeling	Genomic repair and stimulation of the dermal matrix
SIRT-7	Regulation of extracellular matrix (COL I/III)	↑ after peeling	Balance of mature/ immature collagen; long-term stability

Main histochemical, immunohistochemical, and epigenetic markers associated with the effects of phenol–croton peel. Notes: PCNA: proliferating cell nuclear antigen; MPO: myeloperoxidase; MMP: matrix metalloproteinase; TGF-β: transforming growth factor beta; VEGF: vascular endothelial growth factor; NF-κB: nuclear factor kappa B; IL: interleukin; TNF-α: tumor necrosis factor alpha; NETs: neutrophil extracellular traps. *Source: Table prepared by the author (Dr Carolina Marçon)*

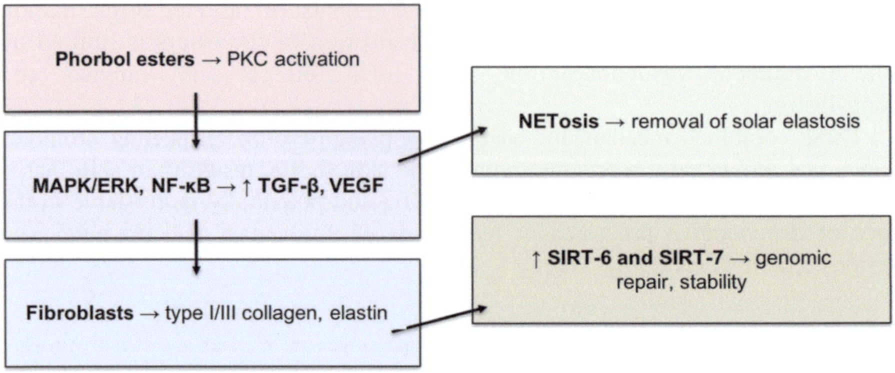

Fig. 7.6 Molecular and epigenetic pathways activated by phenol–croton peel. Molecular cascade induced by phorbol esters from *Croton tiglium* oil, with activation of protein kinase C (PKC) and subsequent induction of the MAPK/ERK and NF-κB pathways, increased inflammatory cytokines, TGF-β and VEGF, activation of fibroblasts, and deposition of collagen I/III. The process also involves NETosis and epigenetic induction of sirtuins (SIRT-6 and SIRT-7), which contribute to the stability and durability of dermal remodeling. *Source: Figure prepared by the author (Dr Carolina Marçon)*

7.7 Final Considerations

The integrated analysis of histological, experimental, and molecular evidence confirms that the phenol-croton oil peel is one of the most potent and long-lasting skin resurfacing procedures available in dermatology. By inducing a deep and controlled chemical injury, this method triggers a sequence of regenerative events that result in the complete replacement of the damaged dermal matrix with new tissue, rich in collagen and reorganized elastic fibers, while preserving tissue elasticity and function.

Epidermal regeneration is rapid and orderly, accompanied by homogeneous redistribution of melanin and reorganization of melanocytic activity, which is responsible for the uniform and sustained lightening of the skin. In the dermis, the balanced deposition of type I and type III collagen, restoration of elastic architecture, and increased mucin confer firmness, flexibility, and hydration. These effects are histologically stable for decades, surpassing in depth and durability those achieved by other deep peels, dermabrasion, or ablative technologies.

At the cellular and molecular level, the procedure activates signaling pathways and gene expression that modulate proliferation, apoptosis, matrix remodeling, and epigenetic regulation, including the activation of sirtuins and growth factors such as TGF-β. This functional reprogramming ensures that repair is not only structural but also qualitative, promoting a more stable cutaneous microenvironment that is resistant to degenerative and pigmentary processes.

The sum of these mechanisms explains not only the marked aesthetic rejuvenation but also the therapeutic efficacy of phenol-croton oil in conditions such as actinic keratoses, Bowen's disease, and chronic hyperpigmentation. When performed with proper technique and by experienced hands, it demonstrates a consistent and predictable safety profile, remaining, after more than six decades of use and study, the gold standard for deep chemical resurfacing, supported by robust scientific evidence.

Sources

1. Hetter GP. An examination of the phenol-croton oil peel: Part I. Dissecting the formula. Plast Reconstr Surg. 2000;105(1):227–39. discussion 249–251
2. Hetter GP. An examination of the phenol-croton oil peel: Part IV. Face peel results with different concentrations of phenol and croton oil. Plast Reconstr Surg. 2000;105(3):1061–83.
3. Justo AS, Lemes BM, Nunes B, Antunes KA, Carletto B, Koga AY, Lipinski LC, Montemor Netto MR, Campagnoli EB, Beltrame FL, Wambier CG. Depth of injury of Hetter's phenol-croton oil chemical peel formula using 2 different emulsifying agents. J Am Acad Dermatol. 2020;82(6):1544–6.
4. Justo AS, Lemes BM, Nunes B, Antunes KA, Capote ACMO, Lipinski LC, Campagnoli EB, Emiliano J, Meurer EC, Ezemma O, Miot HA, Beltrame FL, Wambier CG. Characterization of the activity of Croton tiglium oil in Hetter's very heavy phenol-croton oil chemical peels. Dermatol Surg. 2021;47(7):944–6.
5. Pardoe R, Minami RT, Sato RM, Schlesinger SL. Phenol burns. Burns. 1976;3(1):29–41.
6. Kligman AM, Baker TJ, Gordon HL. Long-term histologic follow-up of phenol face peels. Plast Reconstr Surg. 1985;75(5):652–9.
7. Baker TJ, Gordon HL, Mosienko P, Seckinger DL. Long-term histological study of skin after chemical face peeling. Plast Reconstr Surg. 1974;53(5):522–5.
8. Larson DL, Karmo F, Hetter GP. Phenol-croton oil peel: establishing an animal model for scientific investigation. Aesthet Surg J. 2009;29(1):47–53.
9. Butler PE, Gonzalez S, Randolph MA, Kim J, Kollias N, Yaremchuk MJ. Quantitative and qualitative effects of chemical peeling on photo-aged skin: an experimental study. Plast Reconstr Surg. 2001;107(1):222–8.
10. Zukowski ML, Mossie RD, Roth SI, Giese S, McKinney P. Pilot study analysis of the histologic and bacteriologic effects of occlusive dressings in chemosurgical peel using a minipig model. Aesthetic Plast Surg. 1993;17(1):53–9.
11. Kaminaka C, Yamamoto Y, Yonei N, Kishioka A, Kondo T, Furukawa F. Phenol peels as a novel therapeutic approach for actinic keratosis and Bowen disease: prospective pilot trial with assessment of clinical, histologic, and immunohistochemical correlations. J Am Acad Dermatol. 2009;60(4):615–25.
12. Stegman SJ. A study of dermabrasion and chemical peels in an animal model. J Dermatol Surg Oncol. 1980;6(6):490–7.
13. Brody HJ. The phenol-croton oil peel was originally investigated in the 1980s. Aesthet Surg J. 2009;29(5):446.
14. Lemes BM, da Silva JA, Lin EM, Capote ACMO, Neves AKL, Machinski I, Pereira AV, Koga AY, Lipinski LC, Beltrame FL, Miot HA, Wambier CG. The effects of 35% trichloroacetic acid–croton oil and 35% glycolic acid–croton oil compared with 35% phenol–croton oil Hetter's very heavy formula for deep chemical peel. J Am Acad Dermatol. 2022;87(5):1227–9.
15. Vagotis FL, Brundage SR. Histologic study of dermabrasion and chemical peel in an animal model after pretreatment with Retin-A. Aesthetic Plast Surg. 1995;19(3):243–6.
16. Brown AM, Kaplan LM, Brown ME. Phenol-induced histological skin changes: hazards, technique, and uses. Br J Plast Surg. 1960;13:158–69.
17. Schwartz L, Peck SM. Cosmetics and dermatitis. New York: Paul B. Hoeber; 1946. p. 29–60.
18. MBC M, Mirza FN, Steiner D, Ribeiro F, Landau M, Marçon C, Celidonio TC, Soon SL, Wambier CG, International Peeling Society. Comparative long-term efficacy of phenol-croton

oil chemical peels for persistent melasma at varied *Croton tiglium* oil concentrations. J Am Acad Dermatol. 2024;91(2):336–8.

19. Mao G, Douglas D, Prajapati M, Janardhanam Raghavendra Rao T, Zheng H, Zhao C, Billack B. Investigation of inflammatory mechanisms induced by croton oil in mouse ear. Curr Res Toxicol. 2024;7:100184.

8 Technical Protocols of the Phenol–Croton Oil Peel: Skin and Patient Preparation, Safety, Application, and Post-treatment Care

8.1 Introduction

The safe and effective performance of phenol–croton peel requires a meticulous approach, grounded in standardized technical protocols and a precise understanding of each procedural step. The final outcome, in terms of both efficacy and safety, is directly influenced by the quality of pre-peel skin preparation, careful patient selection, application technique, and appropriate post-procedure management.

While the formulation of the solution determines the depth of penetration and tissue response, clinical experience demonstrates that technical factors such as uniformity of application, control of the amount applied per area, and adherence to safe intervals between regions are equally critical for predictable results and reduction of systemic risks.

Standardization of skin preparation, combined with patient education and conditioning in the weeks preceding the procedure, helps to optimize tissue regeneration and minimize complications such as dyschromia and scarring. Likewise, precise technical execution, together with well-managed post-treatment care, ensures a faster healing process with superior aesthetic and functional outcomes.

This chapter systematically describes the fundamental steps for performing phenol–croton peel, covering pre-procedure patient preparation, skin preparation on the day of the procedure, application technique, and immediate and late post-treatment management. Complications and their management will be addressed in a dedicated chapter, allowing this section to remain focused on technical execution.

8.2 Patient Preparation

8.2.1 Pre-procedure Clinical and Laboratory Assessment

The success and safety of phenol–croton peel depend on rigorous, multifactorial screening that goes beyond the simple exclusion of absolute contraindications.

C. Marçon, C. Wambier, *Phenol-Croton Oil Peel*,
https://doi.org/10.1007/978-3-032-25993-6_8

Assessment should consider not only skin health, but also systemic condition, medical history, and the patient's behavioral profile, identifying factors that may influence the depth of solution penetration, the intensity of the inflammatory response, the quality of healing, and the risk of systemic toxicity.

This is an integrative process in which anatomical and functional aspects of the skin, physiological and laboratory parameters, medication history, emotional profile, social support, logistical conditions, and alignment between expectations and realistic therapeutic possibilities are all analyzed together. The aim is to fully understand the biological and psychosocial context in which the intervention will take place.

Clinical assessment should include a targeted medical history, covering cardiovascular, hepatic, renal, respiratory, immunological and psychiatric backgrounds, as well as careful review of current medications to detect potential interactions that could increase the risk of arrhythmias, bleeding or impaired healing. Detailed skin inspection should consider phototype, skin thickness, integrity of the epidermal barrier, presence of previous scars, and identification of areas anatomically more susceptible to complications. It is also essential to assess the social support network and psychological preparedness, ensuring the patient is able to adhere to pre- and post-operative instructions.

In the dermatological examination, morphofunctional analysis should integrate thorough inspection and palpation and, where available, objective tools such as high-frequency ultrasound or digital optical analysis. Skin thickness and dermal density are decisive factors: thin, atrophic skin is at greater risk of excessive penetration, dyschromia, ulceration and atrophic scarring, while thick, sebaceous skin may show irregular penetration, heterogeneous frosting and a less predictable inflammatory response. Regional variations require special attention—lower eyelids (risk of retraction, ectropion and ulceration), perioral region (predisposition to thick crusts and scarring), glabella and nose (terminal vascularization and increased risk of necrosis), and mandibular line (prone to demarcation lines).

Pigmentary risk should be stratified based on the Fitzpatrick classification, adapted for multiethnic populations, by investigating the history of sunburn, ease of tanning, residual post-inflammatory hyperpigmentation, and tendency to develop pigmentation after trauma or procedures. Tools such as colorimetry and spectrophotometry may complement the assessment, determining the functional phototype and identifying areas with persistent post-traumatic pigmentation. Patients with higher phototypes or clinical signs of risk for PIH should undergo extended preconditioning protocols and more conservative application techniques.

Scarring history and previous facial surgeries must be carefully investigated. A history of keloids, hypertrophic scars, or poor wound healing increases the risk of an exaggerated inflammatory response and disorganized dermal fibrosis. Surgeries such as rhytidectomy, blepharoplasty, and rhinoplasty alter vascularization and may increase the risk of necrosis and demarcation; a minimum interval of 6 months is recommended between facial surgery and deep peeling, with contraindication in previously undermined areas.

Facial architecture analysis includes assessment of laxity, volume, and structural balance. Emaciated faces or those with marked lipodystrophy tend to yield limited or unaesthetic results, with accentuation of thinness, while severe laxity and structural ptosis generally indicate the need for complementary surgical intervention to achieve satisfactory outcomes.

Dermatological screening should exclude active inflammatory dermatoses (such as nodular acne, severe rosacea, intense seborrheic dermatitis, facial psoriasis, and cutaneous lupus) and immune-mediated diseases with the Koebner phenomenon, unless there is a minimum of 3–6 months of clinical stability. Vitiligo constitutes a relative contraindication, requiring at least 6–12 months of stability and individualized assessment. Frontal fibrosing alopecia is considered an absolute contraindication, and active infections—viral, bacterial, or fungal—as well as active cutaneous neoplasms, represent formal contraindications.

The functional support of the skin should be assessed by evaluating the integrity of the epidermal barrier, hydration, sebum regulation, microbiome balance, and degree of cutaneous reactivity. Previous use of oral isotretinoin, systemic or topical corticosteroids, acids, or recent peels should be investigated, in addition to establishing safe intervals with other procedures—6–12 months for CO_2 laser, 3–6 months for medium-depth peels with 35% TCA, 4–8 weeks for mild procedures, and 12–18 months between full-face phenol–croton peels.

Systemic assessment should include cardiovascular examination with ECG and QTc calculation (preferably using Fridericia's formula) for all patients, 24-h Holter monitoring to detect arrhythmias not captured on baseline ECG, and cardiology evaluation in cases of abnormalities or high risk. Hepatic and renal function should be analyzed via ALT, AST, GGT, bilirubin, albumin, urea, creatinine, and eGFR. The metabolic and nutritional profile should include fasting glucose, glycated hemoglobin, electrolytes, full blood count, and markers such as zinc, vitamin D, and iron. Serology for HIV, hepatitis B and C should be requested when indicated. Respiratory assessment is indicated in cases of asthma, chronic bronchitis, respiratory sequelae of COVID-19, and COPD.

Medication review is a critical step in the pre-assessment for phenol–croton peel, and should include consultation of reliable databases such as CredibleMeds® to identify drugs with the potential to prolong the QTc interval and consequently increase the risk of serious ventricular arrhythmias, such as torsades de pointes. These include certain tricyclic antidepressants (e.g., amitriptyline) and some selective serotonin reuptake inhibitors (such as citalopram and escitalopram), typical and atypical antipsychotics (haloperidol, ziprasidone), antimicrobials such as macrolides (azithromycin, clarithromycin) and fluoroquinolones (levofloxacin, moxifloxacin), systemic azole antifungals (fluconazole, voriconazole), and class IA and III antiarrhythmics (amiodarone, sotalol). In addition, other medications should be evaluated for their potential to indirectly affect the safety of the procedure: beta-blockers (such as propranolol and atenolol), which may exacerbate phenol-induced bradycardia and mask early signs of cardiovascular toxicity; calcium channel blockers (such as verapamil and diltiazem), which may potentiate hypotension and depression of myocardial contractility; and immunosuppressants (such as

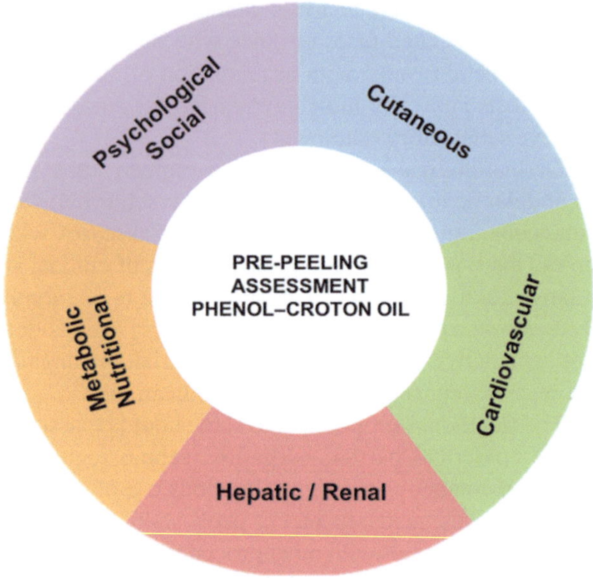

Fig. 8.1 Multidimensional pre–phenol–croton peel assessment wheel. Multidimensional assessment wheel for pre-peel screening with phenol–croton, organized into the following domains: cutaneous, cardiovascular, hepatic/renal, metabolic/nutritional, and psychological/social. (*Source: Figure created by the author (Dr Carolina Marçon)*)

ciclosporin, methotrexate, and biological agents), which impair healing and increase susceptibility to opportunistic infections. The analysis should always consider the possibility of temporary substitution, dose adjustment, or enhanced monitoring, in coordination with the patient's attending physicians, to reduce risks and optimize the safety of the peel.

Nutritional and hydration assessment should identify and correct protein, vitamin, and mineral deficiencies, ensuring adequate systemic hydration. Psychological and social evaluation should investigate dysmorphic disorders, severe depression, anxiety, and unrealistic expectations, confirm the availability of home support in the initial days, and ensure that the patient understands and accepts the required downtime and recovery period (Fig. 8.1).

The final decision to proceed with the peel should result from a comprehensive analysis that balances benefits and risks, considering the possibility of postponing the intervention to optimize clinical or nutritional status, adjust medications, or stabilize chronic diseases. This process, duly documented and formalized in the informed consent, ensures that the procedure is performed only under conditions that maximize the predictability of outcomes and minimize the risk of complications (Table 8.1).

8.2.2 Nutritional and Fluid Preparation

Phenol-croton oil peeling triggers intense protein denaturation and controlled necrosis, resulting in a complex and metabolically demanding healing process. The patient's nutritional status, often overlooked, is crucial for the speed and quality of

Table 8.1 Pre-peel screening: essential clinical and laboratory criteria

Domain	Items to check	Risk finding	Management/ postponement
Cutaneous	Phototype, skin thickness, scars, anatomical risk areas	Very thin or thick skin, atrophic/keloid scars, risk in eyelids/nose	Postpone, adjust protocol or contraindicate in specific areas
Cardiovascular	ECG, QTc, Holter, cardiac history	QTc ≥ 470 ms, arrhythmias, uncontrolled heart disease	Cardiology assessment, clinical correction or stabilization/ contraindicate
Hepatic/renal	ALT, AST, bilirubin, creatinine, eGFR	Moderate/severe insufficiency	Optimize function before peeling/contraindicate
Metabolic/ nutritional	HbA1c, full blood count, iron, zinc, vit D, proteins	HbA1c > 7%, nutritional/ protein deficiencies	Correct deficiencies, optimize nutrition and hydration
Psychological/ social	Body dysmorphic disorders, severe depression, home support	Unrealistic expectations, lack of social support	Refer for psychological assessment and support/ contraindicate

Pre-peel screening: essential clinical and laboratory criteria. The table summarizes the main domains assessed in the pre-phenol-croton oil peel stage, highlighting items to be checked, risk findings, and recommended management. (*Source: Table created by the author (Dr Carolina Marçon)*)

this repair, directly impacting the risk of complications and the durability of the results achieved.

Dermal regeneration following a deep peel depends on efficient protein synthesis for the production of collagen, elastin, and other components of the extracellular matrix; immunocompetence for inflammation control and infection prevention; redox balance to neutralize free radicals generated during the inflammatory phase; and adequate availability of key micronutrients—such as zinc, iron, selenium, copper, and vitamins A, C, D, E, and the B complex—which act as essential enzymatic cofactors in tissue repair processes.

Patients with nutritional deficiencies are at an increased risk of delayed re-epithelialization, persistent inflammation, post-inflammatory dyschromia, and the formation of atrophic or hypertrophic scars. Therefore, nutritional screening should ideally be performed at least 4 weeks prior to the procedure, including clinical and dietary history (with attention to recent weight loss, restrictive diets, vegetarianism or veganism without adequate supplementation, and the presence of chronic diseases), targeted physical examination (assessment of muscle mass, skin turgor, mucous membranes, nails, and hair), and, when indicated, laboratory tests such as full blood count, albumin, prealbumin, ferritin, serum iron, vitamin B12, folate, vitamin D, zinc, and selenium.

Nutritional preparation should preferably begin at least 4 weeks in advance, ensuring adequate protein intake—between 1.2 and 1.5 g/kg/day, adjusted according to age, physical activity level, and renal/hepatic function—supplementation of critical micronutrients (vitamin C between 200 and 500 mg/day for collagen synthesis and antioxidant function; vitamin A between 5000 and 10,000 IU/day, in the absence of contraindications, for epithelial differentiation; vitamin D with a target 25-OH level between 30 and 40 ng/mL for immunomodulation; zinc between 8 and 11 mg/day and copper 0.9 mg/day as cofactors for collagen synthesis; selenium 55 μg/day for antioxidant defense), systemic hydration adjusted to body weight (approximately 35 mL/kg/day, considering renal function and clinical conditions), and strict glycemic control, with HbA1c below 7% to optimize wound healing and reduce infection risk.

In addition to adequate intake of macronutrients and micronutrients, optimizing systemic hydration in the days preceding phenol–croton oil peeling is essential to maintain renal perfusion, reduce the risk of acute kidney injury, and promote optimal wound healing. Studies indicate that patients who are dehydrated preoperatively have a higher incidence of postoperative acute kidney injury, even in non-renal surgeries, with up to a fourfold increased risk compared to adequately hydrated individuals. This effect is related to reduced renal blood flow, decreased medullary perfusion, and activation of deleterious neurohormonal responses, which can be mitigated by appropriate preoperative hydration.

When clinically indicated—especially in patients with renal dysfunction, hypotension, or increased cardiovascular risk—controlled intravenous hydration may be considered in the hours preceding the procedure, always under medical supervision.

With regard to fasting, the updated guidelines of the American Society of Anesthesiologists (ASA) recommend that, in healthy patients undergoing elective procedures, the intake of clear fluids (water, tea, or carbohydrate solutions) is permitted up to 2 h before anesthetic induction. Evidence from randomized studies and meta-analyses shows that this practice does not increase the risk of bronchial aspiration, does not significantly alter gastric volume or acidity, and furthermore, improves comfort, reduces postoperative nausea and vomiting, and contributes to hemodynamic stability.

For solid foods, the recommendation remains a minimum interval of 6 h for light meals (such as toast or fruit) and 8 h for full meals, especially those high in fat, which delay gastric emptying.

However, these recommendations do not apply to patients with risk factors for delayed gastric emptying—such as diabetic gastroparesis, severe gastro-esophageal reflux, use of GLP-1 receptor agonists (e.g., semaglutide, liraglutide, tirzepatide)—or in urgent/emergency settings. In such cases, prolonged fasting remains indicated.

Given that phenol–croton oil peeling is a procedure with higher potential risk, the safest strategy is to individualize management and determine fasting duration in conjunction with the responsible anesthetist, weighing risks and benefits. Thus, allowing clear fluids up to 2 h before should only be adopted when there has been careful assessment and clinical safety is assured.

Identified deficiencies should be corrected on an individual basis, under medical or nutritional supervision. In addition, it is essential to discontinue aggressive hypocaloric diets or prolonged fasting protocols in the weeks preceding the peeling, encourage balanced meals with sources of lean protein, a variety of vegetables, antioxidant-rich fruits, and high-quality fats (mono- and polyunsaturated), reduce alcohol consumption—which impairs hepatic metabolism of phenol and wound healing—and avoid excessive intake of simple sugars, which promote glycation of the dermal matrix.

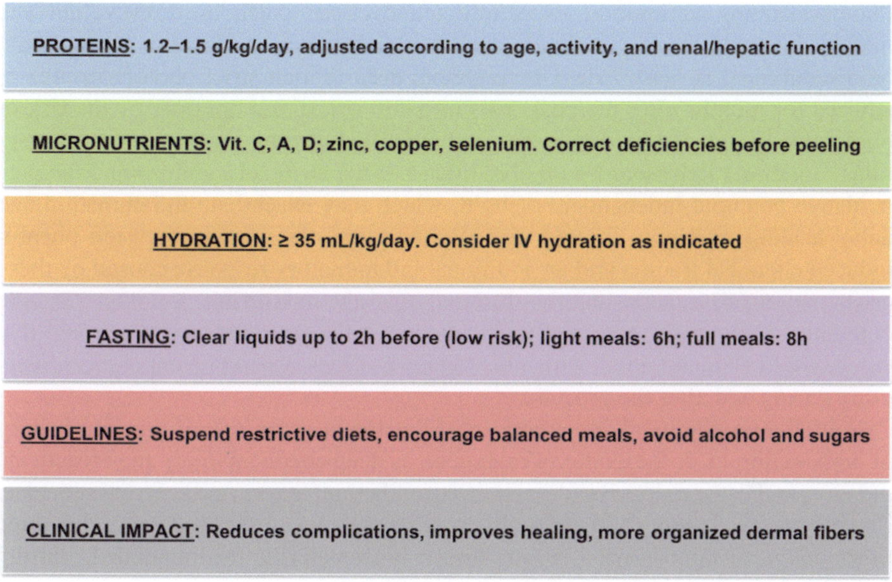

Fig. 8.2 Infographic—nutritional and fluid preparation prior to phenol–croton oil peeling. Infographic summarizing the main pillars of nutritional and fluid preparation prior to phenol–croton oil peeling. The essential axes are highlighted: proteins, micronutrients, hydration, fasting, additional guidance, and the expected clinical impact. Proper preparation helps reduce re-epithelialization time, improve wound healing quality, organize collagen and elastic fibers, and decrease the risk of pigmentary and scarring complications. (*Source: Figure prepared by the author (Dr Carolina Marçon)*)

When properly managed, preoperative nutritional and fluid preparation for phenol–croton oil peeling contributes to reduced re-epithelialization time, less intense postoperative erythema and edema, improved quality and organization of collagen and elastic fibers, and reduced risk of pigmentary and scarring complications (Fig. 8.2).

8.3 Pre-procedure Guidance

In the period preceding phenol–croton oil peeling, certain measures should be adopted to reduce risks and optimize recovery, including the temporary discontinuation of drugs and supplements that interfere with coagulation or wound healing, antiviral prophylaxis, adjustment of topical treatments, psychosocial guidance, and standardized photographic documentation. These measures complement prior clinical and laboratory assessment and are part of the procedure's safety protocol.

The discontinuation of medications that may negatively interfere with the procedure should be planned in advance. It is recommended to stop non-steroidal anti-inflammatory drugs, natural anticoagulants, and herbal supplements such as ginkgo biloba, ginseng, vitamin E, omega-3, and turmeric at least 10 days prior, as all are associated with antiplatelet effects and a potential increased risk of bleeding.

Photosensitizing antibiotics, especially tetracyclines (such as doxycycline and minocycline) and fluoroquinolones (such as ciprofloxacin and levofloxacin), should be discontinued at least 7 days beforehand, even though strict photoprotection is advised for months after the peel. This measure is justified not only by the risk of phototoxicity induced by direct solar radiation, but also by the possibility of reactions to indirect light sources (visible light, intense artificial lighting) and the pro-oxidative potential independent of light, which may exacerbate inflammation and delay healing in deeply injured skin. Furthermore, the overlap between phenol-induced chemical trauma and an additional inflammatory response caused by these drugs may result in persistent dyschromia, unaesthetic scarring, and unpredictable outcomes. Conversely, essential medications for the management of chronic diseases should be maintained, with adjustments as necessary to prevent clinical instability during and after the procedure.

Antiviral prophylaxis is mandatory for all patients, regardless of previous history of herpes simplex or the extent of treatment, as deep chemical injury may reactivate the virus and cause extensive ulceration, secondary infection, and scarring sequelae. The use of valaciclovir (500 mg orally, twice daily), acyclovir (400 mg orally, three times daily), or famciclovir (250 mg orally, twice daily) is recommended, starting 1–2 days before the peel and continuing for 7–10 days.

Continuous use of tretinoin and other exfoliating acids, such as glycolic, mandelic, lactic, or salicylic acid, increases epidermal permeability and may lead to excessive and uneven penetration of phenol, raising the risk of overtreatment and scarring complications. Therefore, it is recommended to discontinue these agents 4–5 days before the procedure. In patients with higher phototypes, hydroquinone may be continued until the day before, provided it is well tolerated, but all exfoliating acids should be withdrawn.

Given the depressant effect of phenol on cardiac electrical conduction, prophylaxis for arrhythmias with oral magnesium may be indicated in selected cases, especially in the presence of QTc $\geq$ 450 ms, concomitant use of QTc-prolonging drugs, a history of arrhythmias, or high cardiovascular risk. Although there are no specific studies in the context of chemical peels, evidence from cardiac surgery demonstrates that magnesium, administered orally or intravenously, reduces the incidence of postoperative arrhythmias by stabilizing the cell membrane and modulating myocardial electrical conduction. When indicated, elemental magnesium 400 mg may be given orally two to three times daily, starting 2–3 days before and continuing up to 5 days after the procedure, always with prior cardiological assessment and avoiding use in cases of moderate to severe renal insufficiency or untreated advanced heart block.

Psychosocial guidance is an essential part of preparation. The patient should be clearly informed about the postoperative characteristics, including the need for social and work withdrawal for up to 15 days, the presence of significant edema, intense erythema, and crusting in the first days, as well as the possibility of persistent residual erythema for weeks or months. Photographs of different stages of the process should be shown to align expectations. The family or support network should also be prepared to assist with hygiene, nutrition, medication administration, and emotional support in the initial days. Therapeutic success depends not only on the technique applied but also on the patient's active collaboration in following instructions, attending follow-up appointments, and promptly reporting any unusual symptoms.

Standardized photographic documentation is mandatory for both clinical and ethical/medico-legal purposes. It should be performed in an environment with uniform lighting, a neutral background, and controlled color temperature, recording the patient in frontal, oblique, and profile projections, always at the same camera distance and height. It is essential in the immediate pre-procedure period and at all follow-up visits to monitor progress, complications, and outcomes.

The Informed Consent Form (ICF) must be specific for phenol-croton oil peel, covering the nature and depth of the procedure, local and systemic risks, including serious adverse events such as arrhythmias and toxicity, available therapeutic alternatives, and the estimated recovery time with its temporary limitations. It must be signed by both patient and physician, filed in the medical record, and, whenever possible, accompanied by illustrative images to aid understanding (Table 8.2).

Table 8.2 Pre-procedure guidance for phenol-croton oil peel

Domain	Conduct	Practical example	Suspension/ initiation period	Remarks
Discontinuation of drugs/ supplements	Discontinue anti-inflammatories, natural anticoagulants, herbal medicines, and photosensitizing antibiotics	Aspirin, ginkgo biloba, turmeric, vitamin E, doxycycline	7–10 days prior	Risk of bleeding, phototoxicity, or exacerbated inflammation
Antiviral prophylaxis	Start antivirals regardless of herpes history	Valaciclovir 500 mg every 12 h	1–2 days before until 7–10 days after	Reduces risk of ulceration and scarring
Discontinuation of topical acids	Discontinue tretinoin and alpha-hydroxy acids	Tretinoin, glycolic, lactic, mandelic acids	4–5 days prior	Hydroquinone may be continued until the day before in higher phototypes
Antiarrhythmic prophylaxis (when indicated)	Start oral magnesium in selected cases	Elemental magnesium 400 mg PO	2–3 days before until 5 days after	Assess cardiac function
Psychosocial guidance	Align expectations and prepare support network	Pre- and post-procedure comparative photographs	Up to 2 weeks prior	Reinforce initial social/ occupational withdrawal
Photographic documentation	Record using a standardized protocol	Frontal, profile, and oblique projections	Immediately pre-procedure	Essential for follow-up and ethical-legal aspects
Informed consent	Signature of specific informed consent form	Risks, alternatives, recovery time	Before the procedure	Show illustrative images when possible

Pre-procedure guidance for phenol-croton oil peeling. Summary of the main preparatory measures adopted before the procedure, with practical examples, recommended timeframes, and relevant clinical notes. (*Source: Table prepared by the author (Dr Carolina Marçon)*)

8.4 Skin Preparation: *Skin Conditioning*

Skin conditioning, or pre-peel cutaneous preparation, is a fundamental step to optimize the uniform penetration of the phenol-croton oil solution, reduce the risk of complications, and accelerate healing. This approach goes far beyond the isolated use of retinoids or depigmenting agents: it involves reconstruction of the cutaneous bed and active modulation of the inflammatory microenvironment and extracellular matrix, preparing the skin to respond more efficiently and predictably to controlled chemical injury.

From a pathophysiological perspective, cutaneous preparation acts in an integrated manner across four complementary axes. The first is the clearance of senescent and fragmented extracellular matrix (ECM), removing by-products that disrupt cell-matrix cross-talk, such as collagen and elastin fragments, oxidized proteins, and advanced glycation end products (AGEs). By reducing this "molecular noise," mechanochemical signaling between keratinocytes, fibroblasts, and the ECM is restored, promoting cell adhesion, orderly migration, and synthesis of new structural polymers. This process also includes the removal of brittle elastic fibers, such as fragmented fibrillin, and gelatinous collagen aggregates that hinder fibrillar alignment.

The second axis is the stimulation of autophagy and enhancement of macrophage efficiency, with potentiation of cellular recycling pathways (autophagy/lipophagy) and phagocytosis of protein and lipid debris. This modulation reduces the burden of damage-associated molecular patterns (DAMPs), which perpetuate inflammasomes such as NLRP3, resulting in less sustained sterile inflammation, improved debris clearance, and a microenvironment more conducive to tissue repair.

The third axis involves optimizing the inflammatory response with regulated transition via interleukin-6 (IL-6), promoting sufficient initial activation (IL-6, TNF-α) for clearance and defense, followed by an early shift towards a resolving profile, with M2/Th2 polarization and increased IL-10. This modulation shortens the effective inflammatory phase, reduces edema and induration, limits disorganized fibrosis, and accelerates the proliferative and remodeling phases, resulting in improved scar quality.

The fourth axis is the functional reactivation of fibroblasts and restoration of dermal architecture, with recovery of the elongated morphology and mechanosensitivity of these cells, which lose their rounded senescent phenotype. This leads to increased neocollagenesis—with long, well-oriented fibers—and mature elastogenesis, with a "chandelier" architecture. The dermis thus regains its capacity to support rapid re-epithelialization, maintain the newly synthesized matrix, and provide more stable and natural results after peeling.

Histological and clinical studies reinforce the benefits of this strategy. Biopsies after 2–3 weeks of formulations containing matrikine peptides, antioxidants, and phosphatidylserine show up to a 30% increase in superficial collagen and up to 90% in elastin, epidermal thickening, and restoration of the basal layer with viable cuboidal cells. In clinical trials, in the context of ablative and fractional resurfacing, preconditioning reduced epithelialization time, erythema, and immediate post-procedural pain, with improved texture and uniformity at 84 days. In surgeries such as blepharoplasty and rhytidoplasty, the preconditioned side showed longer, less fragmented elastic fibers and reduced solar elastosis in biopsies taken during the procedure.

Key active ingredients involved in skin conditioning include matrikine peptides, such as palmitoyl tripeptide-1, which stimulates type I and III collagen synthesis and promotes fibrillar organization, and palmitoyl hexapeptide-12, which stimulates elastogenesis via TGF-β3 and improves the elastic properties of the dermis. Phosphatidylserine facilitates autophagy and phagocytosis of ECM debris, while antioxidants reduce oxidative stress, protect intact collagen, and limit glycation. Niacinamide and hyaluronic acid contribute to barrier function restoration and skin hydration. Retinoids, such as tretinoin 0.05–0.1%, increase epidermal turnover and receptivity to phenol, and hydroquinone (2–4%) is indicated in phototypes III and IV to prevent post-inflammatory hyperpigmentation.

In clinical practice, pre-peeling should be initiated 2–4 weeks before the procedure, with nightly retinoid use (5–6 times per week), hydroquinone as indicated and tolerated, antioxidants, matrikine peptides, niacinamide, and physiological moisturizers, always combined with strict photoprotection and avoidance of sun exposure. Post-peeling, for 4–10 weeks, antioxidants, matrikine peptides, and barrier-restoring agents should be maintained, avoiding strong acids in the initial weeks and ensuring strict photoprotection.

Expected clinical benefits include more uniform penetration of the phenol-croton oil solution, reduced risk of post-inflammatory hyperpigmentation and demarcation lines, faster healing with less edema and induration, and improved histological quality of the repaired tissue, with long collagen fibers and mature elastin. Although promising and supported by histological and clinical studies, part of the literature on skin conditioning derives from narrative reviews and industry-sponsored research, requiring that indications be individualized, considering phototype, skin condition, healing history, and pigmentary risk (Table 8.3).

Table 8.3 Pre-peeling skin conditioning: pathophysiological axes, active ingredients, and expected clinical benefits

Pathophysiological axis	Main mechanisms	Recommended actives	Expected clinical benefits
Extracellular matrix (ECM) clearance	Removal of fragmented collagen/elastin, AGEs, and oxidized proteins; restoration of cell-matrix signaling	Retinoids, antioxidants, matrikine peptides	Improved cell adhesion/migration; organized matrix for predictable healing
Stimulation of autophagy and macrophage efficiency	Activation of cellular recycling pathways; reduction of DAMPs and NLRP3 inflammasome	Phosphatidylserine, antioxidants	Reduction of chronic sterile inflammation; more favorable environment for repair

(continued)

Table 8.3 (continued)

Pathophysiological axis	Main mechanisms	Recommended actives	Expected clinical benefits
Optimization of the inflammatory response	Initial activation (IL-6, TNF-α) followed by early shift to a resolving profile (IL-10, M2/Th2 polarization)	Antioxidants, niacinamide	Reduced edema/induration; rapid transition to the proliferative phase; improved quality of healing
Reactivation of fibroblasts and dermal restoration	Fibroblasts regain elongated morphology; increased neocollagenesis and mature elastogenesis	Palmitoyl tripeptide-1, palmitoyl hexapeptide-12, hyaluronic acid	Organized neocollagen and elastin; rapid epithelialization; stable and natural results

Summary of the four pathophysiological axes of pre-peeling skin conditioning, with respective mechanisms, associated topical agents, and expected clinical benefits. (*Source: Table prepared by the author (Dr Carolina Marçon)*)

8.5 Analgesia and Sedation

Pain management in phenol-croton oil peel presents unique characteristics that distinguish it from other deep ablative procedures. During application, pain is minimal, a phenomenon attributed to the intrinsic anesthetic action of phenol, which induces local neural blockade by denaturing membrane proteins and inactivating voltage-gated sodium channels, thereby interrupting nerve impulse conduction in dermal sensory endings and providing rapid analgesia. The low pain intensity during application contrasts with the significant postoperative discomfort, which tends to peak around 30 min after the procedure and lasts on average 8–12 h. This critical period requires effective strategies to ensure patient comfort, reduce anxiety, and enable adequate recovery.

The delayed painful period is related to chemical necrosis and the subsequent tissue inflammatory response, with the release of prostaglandins, bradykinin, histamine, and pro-inflammatory cytokines, which are responsible for peripheral and central sensitization of pain pathways. Thus, the analgesic strategy should address two distinct phases: maintenance of comfort during application—already ensured by the local anesthetic effect of phenol—and prevention and control of subsequent pain, which requires pre-emptive and maintenance measures in the immediate postoperative period.

Numerous pharmacological approaches have been described, including opioids, non-steroidal anti-inflammatory drugs (NSAIDs), and benzodiazepines. An appropriate protocol should balance analgesic efficacy, cardiovascular and respiratory safety, and optimal conditions for intraoperative monitoring. Sedation, when indicated, should provide anxiolysis, perioperative analgesia, and amnesia, while maintaining spontaneous ventilation, protective reflexes, and responsiveness to verbal and light physical stimuli. It should be administered exclusively in a hospital setting, with continuous cardiac monitoring and ventilatory support available.

Routine sedation is not highly recommended, as it is unnecessary during application and may mask early signs of systemic phenol toxicity, such as confusion, vertigo, tinnitus, nystagmus, psychomotor agitation, tremors, and seizures, as well as reduce natural protective reflexes (lacrimation, cough), which are useful for detecting inadvertent exposure to chemicals in the conjunctiva or airways, thus hindering the detection of complications. Sedation also interferes with the patient's ability to follow important safety commands given by the surgeon. Furthermore, several drugs used in this context may prolong the QT interval and trigger torsades de pointes (TdP), especially in predisposed patients, including high-dose benzodiazepines, methadone, high doses of fentanyl, ondansetron, droperidol, and ketamine combined with central nervous system depressants. Therefore, conscious sedation should be reserved for selected cases, conducted by an experienced anesthetist, with hemodynamic and electrocardiographic monitoring. In well-selected patients, conscious sedation combined with pre-emptive intravenous analgesia using midazolam, diazepam, fentanyl, or ketamine in titrated doses, with continuous monitoring, may be considered. The aim should be solely to control anxiety and provide mild sedation, avoiding deeper levels.

The drugs most commonly used for sedation and analgesia in phenol-croton oil peel have complementary mechanisms of action. Propofol is the hypnotic agent of choice due to its rapid induction and recovery, resulting from high plasma clearance and large volume of distribution, providing titratable sedation and anxiolysis, but without intrinsic analgesic effect, which is why it is often combined with opioids. Fentanyl, a potent μ-opioid agonist, modulates nociceptive transmission at spinal and supraspinal levels, offering rapid-onset, short-duration analgesia, with hemodynamic stability and minimal impact on the QT interval, as do its short-acting analogs remifentanil and alfentanil. Midazolam, a short-half-life benzodiazepine, exerts anxiolytic, sedative, and amnestic effects by potentiating the neurotransmitter GABA, and is safe for conscious sedation as it does not significantly prolong the QT interval; it may be combined with dexmedetomidine, an α2-adrenergic agonist with sedative and analgesic properties, provided there is strict monitoring to prevent bradycardia. Ketamine acts predominantly as a non-competitive NMDA receptor antagonist, with a potent analgesic effect even at subanesthetic doses, reducing the need for additional opioids and preserving spontaneous ventilation, and also acts on opioid receptors as a secondary mechanism.

An effective approach to pain management in phenol-croton oil peeling, without the need for sedation, involves the pre-emptive combination of dipyrone (1 g orally or intravenously), ketorolac tromethamine (100 mg sublingually), and prolonged-release tramadol (100 mg orally), administered approximately 1 h prior to the procedure. This combination acts synergistically at different points along the nociceptive pathway: dipyrone exerts multimodal analgesic and antipyretic effects, involving central and peripheral cyclooxygenase inhibition, modulation of the nitric oxide pathway, and activation of endocannabinoid systems; ketorolac, a potent non-steroidal anti-inflammatory drug, inhibits prostaglandin synthesis—key mediators in peripheral sensitization—and provides analgesia comparable to opioids in moderate to severe acute pain, without the risk of respiratory depression; and tramadol, an atypical opioid, combines μ-opioid receptor agonism with inhibition of serotonin and noradrenaline reuptake, modulating descending nociceptive transmission. This multimodal analgesia allows for lower doses of each drug, reducing the likelihood of adverse effects, preventing central sensitization, and minimizing secondary hyperalgesia. Regarding cardiovascular safety, dipyrone and ketorolac are not significantly associated with QT prolongation at therapeutic doses, while tramadol, although rarely implicated in this effect, may cause it in cases of overdose or individual predisposition.

Complementary strategies include loco-regional blockade with 2% lidocaine, which is useful in selected cases but should be used with caution to avoid cardiac toxicity when combined with phenol; and the use of potent topical anesthetics (7% lidocaine and 7% tetracaine under occlusion with a plastic mask), which may increase initial comfort but also raise the risk of cardiotoxicity. Intramuscular administration of methadone at the end of the procedure can prolong analgesia, but it is the main drug associated with QT prolongation, with significant risk even at low doses or with short-term use. Intravenous vitamin C (1–3 g/day) has been studied as an analgesic adjuvant in the postoperative period, with benefits attributed to its antioxidant action, modulation of neuronal excitability, and reduction of central sensitization, leading to decreased pain intensity and lower opioid consumption. However, in the context of phenol-croton oil peeling, there is a theoretical concern that early administration of antioxidants may attenuate the initial inflammatory response, which is fundamental for stimulating neocollagenesis. Thus, when used, it is recommended that it be administered only after the first few postoperative hours, once the inflammatory cascade has been triggered. Additional measures include the use of a fan to promote thermal comfort and reduce the burning sensation during the first 6–8 h, and the application of cold compresses.

The use of systemic corticosteroids during anesthetic or sedative management in phenol-croton oil peeling should be carefully considered, as their potent anti-inflammatory action may interfere with the fundamental biological mechanisms of dermal remodeling induced by the procedure. The inflammatory cascade triggered by deep peeling involves controlled release of pro-inflammatory cytokines (IL-1, IL-6, TNF-α) and growth factors such as TGF-β, which are essential for the recruitment and activation of fibroblasts and myofibroblasts. Corticosteroids, by inhibiting phospholipase A_2 and consequently the production of pro-inflammatory eicosanoids (prostaglandins and leukotrienes), reduce neutrophil and macrophage chemotaxis, suppress the expression of adhesion molecules, and directly inhibit fibroblast proliferation and secretory activity. In addition, they negatively modulate the expression of TGF-β and metalloproteinases, significantly impacting the synthesis and maturation of newly formed collagen. While this effect may be desirable for attenuating edema or post-procedural discomfort in certain situations, it can compromise the regenerative response and, therefore, the final aesthetic outcomes of deep peeling. Thus, in clinical practice, corticosteroids should be reserved for specific cases, such as exacerbated inflammatory reactions or risk of systemic complications, always with a careful assessment of the risk-benefit ratio.

The choice of sedative and analgesic agents should consider the potential for QT prolongation. The most common mechanism of this effect is inhibition of the IKr potassium channel (HERG/KCNH2), which delays ventricular repolarization and favors TdP. The risk increases with pro-arrhythmic polypharmacy, genetic predisposition, electrolyte disturbances, bradycardia, and the use of tricyclic antidepressants, first-generation antihistamines, macrolides, and fluoroquinolones. Among general anesthetics, volatile agents such as sevoflurane, isoflurane, and desflurane prolong the QT interval modestly and reversibly, but this is relevant in high-risk patients. Propofol is generally safe and may antagonize volatile-induced prolongation. Etomidate and thiopental have little impact; ketamine does not significantly alter the QT interval but increases sympathetic activity. Among neuromuscular blockers, suxamethonium prolongs the QT interval and should be avoided in high-risk patients; rocuronium, vecuronium, and atracurium have no significant impact. Other potentially pro-arrhythmic oral agents include certain neuroleptics, such as droperidol, whose oral use is rare and restricted in several countries due to warnings of risk for ventricular arrhythmias. Among opioids, only methadone is relevant for QT prolongation, with no significant effect for fentanyl, sufentanyl, alfentanil, remifentanil, morphine, or codeine. Tramadol may prolong the QT interval at high doses. Among adjuvants and antiemetics, droperidol and ondansetron have a dose-dependent effect, while haloperidol, chlorpromazine and metoclopramide have torsadogenic potential. Dexamethasone, scopolamine and aprepitant are safe alternatives.

To optimize safety, it is essential to correct electrolyte disturbances prior to induction ($K^+ > 4.0$–4.5 mmol/L; $Mg^{2+} > 2.0$ mg/dL), maintain normothermia, avoid proarrhythmic polypharmacy, prefer drugs with minimal QT impact, and ensure continuous cardiac monitoring during and after the procedure, especially in high-risk patients.

In summary, analgesic and sedative management in phenol-croton oil peeling should balance patient comfort, cardiovascular safety, and preservation of tissue regeneration mechanisms. The lack of widely validated protocols in the literature underscores the importance of close collaboration between dermatologists and anesthetists to individualize management, selecting drugs with low proarrhythmic risk, employing multimodal analgesia, and maintaining rigorous monitoring during and after the procedure to ensure optimal clinical and histological outcomes (Tables 8.4 and 8.5).

Table 8.4 Multimodal analgesia without sedation: suggested protocol

Drug	Dose	Timing of administration	Key mechanism	Notes (QTc/renal/hepatic)
Dipyrone	1 g PO or IV	1 h before peeling	Central/peripheral COX inhibition; NO/endocannabinoid modulation	Safe for QT; adjust in hepatic dysfunction
Ketorolac tromethamine	100 mg SL	1 h before peeling	Potent prostaglandin synthesis inhibitor	Avoid in renal insufficiency; no significant QT impact
Tramadol (extended release)	100 mg PO	1 h before peeling	μ-Opioid agonist; serotonin/noradrenaline reuptake inhibition	Rare risk of QT prolongation at high doses; caution in epilepsy
Vitamin C (optional adjuvant)	1–3 g IV/day	Start after the first postoperative hours	Antioxidant action; modulation of neuronal excitability	May attenuate initial inflammatory response; use only after 6–12 h
Physical measures	–	First 6–8 h post-procedure	Fan, cold compresses	Reduce thermal discomfort and burning sensation

Suggested protocol for multimodal analgesia in phenol-croton oil peeling, with pre-emptive combination of dipyrone, ketorolac and tramadol, as well as pharmacological and physical adjuvant measures. (*Source: Table prepared by the author (Dr Carolina Marçon)*)

Table 8.5 Analgesic and sedative agents: safety profile in phenol-croton oil peeling

Class/agent	Main mechanism	QTc impact	Benefits	Risks/notes
Propofol	GABAergic hypnotic	Neutral/antagonizes volatiles	Rapid induction/recovery; titratable sedation	No intrinsic analgesia; risk of hypotension
Fentanyl and analogs (remi/alfentanil)	μ-Opioid agonists	QT neutral	Potent analgesia, rapid onset, short duration	Respiratory depression at high doses
Midazolam	Benzodiazepine; GABA-A agonist	Minimal impact on QT	Anxiolysis, conscious sedation, amnesia	Risk of respiratory depression at high doses
Dexmedetomidine	α2-adrenergic agonist	No significant impact on QT	Cooperative sedation; adjunct analgesic effect	Bradycardia and hypotension; strict monitoring required
Ketamine	NMDA antagonist; partial opioid agonist	Does not prolong QT	Potent analgesia; preserves spontaneous ventilation	May cause hypertension, tachycardia, and hallucinations
Methadone	μ-Opioid agonist; serotonin/ noradrenaline reuptake inhibitor	Prolongs QT	Prolonged analgesia	High torsadogenic risk; avoid even at low doses
Ondansetron	5-HT3 antagonist	Prolongs QT (dose-dependent)	Effective antiemetic	Risk of TdP in predisposed individuals
Droperidol	Dopaminergic-blocking neuroleptic	High risk of QT prolongation	Antiemetic and sedative	Restricted in many countries due to ventricular arrhythmias
Lidocaine (regional block)	Sodium channel blocker	Neutral	Regional pain control	Risk of cardiac toxicity if combined with phenol

Main analgesic and sedative agents used in the context of phenol-croton oil peel, with respective mechanisms of action, impact on QTc, clinical benefits, and associated risks. (Source: *Table prepared by the author (Dr Carolina Marçon)*)

8.6 Safety and Environmental Control

The handling of solutions containing phenol and other chemical compounds used in phenol-croton oil peel requires strict safety and environmental control protocols, which are essential to protect the patient, the team, and the environment. Phenol, in addition to its caustic potential and systemic toxicity, is highly volatile, necessitating specific measures to minimize vapor inhalation and prevent accidents. The handling of phenol and croton oil, as well as the preparation of the peeling solution, involves significant chemical risks—particularly phenol, whose toxicity manifests via both cutaneous and inhalational routes.

According to regulatory bodies such as the *Occupational Safety and Health Administration* (OSHA) and the *National Institute for Occupational Safety and Health* (NIOSH), the occupational exposure limit for phenol vapors is 5 ppm, with a *skin* notation, indicating that dermal absorption contributes significantly to systemic load. Given this risk profile, all handling must be performed in a controlled environment with efficient ventilation, using appropriate and complete Personal Protective Equipment (PPE), and following protocols for segregation, containment, and environmentally appropriate disposal of generated chemical waste.

8.6.1 Waste Management and Disposal

The management of waste generated during the preparation and application of phenol-croton oil peel must follow strict biosafety and environmental protection protocols, as established by ANVISA RDC No. 222/2018 and complementary technical standards. All materials contaminated by phenol or other chemical agents used in procedure—such as gloves, gauze, cotton-tipped applicators, absorbent papers used for cleaning spills, and residues present in bottles or containers—must be classified as hazardous chemical waste, Group B.

Segregation of this waste must occur at the exact moment of its generation. Storage should be in rigid, leak-proof, chemically resistant, and properly sealed containers. Identification must follow the orange color standard, bearing the chemical hazard symbol and the inscription "Chemical Waste—Group B," in accordance with Annex II of RDC No. 222/2018 (Fig. 8.3). Final disposal must be carried out by a licensed company, using environmentally appropriate methods and considering the hazardousness and chemical incompatibilities described in Annexes IV and V of the resolution.

In the context of phenol-croton oil peel, the following are classified as Group B:

- Residues of solutions containing phenol and croton oil.
- Contaminated gloves, gauze, cotton, applicators, and absorbent papers.
- Bottles, cups, containers, and reusable applicators that are damaged or cannot be decontaminated.
- Solutions used for cleaning and decontaminating surfaces or instruments that contain traces of phenol.

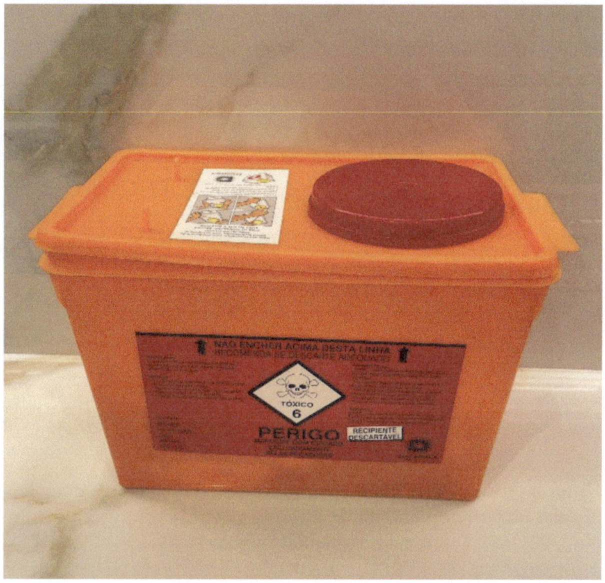

Fig. 8.3 Rigid box for disposal of hazardous chemical waste, Group B, in accordance with ANVISA RDC No. 222/2018. Used for the storage of materials contaminated with phenol and croton oil (gloves, gauze, applicators, containers, and cleaning solutions), properly identified with orange color and chemical hazard symbol. (Source: *Photographic image produced by the author, exclusively for this publication, in accordance with ANVISA RDC No. 222/2018*)

Specifically, regarding bottles, cups, or other containers used for the preparation of phenol-croton oil peel, it is recommended that they are not washed and reused in clinical practice. Both phenol and croton oil have a high capacity for impregnation and persistence on surfaces, with phenol being a caustic and toxic agent with rapid dermal absorption, and croton oil containing phorbol esters with potent biological activity. Even after superficial washing, active residues may remain, posing a risk of cross-contamination, occupational exposure, and instability of the formulation in subsequent preparations. Although chemical decontamination is possible through specific neutralization—for example, using polyethylene glycol 400 or glycerin for phenol—this process must be carried out exclusively in equipped laboratories, with fume hoods, full PPE, and by trained professionals, which is neither feasible nor safe in the outpatient setting. Thus, according to ANVISA RDC No. 222/2018 and good biosafety practices, containers holding residues of phenol or croton oil that cannot be immediately and reliably decontaminated must be mandatorily disposed of as hazardous chemical waste, Group B, in rigid, leak-proof, orange-labeled containers, together with other contaminated materials.

Temporary storage of this waste must take place in a ventilated area, protected from direct sunlight, heat, and sources of ignition, avoiding excessive accumulation. Internal transport should be carried out in secondary containers that prevent leaks and reduce the risk of accidental exposure.

Sharps, such as needles, blades, and syringes, are classified as Group E, according to the same resolution. Disposal must be immediate, in rigid, leak-proof, puncture-resistant containers, compliant with ABNT NBR 13853, properly identified in yellow and placed at the point of generation. When these sharps are contaminated with phenol—as in the case of syringes and needles used to aspirate

Table 8.6 Management and disposal of chemical waste in phenol-croton oil peel

Waste category	Practical examples	ANVISA classification	Recommended disposal method	Notes
Phenol and croton oil solutions	Residual formulations	Group B—Hazardous chemical waste	Dispose of in a rigid, leak-proof container, identified in orange	Do not reuse bottles; risk of persistent contamination
Contaminated materials	Gloves, gauze, cotton, applicators	Group B—Hazardous chemical waste	Place in rigid, leak-proof, sealed containers	Replace immediately after splashing
Containers and bottles	Cups or bottles used during handling	Group B—Hazardous chemical waste	Discard; do not wash	High chemical persistence
Sharps	Needles, blades, syringes	Group E—Sharps	Dispose of in a rigid yellow box (NBR 13853)	If contaminated with phenol: inform the collection team for combined treatment

Criteria for segregation, packaging, and final disposal of chemical and sharps waste generated during the preparation and application of phenol-croton oil peel, in accordance with RDC ANVISA No. 222/2018 and related technical standards. (*Source: Table prepared by the author (Dr Carolina Marçon)*)

components of the formula—the sharps disposal criterion prevails for initial disposal, but it is essential that the team responsible for collection and treatment is informed of the presence of hazardous chemical residues. This enables the adoption of treatment methods that neutralize both biological and chemical risks, such as incineration in licensed facilities.

Proper management of waste generated during phenol-croton oil peel is essential not only to protect the occupational health of staff and patient safety, but also to prevent significant environmental impacts. Improper disposal can lead to soil and water contamination, as well as the release of toxic vapors into the atmosphere, compromising public health and ecological balance (Table 8.6).

8.6.2 Personal Protective Equipment (PPE)

The handling and application of phenol-croton oil peel require the mandatory use of specific Personal Protective Equipment (PPE) for hazardous chemicals, ensuring protection against cutaneous, ocular, and respiratory risks. Phenol is a volatile compound and highly toxic by inhalation, making the use of appropriate respirators essential. N95 filtering masks, although widely used in medical procedures, provide protection only against solid particles and aerosols and are not effective against gases and organic vapors. N95 models with activated carbon may reduce odors (nuisance level) but do not replace the appropriate chemical respirator. Effective protection against phenol and croton oil vapors requires the use of a half-face or full-face respirator equipped with a cartridge specific for organic vapors (OV), approved according to NIOSH (USA) or EN 14387 A1/A2 (Europe) standards. In scenarios with simultaneous generation of particles or mists, a combined OV + P95 or N95 filter cartridge is recommended. The use of these respirators must comply with

OSHA 29 CFR 1910.134 guidelines, which include prior medical evaluation, proper selection and fit testing, staff training, and regular maintenance. In clinical practice, the professional responsible for handling and applying the solution must use a respirator with an organic vapor cartridge, while team members not directly involved in handling may use an N95 mask with activated carbon as an additional measure to reduce odors.

Eye protection is equally essential and must be ensured by safety goggles with side shields or a face shield, certified according to ANSI Z87.1 or EN 166, to prevent splashes and ensure mechanical and chemical resistance.

For hand protection, gloves used must provide proven chemical resistance to phenol, in accordance with EN ISO 374, which classifies protective equipment according to permeation time against different agents. For phenol, the most suitable are butyl rubber gloves (thickness 0.3–0.5 mm) and neoprene gloves, which offer prolonged breakthrough time; laminated gloves such as Norfoil® or SilverShield®, which provide high-performance multi-chemical barriers; and high-thickness nitrile gloves, preferably used in triple layers for greater protection, although they offer limited resistance to prolonged phenol contact. In clinical application, the use of triple-layer nitrile gloves is recommended, fitted over the cuffs of the lab coat to prevent drips, with immediate replacement in case of splashing. When handling larger volumes or diluting the solution, butyl rubber or neoprene gloves should be preferred.

For body protection, the use of a long-sleeved lab coat combined with an impermeable apron made of material certified to EN 14605 Type PB[4] (protection against chemical splashes) or chemical protective clothing Type 3/4 (resistance to jets/sprays) is mandatory, also compliant with ASTM F903 (resistance to liquid penetration). The apron must have sealed seams, back fastening, and adequate overlap between cuffs and gloves to prevent splashes from reaching the skin or clothing, and should be made of smooth, impermeable, and easily decontaminated material (Table 8.7) (Fig. 8.4).

Table 8.7 Personal protective equipment (PPE) recommended for handling and application of phenol–croton peel

Category	Example/material	Level of protection	Practical notes
Respiratory protection	Half-face or full-face respirator with OV cartridge (organic vapors), NIOSH standard or EN 14387 A1/A2	High protection against vapors	Simple N95 does not protect against vapors; in cases of mist, use OV cartridge + P95/N95 filter
Eye protection	Safety goggles with side shields or face shield, ANSI Z87.1/EN 166	Prevention of chemical splashes	Must be worn during all preparation and application procedures
Skin protection (hands)	Butyl rubber, neoprene or laminated gloves (Norfoil®/SilverShield®); triple-layer nitrile gloves	High chemical resistance	Replace immediately if splashed; prefer butyl/neoprene for handling larger volumes

(continued)

Table 8.7 (continued)

Category	Example/material	Level of protection	Practical notes
Body protection	Lab coat + impermeable apron (EN 14605 Type PB[4] or chemical protective clothing Type 3/4, ASTM F903)	Barrier against splashes and skin contact	Apron with sealed seams, high collar, and overlap with gloves

The combined and correct use of PPE is essential to reduce occupational exposure and ensure biosafety. *Note. OV = Organic Vapors.* (*Source: Table prepared by the author (Dr Carolina Marçon)*)

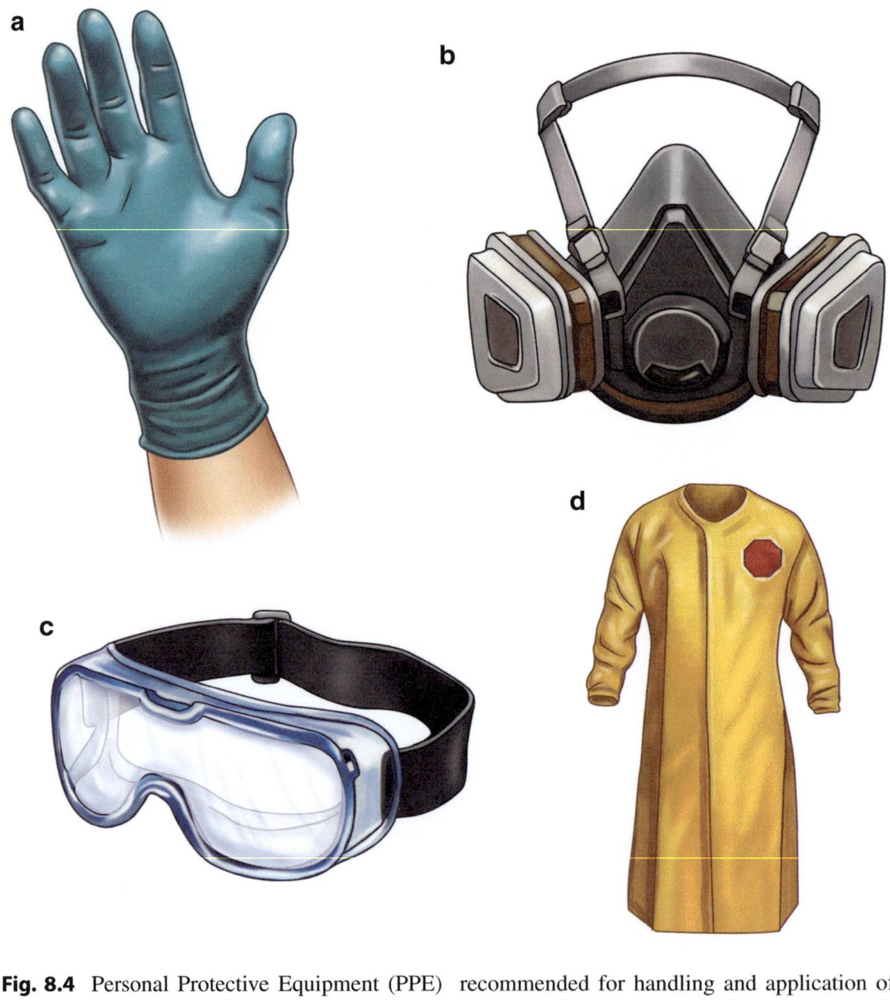

Fig. 8.4 Personal Protective Equipment (PPE) recommended for handling and application of phenol–croton peel. (**a**) Chemical protective gloves (nitrile, butyl, or neoprene), compliant with EN ISO 374, used in layers or of high thickness, resistant to phenol. (**b**) Half-face respirator equipped with organic vapor (OV) cartridges, in accordance with NIOSH/OSHA 29 CFR 1910.134 or EN 14387 A1/A2 standards, essential for protection against toxic vapors of phenol and croton oil. (**c**) Safety goggles with side shields (ANSI Z87.1 or EN 166), providing a barrier against splashes and chemical resistance. (**d**) Long-sleeved impermeable apron, made of certified material (EN 14605 Type PB[4]; ASTM F903), worn over a clinical lab coat, with back fastening and proper overlap with gloves, preventing accidental skin contact. *Illustrative images*

8.6.3 Ventilation and Vapor Control

Phenol is a highly volatile and toxic substance, capable of causing harmful effects both by inhalation and by skin absorption. For this reason, the preparation and application of the phenol–croton solution must take place in an environment with efficient ventilation and strict control of vapor dispersion, in order to keep occupational exposure within the safety parameters established by regulatory agencies.

According to the *Occupational Safety and Health Administration* (OSHA) and the *National Institute for Occupational Safety and Health* (NIOSH), phenol has an occupational exposure limit (PEL/REL) of 5 ppm as a time-weighted average (TWA) for an 8-h work shift, as well as a ceiling limit of 15.6 ppm for up to 15 min, which must not be exceeded. The presence of the *skin* notation indicates that skin absorption contributes significantly to the systemic dose, meaning that even airborne concentrations below the limit may pose a risk if there is direct skin contact.

In practice, 5 ppm corresponds to approximately 19.3 mg of phenol per cubic meter of air. In a 20 m^3 room (for example, 2.5 m high × 2 m wide × 4 m long), this would be equivalent to about 386 mg of phenol dispersed in the environment for continuous exposure over 8 h. This level can be reached quickly in small, poorly ventilated spaces, as phenol volatilizes significantly even at room temperature. The ceiling limit of 15.6 ppm is equivalent to about 60 mg/m^3, and upon reaching this concentration, immediate health risks—such as severe airway irritation, neurological disturbances, and cardiovascular collapse—become critical.

To prevent these levels from being reached, it is essential to implement combined ventilation and exhaust strategies:

- **Local exhaust**: This is the most effective measure for removing phenol vapors directly at the source, before they disperse into the environment. The extraction point should be installed as close as possible to the handling area and kept operational throughout the preparation and application.
- **Chemical fume hood**: Ideal for solution preparation, as it creates a physical barrier and controlled airflow, preventing inhalation of vapors and minimizing environmental contamination.
- **Natural cross-ventilation**: Whenever possible, keep windows open on opposite sides of the room to create a continuous airflow for dilution and removal of vapors.
- **Directional or portable fans**: In the absence of fixed systems, strategically position fans to direct vapors away from the breathing zone of both staff and patient.
- **Ambient temperature control**: Lower temperatures slightly reduce the volatilization rate of phenol, contributing to lower airborne concentrations.
- **Avoid confined spaces**: Do not perform the procedure in very small areas without ventilation or without the possibility of frequent air exchange.

Adhering to these measures ensures that phenol concentrations in the air remain well below critical thresholds, preventing acute symptoms such as lacrimation,

Table 8.8 Ventilation and vapor control

Strategy	Practical description	Notes/reference standards
Local exhaust	Direct extraction close to the handling area, continuous operation	Most effective for reducing vapors at the source
Chemical fume hood	Solution preparation in a hood with controlled airflow	Gold standard in biosafety
Natural cross-ventilation	Opening of opposite windows for continuous airflow	Complementary to mechanical exhaust
Directional fans	Redirecting vapors away from the breathing zone	Auxiliary use, does not replace exhaust
Temperature control	Keep the environment cooler to reduce volatilization	Contributes, but effect is limited
Avoid confined spaces	Do not perform the procedure in small rooms or without air exchange	Essential safety requirement

Technical and environmental measures to reduce the concentration of phenol vapors in the environment during the preparation and application of phenol-croton oil peel, based on OSHA/NIOSH regulatory parameters. (*Source: Table prepared by the author (Dr Carolina Marçon)*)

nasal and pharyngeal irritation, dizziness, and headache, as well as avoiding serious complications from prolonged exposure. More than merely complying with legal and regulatory requirements, adequate ventilation is an essential component of biosafety and the preservation of health for both staff and patients.

The combined adoption of these measures—proper disposal, appropriate use of PPE, and adequate ventilation—significantly reduces occupational exposure, prevents accidents, and ensures compliance with health, environmental, and occupational safety regulations. In addition to protecting the health of staff and patients, these protocols ensure the quality of care and the socio-environmental responsibility of medical practice (Table 8.8).

8.7 Patient Safety

The performance of phenol-croton oil peel, especially on extensive areas such as the *full face*, requires absolute technical rigor and a thorough understanding of its mechanisms of action, potential complications, and preventive measures. It is a highly effective procedure, but carries an inherent risk of systemic toxicity—both from phenol and from *Croton tiglium* oil—as well as local complications that may have serious consequences if not properly managed.

For this reason, only physicians who are trained and familiar with the pharmacology of the substances used, the pathophysiology of cutaneous and systemic reactions, and intraoperative monitoring techniques should perform the procedure. Safe practice demands not only technical skill, but also the adoption of scientifically validated protocols, encompassing everything from screening and preoperative assessment to postoperative follow-up.

Pre-procedure assessment—already discussed in detail in previous chapters—is a mandatory step for risk stratification and prevention of complications. This stage should include a thorough medical history, targeted physical examination, complementary tests (renal and hepatic function, full blood count, metabolic profile, electrocardiogram and, ideally, 24-h Holter monitoring), as well as a careful review of current medications. Patients with a history of QT interval prolongation, arrhythmias, decompensated heart disease, or use of drugs that interfere with cardiac electrical conduction require heightened vigilance.

For full-face phenol–croton peels, continuous cardiac monitoring is mandatory and the procedure must be performed in a setting with full support for clinical emergencies, including immediate availability of cardiopulmonary resuscitation resources. Localized peels, limited to a single cosmetic facial unit, may be performed without cardiac monitoring, provided the patient has no additional risk factors.

In addition to patient preparation, procedural safety is intrinsically linked to other pillars, which are detailed below:

- Adherence to the maximum treated body surface area (BSA).
- Observance of safety pauses to avoid serum phenol peaks.
- Ensuring adequate hydration to facilitate renal excretion of the substance.
- Continuous and prolonged monitoring in indicated cases.
- Use of standardized formulations, precisely compounded and applied by experienced professionals.

Systematic adoption of these measures is essential for phenol–croton peels to maintain a high safety profile and predictable outcomes, protecting patients from potentially serious adverse events (Table 8.9).

Table 8.9 General safety recommendations for phenol–croton peeling

Pillar	Practical recommendation	Rationale
Patient selection	Comprehensive clinical and laboratory assessment (history, physical examination, renal/hepatic function, full blood count, metabolic profile, ECG ± 24 h Holter). Review medications and cardiac history	Identification of cardiovascular, renal and pulmonary risk; prevention of serious complications
Body surface area (BSA)	Do not exceed 5% of BSA in a single session (≈ face + anterior neck). Use the thumb rule for calculations	Direct relationship between treated area and systemic absorption; reduces risk of toxicity
Safety pauses	10–15 min intervals for every 0.5% of BSA treated	Reduces serum phenol peaks, allows urinary clearance and QTc recovery
Monitoring	Continuous multiparametric monitoring if >1.5% BSA or >30 min application; intermittent for 0.75–1.5%; clinical for ≤0.5%	Early detection of arrhythmias, hemodynamic instability and neurological changes

(continued)

Table 8.9 (continued)

Pillar	Practical recommendation	Rationale
Hydration	Oral for small areas (≤0.5% BSA); IV mandatory for >1.5% BSA (ringer's lactate 500 mL pre + 500 mL per 1.5% BSA or 30 min)	Promotes renal excretion of phenol, reduces toxicity and maintains hemodynamic balance
Formulations	Use only validated formulas (Hetter/Baker); certified ingredients (COA/SDS); immediate preparation by the physician	Ensure purity, chemical stability, and dose predictability
Infrastructure and team	Hospital or outpatient setting with full support; multiparametric monitor, AED, airway, oxygen, emergency drugs; physician trained in ACLS	Ensure immediate response to severe complications (arrhythmias, cardiac arrest, respiratory failure)
Emergency management	Clear protocols for CPR, arrhythmias, and decontamination (PEG/glycerin in case of skin contact)	Minimize morbidity in systemic or accidental complications

Summary of the main safety pillars (patient selection, maximum body surface area, safety pauses, monitoring, hydration, formulations, infrastructure/team, and emergency management), with corresponding practical recommendations and pathophysiological justifications. *Note: BSA = Body Surface Area; ECG = Electrocardiogram; BP = Blood Pressure; HR = Heart Rate; SpO_2 = Peripheral oxygen saturation; IV = Intravenous; RL = Ringer's Lactate; AED = Automated External Defibrillator; CA = Cardiac Arrest; CPR = Cardiopulmonary Resuscitation; PEG = Polyethylene Glycol; SDS = Safety Data Sheet; COA = Certificate of Analysis. (Source: Table prepared by the author (Dr Carolina Marçon))*

8.7.1 Recommended Maximum Body Surface Area and Safety Criteria According to the Treated Area

Accurate calculation of the body surface area (BSA) to be treated is a fundamental step for safety in phenol-croton oil peel, since the systemic toxicity of phenol is directly related to the extent of skin exposure.

Limiting the BSA treated in a single session is based on the direct relationship between the skin area exposed to phenol and the amount absorbed by the body. The larger the treated surface, the greater the volume of phenol that crosses the skin barrier and reaches the systemic circulation, increasing the risk of plasma concentrations capable of causing cardiovascular, renal, and neurological effects. The safety threshold of 5% BSA was established to create a margin that allows the aesthetic benefits of the procedure without exceeding the threshold at which absorption becomes dangerous. This restriction also allows the treatment to be divided into staged sessions, distributing the systemic load over time and avoiding peaks in blood concentration—an essential strategy to preserve patient safety without compromising results.

To minimize this risk, it is recommended that no more than 5% of the BSA be treated in a single day. According to the Lund and Browder chart, 5% of the BSA corresponds approximately to the face and anterior neck. Thus, treating the entire face in a single session is, in terms of BSA, close to the maximum safety limit.

Table 8.10 Estimated body surface area (BSA) by facial cosmetic units and the thumbprint method

Region/unit	Approximate % of BSA	Thumbprints	Notes
Entire face	≈ 3–4% (up to 5% with anterior neck)	≈ 90–120 (face) I 150 (face + neck)	Maximum recommended limit per session
Zorro mask	≈ 1.5–2%	≈ 45–60	Includes eyelids, glabella, upper cheeks
Perioral	≈ 1%	≈ 30	Lips + nasolabial fold and chin
Isolated nose	≈ 0.5%	≈ 15	Small cosmetic unit
Full cheek	≈ 1.5% each	≈ 45	Each side
Thumbprint	≈ 0.0333%	1	Method validated by Dargan et al.

Approximate distribution of BSA for different facial regions and equivalence using the thumbprint method, applicable to safe planning of phenol–croton peel. *Note: BSA = Body Surface Area. (Source: Table prepared by the author (Dr Carolina Marçon))*

When the treatment is segmental, the area should be calculated proportionally: the "Zorro mask" (periorbital, including eyelids, glabella, and upper cheeks) corresponds to 1.5–2% of the BSA; the perioral region (lips and surrounding area up to the nasolabial fold and chin), approximately 1%; the nose alone, about 0.5%; and a full cheek, about 1.5%. This proportionality is essential for planning combined treatments and staging sessions, ensuring that the sum of the areas does not exceed the safety limit.

Procedures involving less than 0.5% of the BSA result in minimal systemic absorption and generally do not require continuous cardiac monitoring, except in patients with comorbidities or those taking drugs that prolong the QTc interval. Interventions between 0.75% and 1.5% require closer surveillance, which may include venous access and intermittent monitoring. When the treated area exceeds 1.5% of the BSA, or the application time exceeds 30 min, continuous multiparametric monitoring becomes mandatory, along with intravenous hydration and safety pauses (Table 8.10).

8.7.1.1 Thumbprint Method

To measure small skin areas practically and accurately, Dargan et al. proposed using the thumb pulp as a unit of measurement: each print corresponds, on average, to 0.0333% of the BSA (1/30 of 1%). A whole adult hand is equivalent to about 2.66% of the BSA (80 prints), with the palmar surface alone representing 0.5% of the BSA (15 prints).

Wambier and King applied this concept to the scalp, demonstrating that the thumb projection corresponds to approximately 1% of its total surface area. Although originally intended for alopecia, the method is perfectly adaptable to aesthetic dermatology, allowing precise mapping and planning for facial areas as well.

In the adaptation for phenol–croton peel, each cosmetic unit can be "mapped" by thumbprints, converting the total obtained into a percentage of the BSA. For example, an area accommodating 30 prints is equivalent to 1% of the BSA; treatment of both cheeks and the perioral region, totaling 150 prints, corresponds to about 4% of the BSA.

Rajan and Bhardwaj highlight that thumb size varies with age, sex, and body habitus, which may lead to over- or underestimation of the actual area. For greater accuracy, it is recommended to use the patient's own thumb, analogous to burn calculations, where the palm represents 1% of the individual's BSA. The print template can be recorded and reused in subsequent consultations, ensuring objective documentation.

8.7.1.2 BSA Stratification and Operational Protocols

Stratifying the procedure by treated BSA allows alignment of expected risk with safety measures, standardizing protocols and reducing technical variability. A maximum limit of 5% of the BSA per session is adopted (≈ face + anterior neck). For practical estimates: 1 print = 0.0333% of the BSA; 30 prints = 1%; safety pauses every 0.5% of the BSA (≈ 15 prints) (Table 8.11).

Up to 0.5% of BSA (Low Risk)

Examples: isolated warts; guttate leukoderma in small areas; localized alopecia areata; ingrown toenail; small pilonidal cysts; restricted scars; very limited facial areas.

- **Risk:** minimal absorption; systemic toxicity unlikely.
- **Conditions:** outpatient setting with hospital-grade support, with adequate ventilation; oxygen, AMBU, and AED available.
- **Monitoring:** not continuous, except in at-risk cases; record baseline vital signs.
- **Clinical observation:** assess speech, level of consciousness, attention, orientation, and comfort, as well as subjective complaints (dizziness, nausea, palpitations).
- **Venous access:** not required; oral hydration before and after the procedure.
- **Pauses:** 10–15 min upon reaching 0.5% of BSA.
- **Analgesia/sedation:** prefer simple analgesia (e.g., dipyrone/ketorolac tromethamine) 30–60 min beforehand; cryoanalgesia (cold air/fan) and breathing/verbal support techniques. Avoid deep sedation; if there is significant anxiety, use only mild anxiolytics, keeping the patient fully responsive. Avoid thick layers or occlusive topical anesthetics and avoid infiltrations/nerve blocks that distort the facial surface, as this impairs the uniformity of the peel.
- **Discharge:** observe for 30–60 min, discharge only if clinical and mental parameters are stable. Advise on warning signs for immediate return: palpitations, severe dizziness, shortness of breath, confusion, chest pain, cold sweats, persistent vomiting, or sudden weakness.

Table 8.11 Risk stratification and operational recommendations according to the body surface area (BSA) treated in phenol–croton peel

BSA treated	Area examples	Expected risk	Monitoring	Hydration	Pauses	Observation/ discharge
Up to 0.5% (low risk)	Isolated warts, guttate leukoderma, nose, small scars	Minimal absorption; toxicity unlikely	Baseline vital signs; clinical	Oral	Upon reaching 0.5% (10–15 min)	Discharge after 30–60 min if stable
0.75–1.5% (intermediate)	Upper third of the face, perioral region, isolated cheek	Moderate absorption; intermediate risk	Intermittent (BP, HR, SpO_2 every 10–15 min); baseline ECG if at risk	Oral ± IV	Every 0.5% of BSA	Discharge after 60–120 min
1.5–5% (high risk)	Full face, wide Zorro mask, extensive combinations	High absorption; increased risk of arrhythmias	Continuous multiparametric (ECG, BP, HR, SpO_2)	IV mandatory (RL)	Every 0.5% of BSA	Minimum observation 2–4 h

Summary of risk levels (low, intermediate, and high) according to treated BSA, with examples of areas, monitoring, hydration, safety pauses, and recommended observation times. *Note: BSA = Body Surface Area; BP = Blood Pressure; HR = Heart Rate;* SpO_2 *= Peripheral Oxygen Saturation; ECG = Electrocardiogram; IV = Intravenous; RL = Ringer's Lactate. (Source: Table prepared by the author (Dr Carolina Marçon))*

Between 0.75% and 1.5% of BSA (Intermediate Risk)

Examples: upper third of the face; perioral region; periorbital with feathering; isolated full cheek.

- **Risk:** moderate absorption; requires increased vigilance for early detection of toxicity signs.
- **Conditions:** ventilated procedure room, equipped with a complete emergency kit (oxygen, suction, AMBU, AED/defibrillator, supportive medications).
- **Monitoring:** intermittent (BP, HR, SpO_2) at the start and every 10–15 min; continuous in patients with risk factors (history of arrhythmia, use of QTc-prolonging drugs).
- **Clinical observation:** throughout the procedure, assess speech, level of consciousness, orientation, attention, and comfort, as well as subjective complaints (dizziness, nausea, palpitations).
- **Venous access:** recommended; IV hydration is optional, particularly in prolonged sessions or in patients with reduced oral fluid intake.
- **Breaks:** 10–15 min for every 0.5% of BSA.
- **Analgesia/sedation:** multimodal non-opioid analgesia (metamizole ± NSAID if not contraindicated) + cryoanalgesia. Avoid deep sedation; if necessary, use a mild anxiolytic or short-acting opioid titrated by a qualified professional, ensuring the patient remains responsive. If pharmacological sedation is used, consider enhanced monitoring (including capnography, when available).
- **Discharge:** observe for 60–120 min; discharge only if clinical and mental stability are maintained. Advise on warning signs requiring immediate return: palpitations, severe dizziness, shortness of breath, confusion, chest pain, cold sweats, persistent vomiting, or sudden weakness.

Between 1.5% and 5% of BSA (High Risk)

Examples: full face; extensive "Zorro mask"; large combined areas.

- **Risk:** high absorption, with increased likelihood of serum peaks and arrhythmias; requires strict monitoring and immediate response to any signs of toxicity.
- **Conditions:** continuous multiparametric monitoring (ECG, non-invasive BP, HR, and SpO_2) from start to finish; venous access throughout the procedure; mandatory intravenous hydration, adjusted to session duration and clinical status; well-ventilated environment with local exhaust or cross-ventilation to minimize vapor inhalation.
- **Team:** trained in emergency care, with oxygen, suction, AMBU, AED/defibrillator, airway equipment, and cardiovascular support drugs immediately available.
- **Clinical observation:** continuously monitor speech, level of consciousness, attention, orientation, and comfort, as well as subjective symptoms such as dizziness, nausea, palpitations, or sudden malaise, which may indicate early toxicity.
- **Breaks:** 10–15 min for every 0.5% of BSA.
- **Analgesia/sedation:** prioritize non-opioid multimodal IV analgesia. Avoid long-acting opioids and deep sedation. If sedation is essential, maintain minimal to

moderate sedation, with a dedicated professional for airway management, capnography, and targets of a responsive and communicative patient. Avoid infiltrations/blocks that alter perfusion or distort the surface; maintain continuous cryoanalgesia.
- **Discharge:** minimum observation of 2–4 h, which may be extended depending on clinical status and treated area; discharge only if clinical and mental stability are maintained. Advise on warning signs for immediate return: palpitations, chest pain, shortness of breath, severe dizziness, confusion, cold sweats, persistent vomiting, sudden weakness, or any sudden change in general condition.

General Recommendations
- Always use the patient's thumb to estimate areas.
- Record in the medical notes the number of applications, treated areas, and total application time.
- Never speed up the application on large areas; adhere to scheduled breaks.
- Review medications and avoid combinations that prolong QTc.
- Explain to the patient the rationale for the BSA limit and document consent.
- Stagger sessions when the total area exceeds 5%, prioritizing regions with the greatest benefit.

Classification by BSA provides an objective model for decision-making, anchoring practice in measurable parameters (fingerprints, time, breaks) and linking each treated area range to proportional safety measures. This approach supports responsible execution of phenol-croton oil peeling, preserving efficacy and minimizing systemic risks (Fig. 8.5).

8.7.2 Safety Pauses

Safety pauses consist of a planned interruption of the procedure for a period of 10–15 min after treating each 0.5% of the total body surface area (BSA), or after each equivalent cosmetic unit. This practice is supported by physiological and pharmacokinetic evidence and is recognized as an essential measure to reduce systemic toxicity during phenol-croton oil peel procedures.

The purpose of these pauses is to allow partial elimination of phenol absorbed through the skin, predominantly via the urinary route, before application to a new area. During this interval, significant plasma clearance of the substance occurs, attenuating serum peaks and reducing the risk of cardiovascular, renal, and neurological adverse effects. In addition, the pause allows the transient prolongation of the QTc interval induced by phenol to return to baseline before the procedure continues, minimizing the likelihood of ventricular arrhythmias. This approach is particularly important in patients with a history of cardiac conduction disorders, those taking QTc-prolonging medications, or those with increased cardiovascular vulnerability.

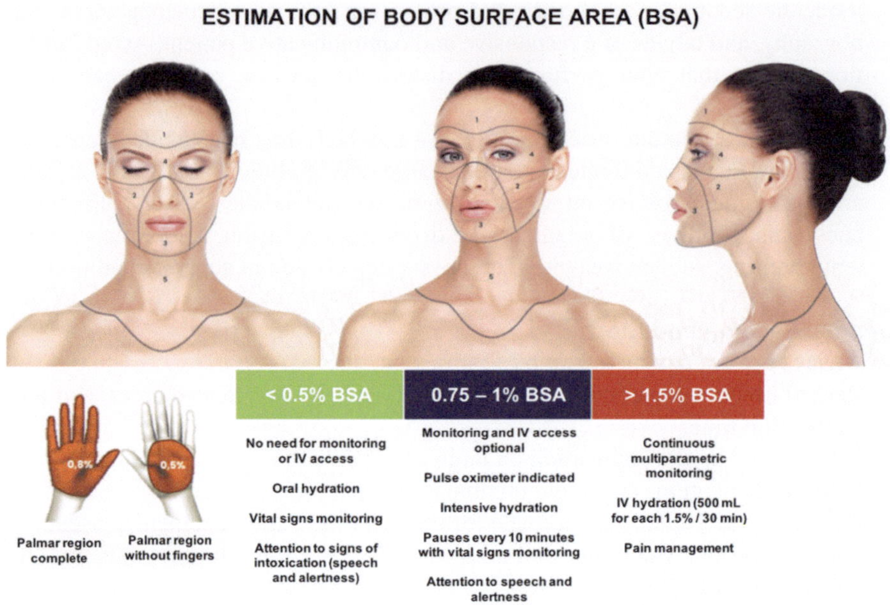

Fig. 8.5 Division of the face into five cosmetic units for segmented and intervalled application of phenol-croton oil peel, ensuring procedural safety. Each unit represents 0.5–1.5% of total body surface area (BSA). The entire face plus the portion of the anterior neck represent 5% of the BSA. The perioral region with feathering to the cheek accounts for 1% of BSA, and the periocular region ("Zorro Mask") for 1.5% of BSA. For procedures involving more than 1.5% of BSA, the patient must be monitored with multiparametric monitoring, safety pauses must be strictly observed, and intravenous hydration should be instituted. (*Source: Photos: Valua Vitaly. Editing and illustration: Ednei Ramos*)

In minor procedures involving up to 0.5% of BSA, a single safety pause at the end of this area already provides a high degree of safety, often allowing continuous multiparametric monitoring to be omitted—although it may still be used in selected patients, at the clinician's discretion.

The absence of scheduled pauses in extensive areas increases the risk of plasma phenol accumulation and cardiac electrical instability. This risk has been well documented by several authors. Truppman and Ellenby demonstrated that procedures performed in less than 30 min and involving 50% or more of the facial area treated were strongly associated with the development of arrhythmias, regardless of the formulation used. Gross observed that 30% of 54 patients undergoing rapid application developed arrhythmias, highlighting that fractionating the application, with intervals for metabolism and excretion, appeared to substantially reduce the risk. Beeson identified arrhythmias in 10 of 43 patients undergoing deep peels, including premature ventricular contractions, bigeminy, paroxysmal atrial tachycardia, and ventricular tachycardia, reinforcing the need for continuous monitoring. More recently, Kadunc and Vanti reported four cases of sustained ventricular tachycardia in 60 patients, even under controlled protocols, concluding that the use of phenol requires strict safety protocols, including scheduled pauses.

The implementation of this measure should be individualized, considering the total area to be treated, the patient's clinical status, the presence of comorbidities, and the estimated application time. Regardless of patient profile, observing a minimum interval of 10 min for each 0.5% of BSA is recommended for all procedures, especially when the total area exceeds 1.5% of BSA (Table 8.12) (Fig. 8.6).

Table 8.12 Safety pauses in phenol–croton peel

Treated area/TBSA	Pause frequency	Recommended duration (min)	Physiological objective	Clinical notes
Up to 0.5% of TBSA	1 pause at the end	10–15	Partial phenol clearance, QTc return	Multiparametric monitoring may be omitted, except in at-risk patients
0.75–1.5% of TBSA	Every 0.5%	10–15	Prevent serum peaks and electrical instability	Important in patients with cardiovascular comorbidities
1.5–5% of TBSA	Strictly every 0.5%	10–15	Minimize risk of arrhythmias and systemic toxicity	Mandatory continuous multiparametric monitoring and intravenous hydration

Recommendations for scheduled intervals according to the treated body surface area (BSA), with a minimum duration of 10–15 min, aimed at reducing phenol serum peaks, allowing urinary clearance, and preventing QTc prolongation and ventricular arrhythmias. *Note: BSA = Body Surface Area; QTc = Corrected QT Interval; IV = Intravenous. (Source: Table prepared by the author (Dr Carolina Marçon))*

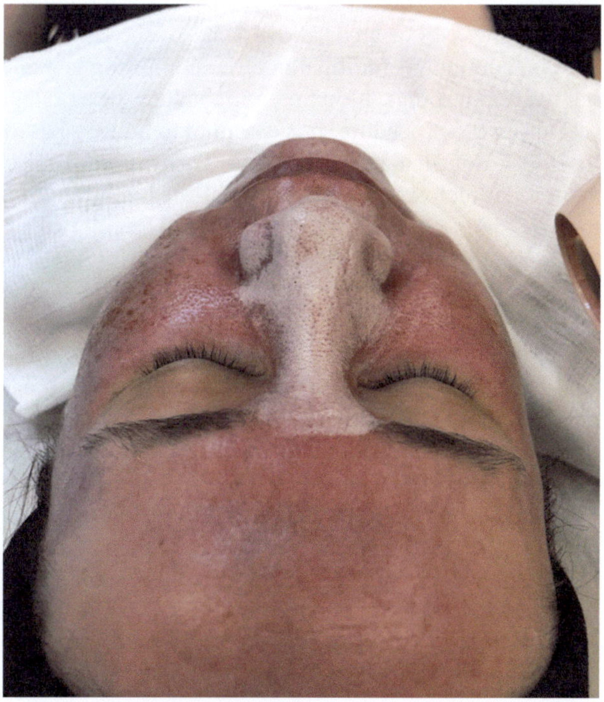

Fig. 8.6 Clinical representation of 0.5% of the body surface area (BSA) treated with phenol-croton oil peel, corresponding to the nasal region. The detail shows the use of a portable fan to provide relief from burning sensation and disperse phenol vapors, reducing their concentration near the patient's nostrils and increasing procedural safety. (*Source: Author's personal archive (Dr Carolina Marçon)*)

8.7.3 Monitoring

Monitoring during phenol peeling is one of the fundamental pillars of safety, as it enables early detection of hemodynamic, respiratory, electrocardiographic, and neurological changes that may precede serious events. The intensity and duration of surveillance should be proportional to the treated body surface area (BSA), total application time, and the patient's risk profile.

Multiparametric monitoring—including continuous electrocardiogram (ECG), blood pressure (BP), heart rate (HR), and oxygen saturation (SpO_2)—is mandatory whenever the treated area exceeds 1.5% of the BSA or when the procedure duration exceeds 30 min. In these situations, systemic absorption of phenol is more significant, increasing the likelihood of arrhythmias and cardiovascular instability. Elderly patients, those on multiple medications or using drugs that prolong the QTc, as well as individuals with comorbidities such as diabetes, hypertension, cardiomyopathies, or depression, require heightened attention and often need prolonged monitoring even after the procedure is completed.

Regardless of the extent treated, all patients should be continuously observed for signs or symptoms of phenol toxicity. This includes changes in vital signs, speech, level of consciousness, and alertness. Ongoing dialogue with the patient is a simple and valuable tool for detecting subtle neurological changes, such as slowed speech, difficulty articulating, or mental confusion.

For procedures involving up to 0.5% of the BSA, clinical monitoring with initial and final BP and HR measurements, direct observation, and, if available, pulse oximetry, is usually sufficient. For 0.75–1.5% of the BSA, periodic measurement of BP, HR, and SpO_2 every 10–15 min is recommended, as well as baseline ECG in at-risk patients. For areas above 1.5% of the BSA or procedures lasting more than 30 min, continuous multiparametric monitoring is mandatory, with constant recording of ECG tracings, blood pressure values, heart rate, and oxygen saturation.

During the procedure, it is essential to know what to observe on the monitor. On the ECG, ventricular arrhythmias (such as frequent extrasystoles, bigeminy, and ventricular tachycardia), paroxysmal supraventricular or atrial tachycardias, symptomatic sinus bradycardia, significant QTc interval prolongation, and conduction blocks should be promptly identified. For BP and HR, sustained hypotension (>20% below baseline), sudden hypertension (>20% above baseline), and abrupt changes in heart rate require immediate investigation. On oximetry, sustained drops in saturation below 94% indicate hypoxemia and demand rapid intervention. Changes in ventilation, such as apnea, irregular or shallow breathing, especially in sedated patients, should be promptly recognized. Neurological changes, such as mental confusion, decreased level of consciousness, dizziness, malaise, or complaints of chest pain and palpitations, are also important warning signs.

In higher-risk patients, the detection of any change, however minimal, should prompt immediate corrective measures, such as extending safety pauses, reinforcing hydration, optimizing analgesia, and maintaining continuous cardiac monitoring for at least 10 min after the end of the application. This step is crucial for early identification of cardiac rhythm changes and prevention of serious complications.

Should arrhythmias, hemodynamic instability, or significant neurological symptoms occur, the procedure must be interrupted immediately and supportive measures instituted according to emergency protocols, including supplemental oxygen, repositioning, fluid resuscitation, and, when necessary, advanced life support.

After this initial surveillance phase, the patient should remain under clinical and multiparametric observation in the post-procedure period, with duration proportional to the treated body surface area. For procedures involving up to 0.5% of the BSA, observation for 30–60 min is recommended; for areas between 0.75% and 1.5%, 60–120 min; and for areas above 1.5%, at least 2–4 h, which may be extended according to clinical evolution. Discharge should only be granted when clinical and mental stability is maintained.

All patients should receive clear instructions regarding warning signs that indicate the need for immediate return, including palpitations, chest pain, severe dizziness, shortness of breath, confusion, sudden weakness, and persistent vomiting.

The selection of a multiparameter monitor for phenol peeling must ensure rapid and accurate detection of cardiovascular and respiratory changes. The ideal equipment should include continuous ECG monitoring with real-time display and the ability to record tracings; non-invasive blood pressure monitoring with automatic measurements at short intervals; and continuous pulse oximetry with configurable audible and visual alarms. In patients under moderate or deep sedation, the addition of capnography enhances safety by allowing continuous monitoring of ventilation. Additional features, such as respiratory rate monitoring derived from the ECG and temperature measurement, may be useful in prolonged procedures. The monitor should be portable, have an internal battery to prevent interruptions, and allow simultaneous display of multiple parameters. It is essential that the device is certified by regulatory agencies (ANVISA in Brazil, FDA or CE in Europe) and complies with electrical safety and performance standards for multiparameter monitors (IEC 60601-1 and IEC 60601-2-49).

This structured and graduated approach to monitoring, combined with the use of safety pauses, is crucial to ensure that phenol peeling is performed effectively and with minimal risk to the patient.

8.7.4 Hydration

Adequate hydration is one of the fundamental pillars in preventing systemic toxicity from phenol, especially in deep or extensive peels. Its role is twofold: to facilitate urinary excretion of absorbed phenol—thereby reducing the systemic concentration of the substance—and to maintain hemodynamic and electrolyte stability during the procedure.

The administration of intravenous fluids before and during the peel helps to minimize metabolic overload and reduce renal toxicity, while also promoting the elimination of phenol via the urinary system. This practice is particularly relevant in prolonged procedures or those involving large areas, where cutaneous absorption is more significant.

8.7.4.1 Choice of Intravenous Solution

Ringer's lactate is the preferred solution for procedures involving phenol due to its balanced composition, which contains not only sodium and chloride but also potassium and calcium—essential for cardiac electrical stability—as well as lactate, which is metabolized to bicarbonate, helping to prevent metabolic acidosis, a condition often associated with systemic absorption of phenol. Unlike 0.9% normal saline, which has high concentrations of chloride and sodium and increases the risk of hypernatremia and hyperchloremic acidosis, Ringer's lactate maintains acid-base balance in a more physiological manner. Although there are no specific comparative studies in phenol peels, the choice of this solution is based on solid clinical and physiological principles, widely adopted in medical practice.

8.7.4.2 General Recommendations (Table 8.13)

- **Segmental procedures involving up to 0.5% of body surface area (BSA):** Oral intake of at least 1 L of fluids (water or isotonic solutions) is recommended in the hours before, during, and after the procedure. This guidance should be initiated in the days prior and maintained in the days following, to ensure adequate hydration and promote phenol elimination.
- **Intermediate procedures (0.75–1.5% of BSA):** Consider the possibility of intravenous hydration in addition to oral, especially in patients with risk factors, prolonged application time, or increased cardiovascular sensitivity.
- **Extensive procedures—especially above 1.5% of BSA or full face:** Intravenous hydration is mandatory. It is recommended to administer 500 mL of Ringer's lactate before starting the procedure and add an additional 500 mL for each 1.5% of BSA treated or for every 30 min of application.

Table 8.13 Hydration recommendations for phenol–croton peel

Treated area/ BSA	Hydration route	Recommended solution	Recommended volume	Notes
Up to 0.5% of BSA (small segment)	Oral	Water or isotonic solutions	≥1 L before, during, and after	Start in the days prior and continue post-procedure
0.75–1.5% of BSA (intermediate)	Oral ± IV	Ringer's lactate	Assess need for an additional 500 mL IV	Indicated for patients with cardiovascular risk or prolonged sessions
>1.5% of BSA or full face (extensive)	IV mandatory	Ringer's lactate	500 mL before + 500 mL for each 1.5% of BSA or every 30 min of application	Multiparametric monitoring; discharge only after clinical and hemodynamic stability

Differentiation of management according to the treated body surface area (BSA), with preference for the use of Ringer's lactate due to its electrolyte profile and protective effect against metabolic acidosis. *Note: BSA = Body Surface Area; IV = Intravenous; RL = Ringer's Lactate. (Source: Table prepared by the author (Dr Carolina Marçon))*

Patient discharge should only be granted after confirmation of clinical and hemodynamic stability. Before discharge, it is essential to provide clear instructions regarding maintenance of oral fluid intake at home and warning signs that warrant immediate return, such as palpitations, dizziness, sudden weakness, chest pain, confusion, shortness of breath, or persistent vomiting. All data related to hydration—type and volume of solution administered, timing, duration, and clinical response—must be recorded in detail in the medical record, ensuring traceability, enabling audits, and contributing to the continuous improvement of safety protocols.

8.7.5 Formulations, Quality Control, and Safe Preparation

It is essential that the physician responsible for performing deep phenol–croton oil peels prepares the formulation immediately before use, following scientifically validated formulas such as those proposed by Hetter or Baker, with a known, standardized, and reproducible composition. Preparation must be the sole responsibility of the physician, in accordance with USP <795> guidelines for non-sterile compounding, reducing occupational risks, preventing errors, and ensuring technical responsibility at all stages.

All raw materials—phenol, croton oil, and emulsifiers—must be sourced from certified suppliers, accompanied by a Certificate of Analysis and Safety Data Sheet (SDS), ensuring traceability, purity, and compliance with current health regulations.

Phenol, which must be of pharmaceutical grade and bear a purity certification seal, should be diluted in absolute alcohol (100%) in a controlled manner. *Croton tiglium* oil, in turn, exhibits high phytochemical variability between different batches and suppliers. Studies using liquid chromatography, mass spectrometry, and HPTLC (High-Performance Thin Layer Chromatography) have shown that many commercial products do not present the same profile of phorbol esters—compounds directly responsible for the depth of action and inflammatory pattern of the peels. Furthermore, stability analyses demonstrate that the oil's composition changes over storage time, with degradation of fatty acids and possible loss of the expected clinical effect (Fig. 8.7).

In this context, the selection of reliable suppliers with up-to-date analytical reports and strict purity control is essential. The current indiscriminate sale of phenol and croton oil, including via the internet and to non-medical professionals, represents a serious public health risk.

The formulation should be prepared in a screw-cap glass bottle, mixed continuously to prevent separation of components, and applied immediately after preparation, minimizing losses due to volatilization and ensuring chemical stability. Regarding the emulsifier, the literature indicates a preference for Novisol®, due to its safety, compatibility with phenol, and its role in emulsion stability, as demonstrated in stability studies of the Hetter formula (Table 8.14).

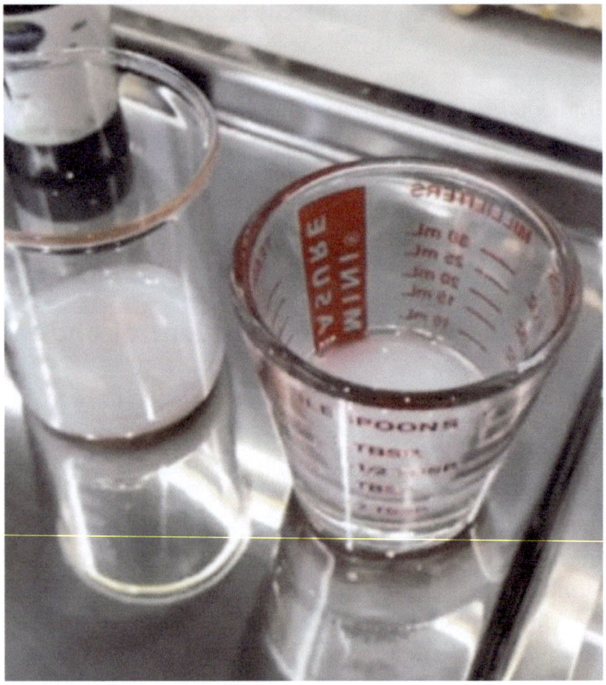

Fig. 8.7 Example of oxidized Hetter solution, evidenced by a pinkish color. The appropriate formulation, prepared immediately before use and mechanically homogenized, should appear white and homogeneous. Color change indicates degradation of components and loss of chemical stability, rendering the solution unsuitable for clinical application. (*Source: Author's personal archive (Dr Carolina Marçon)*)

Table 8.14 Formulations, quality control, and safe preparation in phenol–croton peel

Item	Practical recommendation	Remarks
Responsibility for preparation	Solely the physician's, immediately prior to use	Follow validated formulas (Hetter or Baker) and USP <795> guidelines
Phenol	Pharmaceutical grade, purity certificate	Dilute in absolute alcohol (100%), controlled handling
Croton tiglium oil	Certified suppliers, with up-to-date analytical reports	High phytochemical variability; risk of loss of efficacy with prolonged storage
Emulsifier	Preference for Novisol®	Proven stability in Hetter formulations
Quality control	Technical report (certificate of analysis) + SDS mandatory	Ensure traceability, purity, and regulatory compliance
Storage and preparation	Glass bottle with screw cap, continuous mixing	Apply immediately after preparation to prevent volatilization
Risks of indiscriminate marketing	Online sales and use by non-physicians	Represents a serious health risk and lack of quality control

Formulations, quality control, and safe preparation in phenol–croton peeling. Summary of recommendations for proper handling of solutions, highlighting the importance of medical responsibility, purity of raw materials, and scientific standardization of formulas. *Note: Table prepared by the author (Dr Carolina Marçon) based on data discussed in the text. SDS = Safety Data Sheet for Chemical Products.*

8.7.5.1 What Is the Safe Dose of Phenol for Dermatological Use?

As previously mentioned in an earlier chapter, although the literature lacks precise data on safe cutaneous absorption doses of phenol, several studies demonstrate that its toxicity is considerable at the concentrations and volumes commonly used in dermatological procedures such as phenol–croton peeling. The toxicological literature provides a range for the median lethal dose (LD50) of phenol in humans, varying from 50 to 500 mg/kg body weight, resulting in an estimated dose of 3.5–35 g for a 70 kg individual.

In validated preparations for deep peels, such as the Hetter formula, 10 mL contains approximately 3.5 g of phenol, while the Baker formula contains about 4.9 g of phenol in 10 mL, and an 88% phenol solution contains 8.8 g in 10 mL. Considering that up to 70% of topically applied phenol may be absorbed within 30 min, the absorbed amount would approach lethal doses: 2.45, 3.4, and 6.6 g in 10 mL, respectively.

The presence of ingredients such as croton oil and other additives commonly found in irregularly marketed ready-made formulas, such as olive oil, cresol, sodium salicylate, camphor, glycerin, and soaps, among others, may potentially increase the cutaneous penetration of phenol, exacerbating the risks of systemic toxicity. The total volume of phenol, application methods, and types of dressing are not standardized, representing an additional risk, especially when the procedure is performed by non-medical professionals.

8.7.6 Emergency Interventions and Required Infrastructure

Deep phenol peels must be performed exclusively in a hospital or outpatient setting with full hospital support, fully complying with current technical and health regulations. This includes the availability of equipment, supplies, and a team trained to manage high-complexity clinical complications.

The presence of cardiopulmonary resuscitation equipment is mandatory, including multiparameter monitor, defibrillator, pulse oximeter, surgical aspirator, oxygen supply, oropharyngeal airways, supraglottic devices, materials for orotracheal intubation, mechanical ventilator or manual ventilation system (Ambu®), as well as rapid access to emergency medications (adrenaline, amiodarone, lidocaine, atropine, vasopressors, antiarrhythmics, benzodiazepines, and antagonists).

The responsible physician must have up-to-date training in Advanced Cardiac Life Support (ACLS) and be proficient in cardiopulmonary resuscitation protocols, ensuring immediate and effective response to events such as:

- Ventricular arrhythmias (VF, pulseless VT).
- Symptomatic bradyarrhythmia's.
- Cardiorespiratory arrest.
- Acute respiratory distress syndrome (ARDS) .
- Circulatory collapse secondary to systemic phenol toxicity.

Preparation for emergency situations should include clear protocols and appropriate equipment for immediate decontamination in the event of accidental exposure or excessive chemical injury. Phenol, due to its high toxicity and rapid cutaneous absorption, can cause extensive local damage and potentially fatal systemic effects within minutes of contact.

Initial management should prioritize immediate cessation of exposure, with removal of the individual from the source and prompt disposal of contaminated clothing, shoes, gloves, and accessories. This step must be performed by a professional wearing appropriate Personal Protective Equipment (PPE), including impermeable gloves and gown, to prevent secondary contamination.

Copious and immediate irrigation of the skin with running water should be started without delay and maintained for at least 15 min. However, the low solubility of phenol in water may limit the effectiveness of this measure. For this reason, international guidelines—such as those from the ATSDR (Agency for Toxic Substances and Disease Registry) and NIOSH (National Institute for Occupational Safety and Health)—recommend the use of water-soluble solvents as an additional step.

Polyethylene glycol (PEG 300 or PEG 400) is considered the agent of choice for cutaneous removal, due to its ability to dissolve phenol and reduce dermal penetration. Alternatively, glycerin (glycerol) has similar efficacy and may be used when PEG is unavailable. The application consists of spreading the solvent over the affected area, gently massaging to promote solubilization, followed by further copious irrigation with running water.

In the event of ocular exposure, immediate irrigation with running water or sterile balanced saline solution is recommended for at least 15 min, followed by urgent ophthalmological assessment.

After decontamination, patients with significant exposure should be kept under clinical and laboratory monitoring for early detection of signs of systemic toxicity, such as arrhythmias, neurological changes, or renal or hepatic dysfunction.

The implementation of these protocols, widely recognized by occupational health and clinical toxicology authorities, should be part of the safety routine in services using phenol, integrated into the contingency plan and ensuring a rapid and effective response to serious adverse events.

The safety of the procedure is based on the combination of the following factors:

1. **Careful patient selection**—prior clinical and laboratory assessment, identification of comorbidities, and cardiovascular risk stratification.
2. **Controlled environment**—infrastructure that allows rapid response to medical emergencies.
3. **Rigorous monitoring**—continuous and adapted to the extent and duration of the peel.
4. **Appropriate technique and safe formulation**—handling of substances of proven purity, immediate preparation prior to use, and application according to validated scientific protocols.

Table 8.15 Emergency interventions and required infrastructure for phenol–croton peel

Category	Essential requirements	Practical notes
Environment	Exclusively hospital-based or outpatient with full hospital support	Must fully comply with technical and sanitary regulations
Monitoring	Multiparameter monitor (ECG, BP, HR, SpO_2); capnography if sedation is used	Certified equipment (ANVISA, FDA, CE)
Resuscitation equipment	Defibrillator, oximeter, aspirator, oxygen, AMBU®, mechanical ventilator, complete airway set	Pre-test required; immediate access mandatory
Emergency drugs	Adrenaline, amiodarone, lidocaine, atropine, vasopressors, antiarrhythmics, benzodiazepines, antagonists	Updated stock; doses calculated according to patient's weight
Medical team	Updated ACLS training; mastery of CPR protocols	Emergency simulations recommended periodically
Decontamination protocols	Immediate irrigation with water; use of PEG 300/400 or glycerin	PPE mandatory to avoid secondary contamination
Ocular exposure	Irrigation with sterile balanced saline solution ≥15 min	Immediate referral to ophthalmologist
Post-exposure monitoring	Clinical + laboratory assessment (cardiac, renal, hepatic, neurological)	Keep under observation until stable
Safety pillars	Careful patient selection; controlled environment; strict monitoring; safe formulation; preparedness for emergencies	Structural foundation to reduce severe risks

Summary of essential resources in environment, monitoring, equipment, team, drugs, and decontamination protocols, associated with the five fundamental pillars of procedural safety. *Note: ECG = Electrocardiogram; BP = Blood Pressure; HR = Heart Rate; SpO_2 = Peripheral Oxygen Saturation; ACLS = Advanced Cardiac Life Support; CPR = Cardiopulmonary Resuscitation; PEG = Polyethylene Glycol; PPE = Personal Protective Equipment; CE = Conformité Européenne. (Source: Table prepared by the author (Dr Carolina Marçon))*

5. **Preparedness for management of systemic and local complications**—team training, emergency simulations, and clear pathways for hospital transfer when necessary.

Thus, phenol peeling should be regarded as a highly complex medical procedure, whose success and safety depend both on technical excellence and the ability to respond immediately to potentially fatal adverse events (Table 8.15).

8.8 Application Technique

8.8.1 Skin Preparation and Cleansing

Proper skin preparation prior to deep chemical peeling is a fundamental step to ensure uniform penetration of the solution, optimize clinical outcomes, and reduce the risk of complications. Although there are no formally established universal protocols, both the literature and clinical practice agree on the importance of thorough cleansing and degreasing of the skin.

This step aims to completely remove residues, sebum, cosmetics, and impurities, creating a clean and dry surface that facilitates homogeneous absorption of the peeling solution. Various agents may be used for this purpose:

- **Acetone**—a highly lipophilic organic solvent, considered the gold standard for degreasing, providing rapid and complete removal of surface lipids and making the skin more permeable to the peeling solution.
- **Isopropyl alcohol**—an alternative with moderate degreasing action, which may be used alone or in combination with antiseptics.
- **Antiseptic solutions of chlorhexidine combined with isopropyl alcohol**—such as *ChloraPrep One-Step* (2% chlorhexidine gluconate and 70% isopropyl alcohol) and *Prevantics Maxi Swabstick* (3.15% chlorhexidine gluconate and 70% isopropyl alcohol), FDA-approved for pre-surgical skin preparation, combining antiseptic action with the degreasing effect of alcohol. This combination may be as effective as acetone for removing surface oiliness, although acetone remains superior when complete degreasing is the primary objective.
- **Pure antiseptic solutions based on chlorhexidine**—effective in reducing microbial load, but with limited lipid removal capacity, and should be combined with a degreasing agent when optimizing chemical penetration is desired.
- **Cleansers containing alpha-hydroxy acids or salicylic acid**—recommended as an adjunct preparation for oily or acne-prone skin.

After degreasing, controlled physical removal of the stratum corneum may be performed to enhance solution penetration, using dry gauze or gauze slightly moistened with the degreasing agent, with friction gentle, uniform, and controlled, avoiding excessive trauma that could cause irregularities in penetration and compromise healing.

A crucial point is the complete removal of previously applied topical anesthetics, especially the more potent ones (such as high-concentration lidocaine/tetracaine combinations) used under occlusion with a plastic mask. In such cases, it is essential to remove them entirely—preferably with running water and soap—prior to the application of phenol–croton oil, in order to prevent inadvertent drug delivery and a consequent increased risk of cardiotoxicity.

The choice of agents and steps depends on the patient's profile, phototype, skin thickness, oiliness, sensitivity, availability of supplies, allergy history, and practitioner preference, always prioritizing safety and predictability. Regardless of the chosen approach, complete removal of oil and residues is mandatory, as failure at this stage compromises solution penetration and the uniformity of the result.

The systematic review by Cox et al. reinforces that, although degreasing is widely recommended, robust comparative studies defining the superiority of one method over another are lacking. Nevertheless, clinical experience and international consensus support these practices as the standard for safety and quality.

Although acetone alone is widely recognized as the agent of choice for pre-peel degreasing, some protocols propose its combination with isopropyl alcohol, merging the rapid and deep degreasing action of acetone with the antiseptic effect of alcohol. Despite the theoretical rationale, there is no robust evidence of superiority for this combination in terms of uniformity or depth of penetration in phenol–croton oil peels.

With regard to antisepsis, alcohol and chlorhexidine have distinct mechanisms and profiles. Alcohol (ethyl or isopropyl at 70%) rapidly denatures proteins, providing immediate and broad-spectrum action against bacteria, viruses, and fungi, but with no residual effect after evaporation. Chlorhexidine (0.5%–4%), on the other hand, acts by disrupting the cytoplasmic membrane and precipitating cellular proteins, offering prolonged residual activity—up to 6 h—due to its binding to skin proteins. Evidence indicates that chlorhexidine alone keeps the skin free from bacterial recolonization for longer than alcohol alone, although it has a slower initial action and less degreasing capacity.

Sequential application of acetone followed by chlorhexidine has a strong technical rationale for skin preparation prior to deep phenol–croton oil peeling. Due to its high liposolubility, acetone provides rapid and thorough degreasing, removing lipids, hydrophobic residues, and surface contaminants, leaving the epidermis dry and more permeable, which favors uniform penetration of the chemical solution. However, its antimicrobial effect is limited and lacks significant residual activity. Subsequent application of chlorhexidine, preferably combined with 70% isopropyl alcohol, enhances antisepsis through the sum of distinct mechanisms: immediate and broad-spectrum action against bacteria, viruses, and fungi provided by alcohol, and the prolonged residual effect of chlorhexidine for up to 6 h, resulting from its binding to skin proteins.

Despite these advantages, it should be considered that chlorhexidine residues on the skin surface may interact with the phenol–croton oil solution, altering its wettability and spreading pattern. This interaction may occur either through a physical effect—forming a residual film that modifies surface tension—or through possible chemical interference with formulation components, especially in solutions containing surfactants or lipophilic agents. Therefore, it is recommended to remove excess chlorhexidine completely with a sterile dry or slightly moistened gauze after antisepsis, thus maintaining the residual antimicrobial barrier without compromising the homogeneous absorption of the exfoliating agent.

When correctly performed, this sequence combines maximum degreasing efficiency with immediate and persistent antisepsis, reducing the risk of intra- and post-procedural contamination. Clinical trials, such as that by Darouiche et al. have demonstrated the superiority of the chlorhexidine–alcohol combination over conventional antiseptics in preventing surgical site infection. In more sensitive areas, such as the eyelids, contact with chlorhexidine should be restricted or carefully controlled to prevent irritation or ocular toxicity (Table 8.16).

In the context of phenol–croton oil peeling, this step must be performed exclusively by the physician or under their direct supervision, given its direct influence on penetration depth, inflammatory pattern, and, consequently, the safety and efficacy of the procedure.

Table 8.16 Preparation and cleansing of the skin prior to phenol–croton peel

Agent	Main function	Advantages	Limitations	Practical notes
Acetone	Deep degreasing	Gold standard; rapid and complete removal of lipids	No residual antimicrobial effect	Should always be included in the preparation routine
Isopropyl alcohol	Moderate degreasing + antiseptic	Viable alternative; easily accessible	Less effective than acetone	Can be used alone or in combination
Chlorhexidine + isopropyl alcohol	Immediate antisepsis + prolonged residual effect	FDA approved; efficacy comparable to acetone for superficial removal	May leave residues that interfere with wettability	Remove excess with dry gauze after application
Pure chlorhexidine	Antiseptic with residual effect	Reduces bacterial recolonization for up to 6 h	Low lipid removal	Should be combined with a degreasing agent
Soaps with AHAs or SA	Complementary preparation for oily/acne-prone skin	Helps reduce oiliness and mild desquamation	Insufficient action if used alone	Used as a preliminary preparation, not a substitute

Main agents used in the preparation and cleansing of the skin prior to phenol–croton oil peeling, with their respective functions, advantages, limitations, and practical notes. *Note: Table prepared by the author based on data discussed in the text. AHAs = alpha-hydroxy acids; SA = salicylic acid; FDA = Food and Drug Administration. (Source: Table prepared by the author (Dr Carolina Marçon))*

8.8.2 Marking and Division of the Face into Cosmetic Units

Marking the face prior to deep phenol–croton oil peeling is a critical step, not only to guide the application technique, but also as a safety measure and to ensure predictable outcomes. This step allows the intensity of the treatment to be adjusted according to skin thickness, density of adnexal structures, vascularization, and the photoaging pattern of each region, balancing efficacy and safety.

Historically, Gregory Hetter systematized a facial topographic map based on his extensive clinical experience, delineating zones of tolerance to deep peeling and assigning each a specific concentration of croton oil, decreasing according to tissue fragility and the risk of poor healing. The central logic was clear: thicker areas with deeper rhytids tolerate higher concentrations; thinner, more vascular, fragile regions require lower intensity. Two decades later, Sterling et al. refined this approach by proposing a mapping system coded by depth levels, graded from 1 (deepest) to 6 (most superficial), and subdivided into smaller cosmetic units. This update incorporated millimetric variations in application, enabled greater standardization in segmental treatments, and emphasized the importance of feathering—a smooth transition between areas—to avoid demarcation lines (Fig. 8.8).

The anatomical and functional logic of this division is based on structural differences in facial skin. Dermal thickness is greatest in the lower perioral region, chin, and nasal dorsum, and lowest in the eyelids and preauricular area. The density of skin adnexa, collagen fiber architecture, vascularization, and photoaging pattern also vary significantly between regions, influencing tolerance and response to peeling. Areas with denser collagen and pronounced rhytids, such as the perioral region

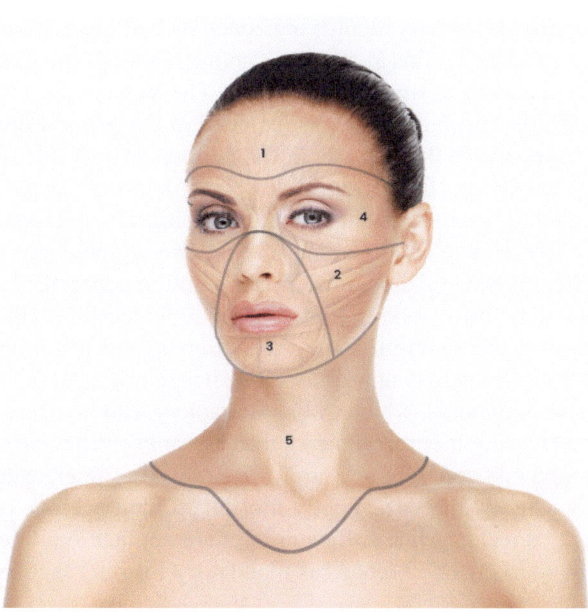

Fig. 8.8 Topographic map of the face for deep phenol–croton oil peeling, based on Hetter's systematization. Division into cosmetic units allows modulation of croton oil concentration and treatment intensity according to skin thickness, density of adnexal structures, vascularization, and photoaging pattern, increasing the predictability of results and the safety of the procedure. (Source: *Photo: Valua Vitaly. Editing and illustration: Ednei Ramos*)

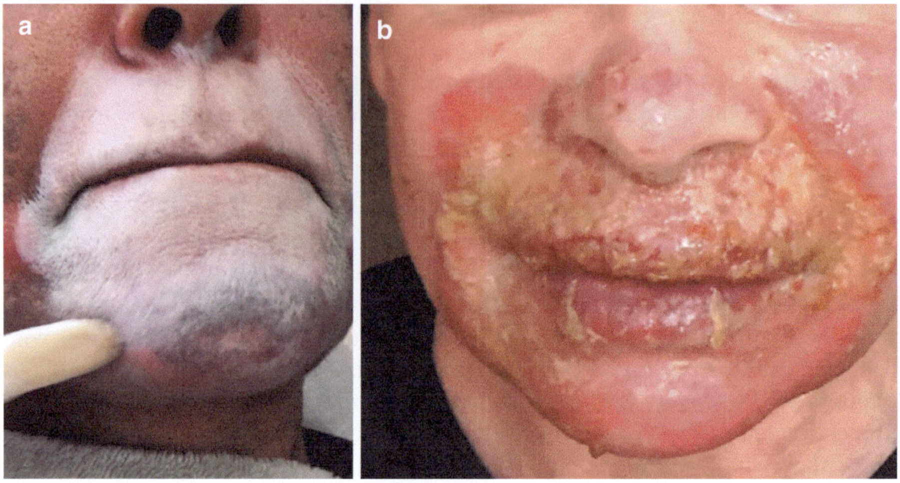

Fig. 8.9 Treatment of the perioral region with feathering towards the cheeks. (**a**) In the first image, solid white frosting is observed, indicating penetration of the solution to the papillary dermis. (**b**) In the second image, clinical evolution on postoperative day 5, characterized by erythema, edema, and intense exudation, consistent with the inflammatory phase of the healing process. (*Source: Author's personal archive (Dr Carolina Marçon)*)

and glabella, tolerate higher concentrations; regions with thin, sensitive skin, such as the periocular area and neck, require gentler approaches.

In practice, marking should be performed with the patient in a seated position; this is essential to ensure correct marking of the mandibular contour region, using a headlamp or surgical light. Cosmetic units are delineated according to anatomical landmarks, clearly identifying zones such as lower perioral, upper perioral, glabella, periocular (eyelids and lateral canthus), cheeks (medial and lateral), forehead, temples, and neck (upper and lower). The nose is not considered a distinct cosmetic unit; the cartilaginous tip is included in the perioral unit, and the bony nasal area is grouped with the glabella in the periocular unit (Fig. 8.9). Transition areas should be marked for feathering, and specific points of deep rhytids or scars may be designated for spot treatment. All markings must be photographed prior to the procedure.

The choice and handling of the dermographic pen during this stage also have a direct impact on the uniformity of solution penetration. Pens with oil- or wax-based ink may form a microscopic hydrophobic barrier on the epidermis, hindering diffusion of the solution in the marked areas and resulting in micro zones of reduced depth, which may appear as subtle irregularities in the final outcome. Even alcohol-based pigments, which evaporate rapidly, can interfere if applied in thick lines. For this reason, it is recommended to use only sterile dermographic pens with alcohol-based ink, applying fine, uniform lines. After degreasing, excess pigment should be removed with gauze lightly moistened with acetone or isopropyl alcohol, leaving only a residual line sufficient to guide application. Photographic documentation of the markings beforehand is mandatory for reference in case of erasure (Fig. 8.10).

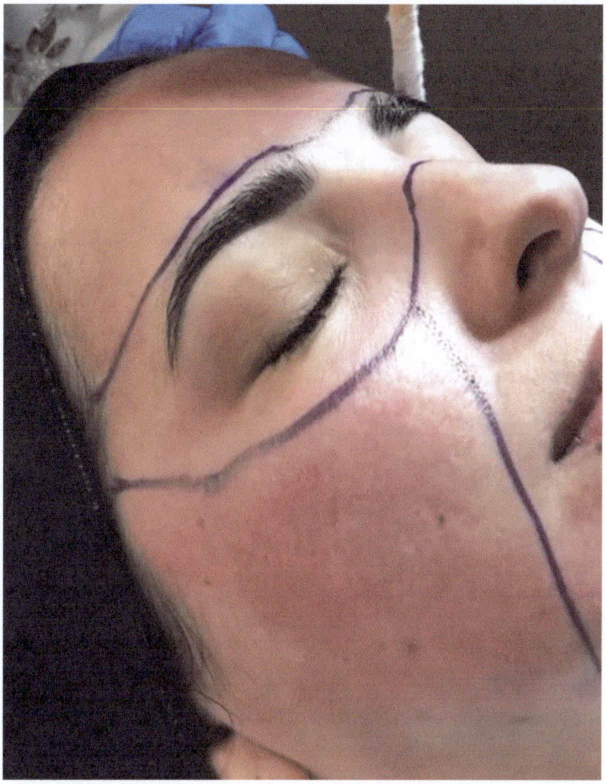

Fig. 8.10 Practical example of facial marking for deep phenol–croton oil peel. The delineation of the *Zorro mask* and other anatomical divisions guiding solution application can be observed, allowing modulation of concentration and treatment intensity according to the thickness and sensitivity of each region's skin. (Source: Author's personal archive (Dr Carolina Marçon))

In advanced protocols, some authors choose to remove all markings before peeling, relying solely on photographic documentation and anatomical knowledge to guide application—an approach that, while eliminating any risk of interference, requires a high level of operator experience.

This division of the face into cosmetic units not only guides the technique but also reduces the risk of demarcation lines, dyschromia, and scarring. It allows adjustment of concentration, volume applied, pressure, and friction time according to the sensitivity and structure of the skin in each area, promoting homogeneous and natural results while preserving facial harmony (Table 8.17).

8.8.3 Practical Application Steps

8.8.3.1 Full-Face Peel

After thorough cleansing` and degreasing, application of the phenol–croton oil solution is initiated. As the preparations tend to separate into two phases about 1 min after mixing, the bottle should remain closed and be shaken vigorously before and during use to maintain a homogeneous emulsion. The depth achieved depends primarily on the technical maneuver: the amount of solution on the applicator, the

Table 8.17 Marking and division of the face into cosmetic units: relative skin thickness, tolerance to croton oil concentrations, and main technical considerations

Cosmetic unit	Thickness/ tolerance	Croton oil concentration (range) (%)	Practical notes
Lower perioral	Thick	0.8–1.6	Deep rhytids; cross the vermilion border slightly; feathering is essential
Glabella	Thick	0.8–1.6	Area of vertical rhytids; requires uniform friction
Periocular	Very thin	0.2–0.4	Higher risk of complications; treat eyelids with caution
Cheeks (medial/ lateral)	Variable (medial > lateral)	0.6–1.0	Good response; attention to transition areas
Forehead	Medium	0.6–1.0	Apply with overlapping passes; careful assessment of frosting
Temples	Thin	0.4–0.6	Scar risk area; treat gently
Neck	Very thin	$\leq$0.4	Avoid high concentrations; risk of dyspigmentation and fibrosis

Facial mapping and division into cosmetic units: relative skin thickness, tolerance to croton oil concentrations, and main technical notes. (*Source: Table prepared by the author (Dr Carolina Marçon)*)

number of passes, pressure/abrasiveness of friction, and contact time per zone are more decisive than isolated variations in concentration. The instrument may be a firm cotton bud, a cotton swab molded onto a wooden stick (chopstick, tongue depressor), or folded gauze; the latter, being more abrasive, achieves greater depth with fewer passes, which is why it is recommended to standardize a single applicator throughout the procedure to avoid inadvertent differences in depth between areas. The procedure is performed by cosmetic units, completing each region before moving on to the next, with an interval of 10–15 min between them; on average, application to each unit takes 10–15 min, allowing for fine assessment of tissue response and control of manipulation time. The non-dominant hand stabilizes the skin while the dominant hand performs overlapping, continuous strokes, re-moistening the applicator as needed but avoiding excessive saturation to prevent dripping. Many physicians prefer cotton-tipped applicators for the control they offer; others opt for folded gauze or a combination of both. The ideal technique includes an initial pass with a more moistened applicator, followed by circular and back-and-forth movements for uniformity. In deep wrinkles or scars, the solution may be rubbed more vigorously or applied focally to enhance penetration (Fig. 8.11).

The application sequence should respect anatomical boundaries and the physiology of vapor dispersion: begin with the forehead, proceed to the lateral face and nose, and leave the periorbital and perioral regions for last, in order to reduce overlapping phenol inhalation; continuous local ventilation with fans or coolers directed to divert vapors from the nostrils is recommended. On the forehead, the solution should slightly cross the anterior hairline and enter the scalp to avoid demarcation. In the periocular region, treat the upper eyelid up to the supratarsal crease and the

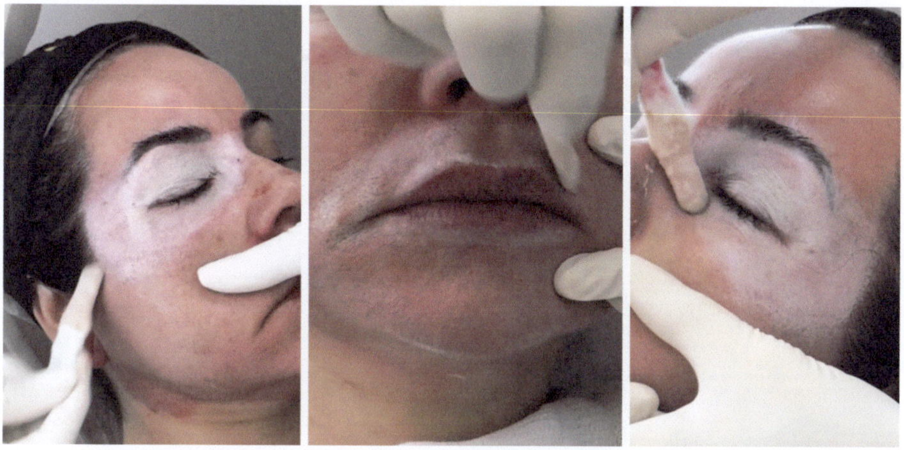

Fig. 8.11 Application of deep phenol–croton peel with a wooden applicator tipped with cotton. After thorough cleansing and degreasing, the solution should be kept homogenized by vigorous shaking during use. The depth achieved depends mainly on the technical maneuver: amount of solution on the applicator, number of passes, pressure/friction, and contact time in each cosmetic unit. The non-dominant hand stabilizes the skin while the dominant hand performs overlapping, continuous movements, re-moistening the applicator as needed. The sequence should respect anatomical boundaries, leaving the periocular and perioral regions for last, always with continuous local ventilation to disperse phenol vapors. (*Source: Author's personal collection (Dr Carolina Marçon)*)

lower eyelid up to 2–3 mm from the lash line, using a minimally moistened applicator; tears should be dried immediately with a cotton bud to prevent reflux of the product into the eyes (phenol opacifies the cornea on contact and should be copiously irrigated if this occurs), and prior application of ophthalmic lubricating ointment may be considered. It is important to observe the peripheral reflex erythema in the treated area to avoid leaving "islands" without coverage when moving to the next region. In the perioral perimeter, cross ~1 mm onto the vermilion for better contour definition and direct friction into the rhytids; the lower limit of treatment reaches the earlobes and extends ~2 cm below the mandibular line, with feathering at the submandibular transition (Fig. 8.12). For eyelids, use a less saturated applicator and gentle pressure to avoid overpenetration; note: taping the eyelids deepens the effect and may promote ectropion when there is no skin excess (Fig. 8.13). The burning sensation is intense for 15–20 s, subsides, and often recurs at ~30 min, persisting for 8–12 h.

Immediate white-opaque frosting indicates epidermal and superficial dermal keratocoagulation and should not be mistaken for the endpoint of a deep peel (Fig. 8.14). The classic endpoint is a thin, homogeneous grey-blue hue, which appears after additional passes and signals controlled penetration to the papillary dermis (Fig. 8.15); in areas treated more aggressively, mild purpura may occur after the white disappears, and vesiculation may develop within the following hour. A shift to a brown-orange color indicates penetration into the reticular dermis and

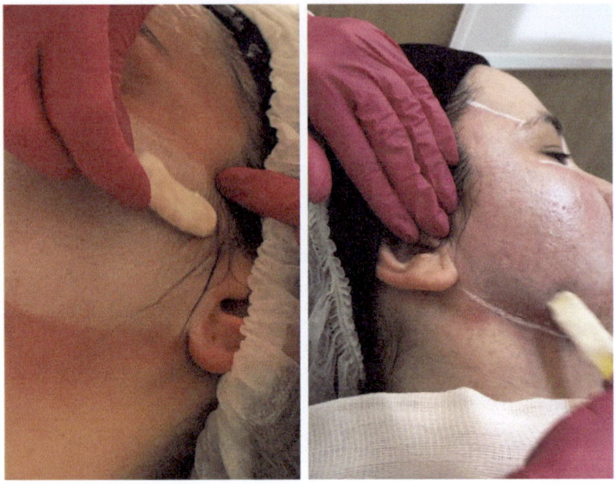

Fig. 8.12 Segmental treatment with deep phenol–croton peel on the cheeks for acne scars. In both images, peripheral reflex erythema is observed, a key clinical sign for assessing the uniformity of solution penetration. On the left, an application with a cotton applicator and onset of solid white frosting. On the right, feathering towards the mandibular contour to prevent demarcation lines. *(Source: Author's personal archive (Dr Carolina Marçon))*

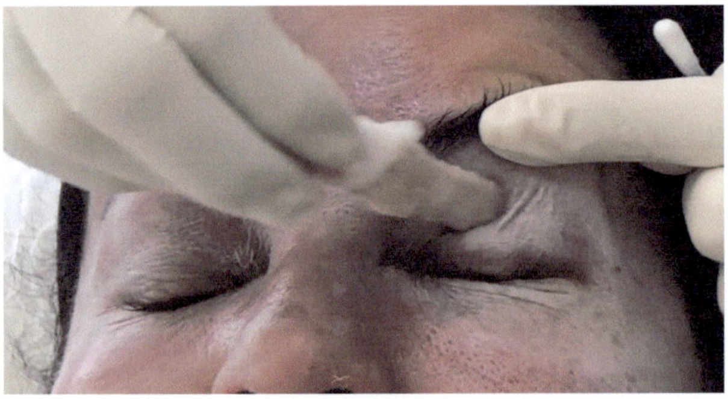

Fig. 8.13 Application of deep phenol–croton peel to the upper eyelid region. Note the use of a lightly saturated cotton applicator, with gentle friction and stabilization of the eyelid by the non-dominant hand. The application is limited to the supratarsal fold, maintaining a distance of 2–3 mm from the lash line to avoid the risk of overpenetration and ocular complications. (*Source: Author's personal archive (Dr Carolina Marçon)*)

necessitates immediate cessation of the procedure (Figs. 8.16 and 8.17). In higher phototypes, attention is required as frosting tends to be subtle. Endpoint assessment also depends on the emulsifier: with classic surfactants, a uniform greyish-white is observed; with others (e.g., Novisol), a diffuse "grey edema" is common, requiring

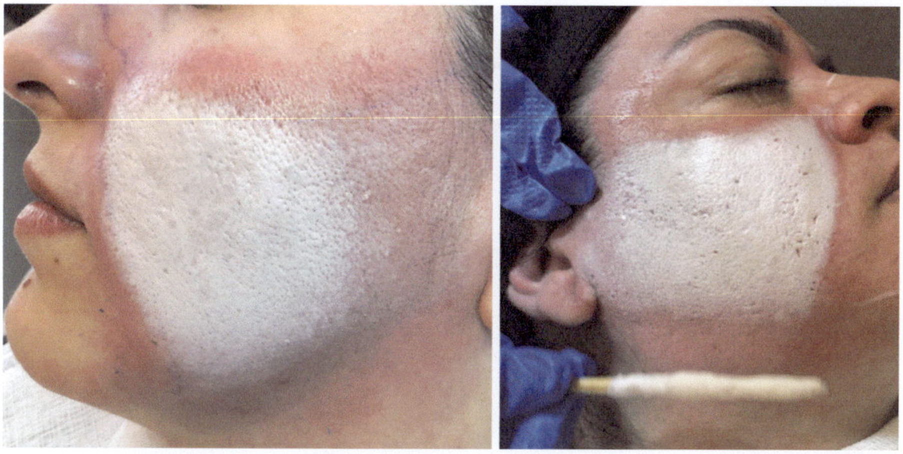

Fig. 8.14 Immediate white-opaque frosting after application of the phenol–croton solution. This appearance reflects epidermal and superficial dermal keratocoagulation, but does not represent the endpoint of a deep peel. (*Source: Author's personal archive (Dr Carolina Marçon)*)

Fig. 8.15 Classic endpoint of deep peel: a thin, homogeneous grey-blue color, indicative of controlled penetration to the papillary dermis. (*Source: Author's personal archive (Dr Carolina Marçon)*)

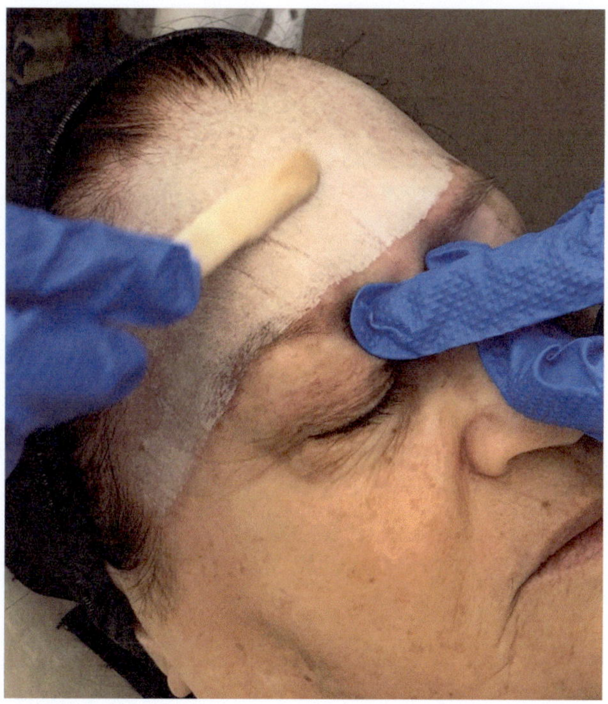

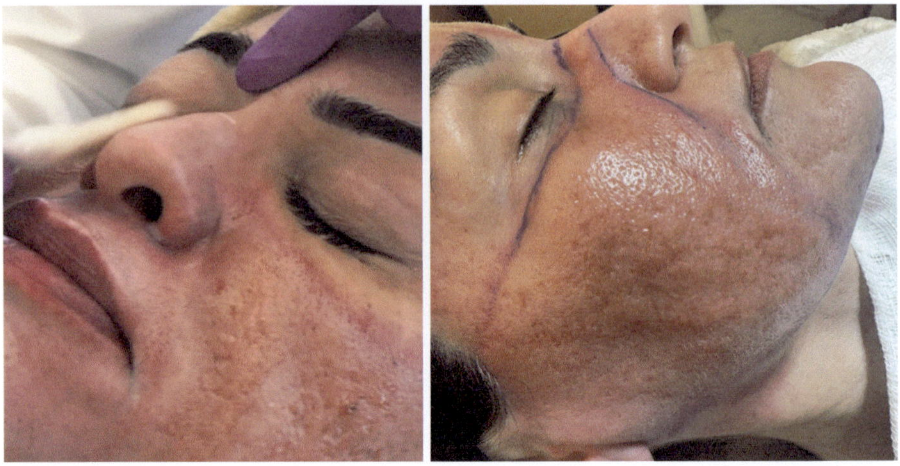

Fig. 8.16 Areas treated more aggressively may develop mild purpura after the disappearance of the white frosting, as well as vesiculation within the first hour. A shift to a brown-orange color indicates penetration into the reticular dermis and requires immediate interruption of the procedure. (*Source: Author's personal archive (Dr Carolina Marçon)*)

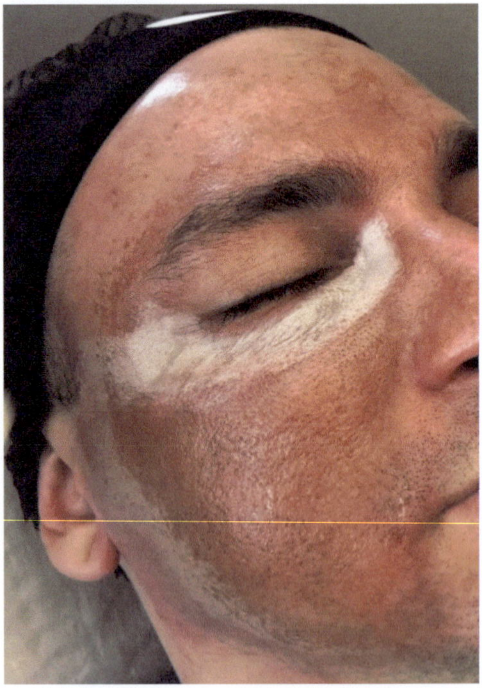

Fig. 8.17 Intermediate clinical aspect during phenol–croton peel. In the malar region, a brown-orange hue is observed, indicative of penetration into the reticular dermis, which necessitates immediate cessation of application to prevent scarring complications. In the lower eyelid and periocular region, initial white-opaque frosting is noted, corresponding to epidermal and superficial dermal keratocoagulation. This differentiation between areas is essential for depth control and procedural safety. (*Source: Author's personal archive (Dr Carolina Marçon)*)

recalibration of pressure and number of passes/layers. In general, timing is not used to determine depth: frost (and chromatic changes) serve as dynamic endpoints, adjusting the number of passes according to local thickness and oiliness. In all scenarios, overlapping and continuous strokes are performed until the planned endpoint is reached, avoiding fluid accumulation in folds and junctions; after each completed zone, the procedure is paused to allow frost stabilization, confirming local absorption and peak action.

Regarding operative parameters, the technique consists of applying the solution uniformly, with firm movements, avoiding excessive friction in areas at higher risk of abnormal scarring (mandibular line, submentum, eyelids—especially lower and lateral and medial corners of the upper lids, borders of cosmetic units, malar and preauricular projections) (Fig. 8.18). The literature emphasizes that application technique is more decisive for outcome and safety than isolated variation in component concentrations. Strict control of application, with the possibility of interrupting the procedure upon reaching the desired depth, is fundamental to minimizc complications and ensure predictable results. The number of passes is a critical

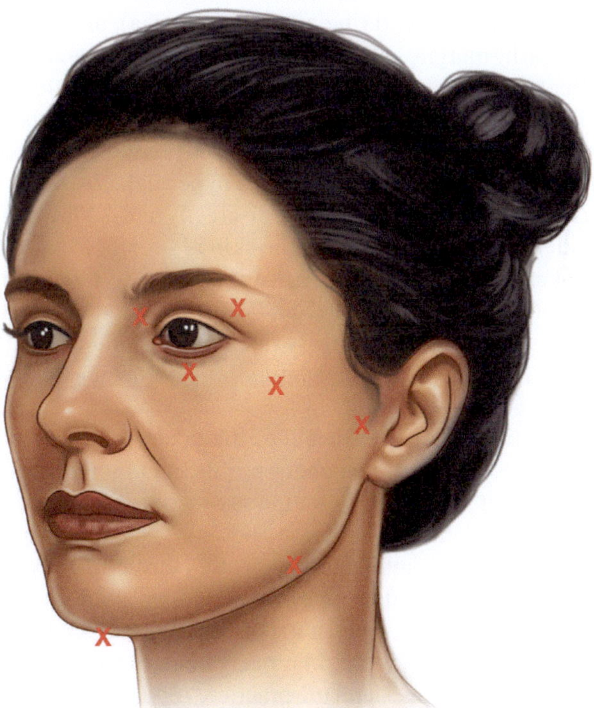

Fig. 8.18 Areas at higher risk for abnormal scarring highlighted in red (*x*). The solution should be applied evenly, with firm and controlled movements, avoiding excessive friction in these areas: mandibular line, submental region, eyelids (especially lower lids and the lateral and medial corners of the upper lids), borders of cosmetic units, malar projection, and preauricular region. (*Source: Figure created by the author (Dr Carolina Marçon), with the aid of artificial intelligence)*

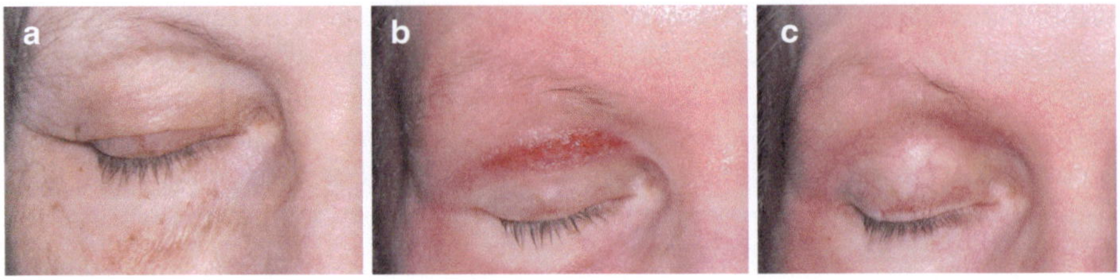

Fig. 8.19 Example of the blepharopeeling technique using phenol–croton oil. (**a**) Pre-treatment, showing fine rhytids and upper eyelid laxity. (**b**) On the seventh day post-procedure, after crust detachment, with persistent erythema and mild, deeper active healing in the area corresponding to the excess skin that would be excised in surgical blepharoplasty. (**c**) Follow-up result, with resolution of erythema, significant improvement in skin texture, reduction in eyelid laxity, and smoothing of rhytids. (*Source: Personal archive of Dr Carlos Wambier)*

intraoperative "control lever": more passes = greater depth; fewer passes = more superficial effect. In practice, formulations of different concentrations are prepared in advance, selected for each area according to thickness and correction needs, or the same formulation is used, varying penetration in different areas through technique. For the eyelid (the most painful area), an almost dry applicator is used up to the lash margin, also treating crow's feet and the entire periorbital region. Blepharopeeling reduces laxity and palpebral rhytids; when performed exclusively chemically, it is applied more deeply in the area that would be excised in upper blepharoplasty (Fig. 8.19); it may cover the entire periocular region or focus on lower eyelids for fine rhytids and hypermelanosis. To avoid a perioral demarcation halo, the vermilion border is discreetly crossed, and the commissures are treated with care. For deep rhytids, the skin is stretched and the tip of a wooden applicator, broken in half, may be used to introduce solution into the furrows. Within a few minutes, the initial white tends to give way to erythema reddish-grey; the skin becomes edematous, with swollen eyelids and a "leathery" sensation to the touch. Adequate analgesia is mandatory for patient comfort and to allow calm and methodical handling.

At the end of deep peeling, the occlusion strategy is chosen according to the objective, treated area, patient profile, and monitoring possibilities. Without occlusion (open technique), continuous inspection is preserved, at the cost of greater microenvironmental variation and more active management of exudate (Fig. 8.20). Occlusion with ointments—typically petroleum jelly, which is inert and non-comedogenic—reapplied every 2–6 h maintains a moist environment, reduces thick crust formation, protects against irritants, facilitates feeding and oral hygiene, and allows painless removal (Fig. 8.21); many centers have historically switched from tape to petroleum jelly as standard practice, reporting equivalent comfort and lower morbidity. Occlusion with tape or an impermeable mask creates a firm seal for 18–48 h and tends to deepen and even out the effect, which is useful for deep static rhytids and complex contours; its drawback is that it does not allow visualization of the skin during recovery, increases edema, and can sometimes be difficult and traumatic to

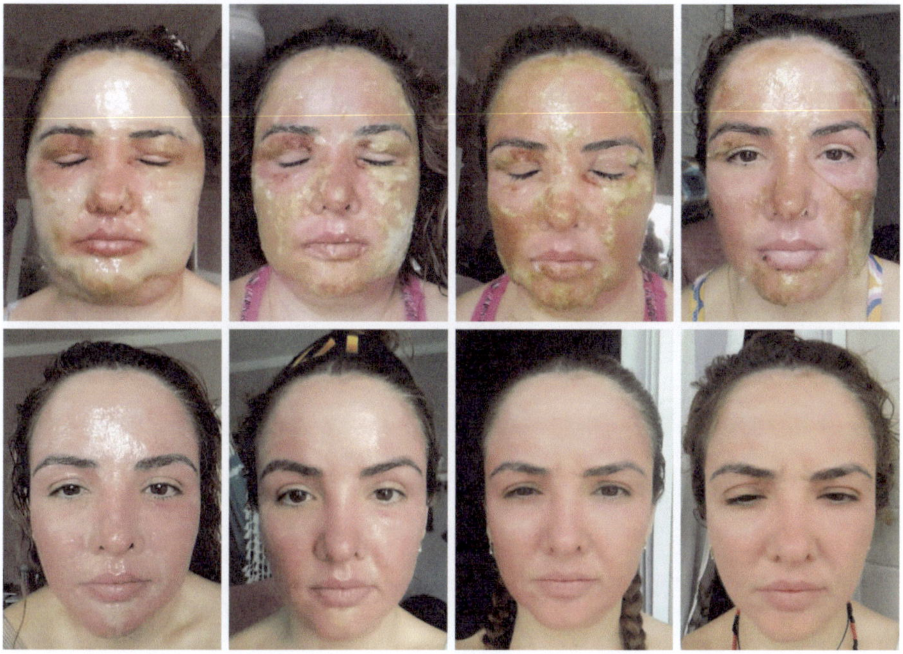

Fig. 8.20 Clinical progression of a patient undergoing deep peeling using the open technique, without occlusion. There is an initial presence of abundant serous exudate and crust formation (top row), followed by progressive detachment and complete re-epithelialization in about 7–10 days (bottom row). The open technique allows continuous inspection of the treated skin, although it requires more active exudate management and more intensive local care. (*Source: Personal archive of the author (Dr Carolina Marçon)*)

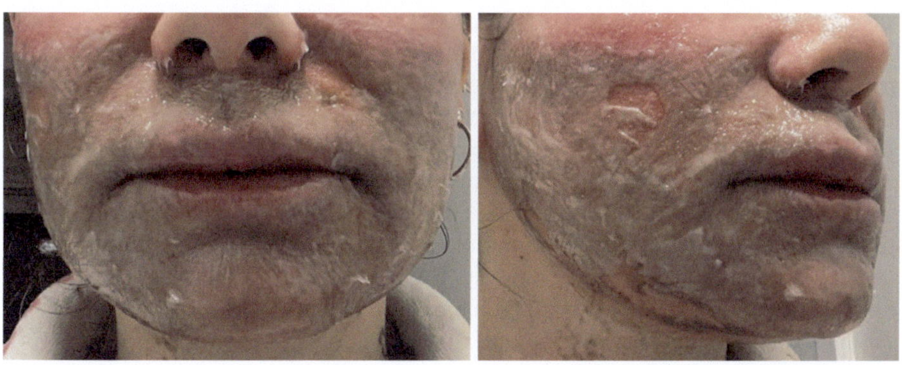

Fig. 8.21 Open technique (without occlusion) on the second postoperative day. The skin surface appears erythematous with characteristic serous exudate, without thick crust formation. The absence of coverage allows continuous inspection, but requires frequent exudate management and greater microenvironmental control. (*Source: Personal archive of the author (Dr Carolina Marçon)*)

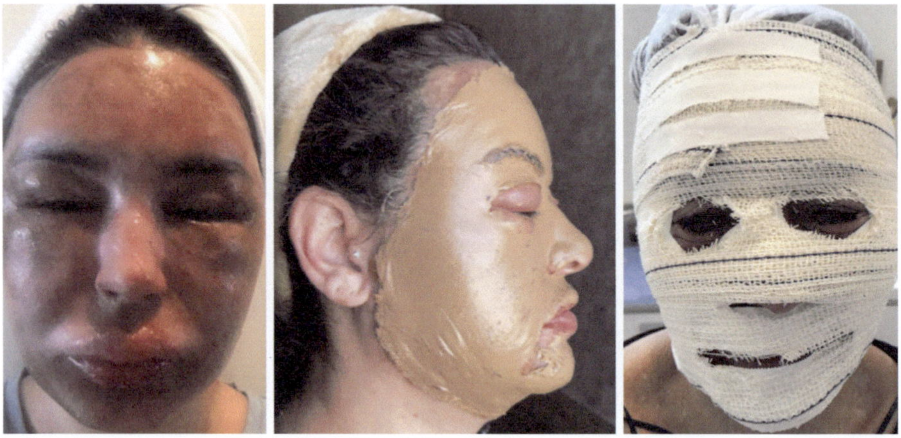

Fig. 8.22 Different occlusion strategies after deep peeling. On the left, occlusion with petroleum jelly reapplied every 2–6 h, which maintains a moist environment, reduces thick crusts, and allows painless removal. In the center, an impermeable plastic mask creates a firm and uniform seal, enhancing the depth of the peel but hindering skin inspection. On the right, classic occlusion with impermeable adhesive strips and elastic bandage, providing homogeneous sealing but with a risk of traumatic removal. (Source: *Author's personal archive (Dr Carolina Marçon))*

remove (Fig. 8.22). When tape is chosen, occlusive plastic strips (vapor-impermeable) are applied parallel to the anterior hairline, molded to the entire face (sparing eyes and mouth), and removed after approximately 48 h; after removal (Fig. 8.23), some protocols dust bismuth subgallate (or thymol iodide) for 7–8 days, starting emollient application on the eighth day to lift the mask. In classic approaches, the occlusive barrier is prepared in advance as an integral part of the technique: specifically, vapour-impermeable plastic adhesive tapes/rubber film (ordinary tape is unsuitable) or latex facial masks molded in plaster and reinforced with gauze are used; fixation is achieved with elastic bandage, covering even the submental area and, when necessary, almost the entire head for uniform sealing. This occlusion prevents exudate evaporation, intensifies maceration, and keeps the active solution at the skin interface for a prolonged period; removal is slow, aided by a wax or petroleum jelly stick, without mechanical debridement. Some authors report a methodological shift after large case series in the 1960s–80s, abandoning tape and adopting petroleum jelly as the routine occlusive with equivalent performance and lower morbidity; others describe a moist dressing based on Crisco (vegetable fat) as a substitute for tape, allowing social reintegration/make-up around day 10 and comparable aesthetic results, which is explained by faster healing in a moist environment. As a general rule, occlusion deepens the effect when used; the choice (or omission) remains a technical and situational decision. Alternatives such as thin

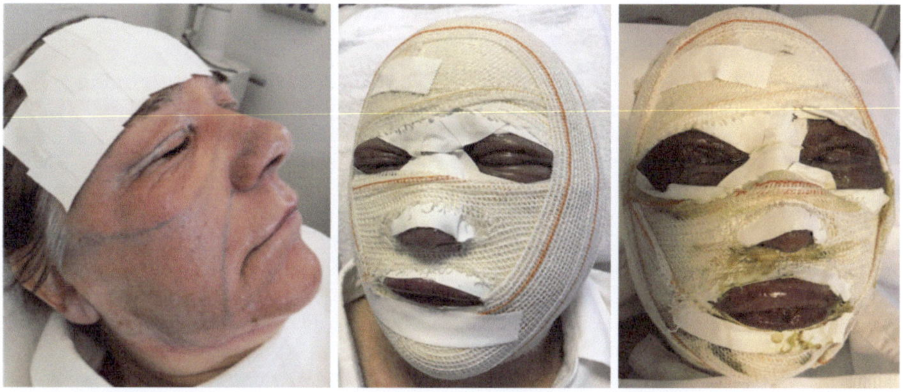

Fig. 8.23 Classic occlusion of the Baker formula with plastic adhesive strips applied parallel to the anterior hairline and reinforced with elastic bandage (left, center, and right). Removal was performed after approximately 48 h. Although the technique provided a firm seal, enhancing and evening out the effect of the peel, it had significant disadvantages, such as increased edema, difficulty in monitoring the skin, and often traumatic removal. These factors led to its gradual disuse in favor of safer alternatives, such as petroleum jelly and semipermeable dressings. (*Source: Author's personal archive (Dr Carolina Marçon)*)

polyurethane films, hydrocolloids, hydrogels, petrolatum gauze, and biosynthetic membranes may improve comfort and exudate control, but when applied too early, they increase local hydration/temperature and may inadvertently deepen the effect; their use should be judicious. Despite widespread use, robust comparative studies establishing unequivocal superiority between methods and ideal timing are lacking.

The most common technical errors are related to excessive application of layers or vigorous friction (deep dermal injury, exacerbated inflammation, fibrosis, and increased risk of scarring, especially on the eyelids), changing the applicator mid-procedure (altering abrasiveness), undertreatment of anatomical transitions (demarcation), and accidental overdose in higher phototypes when frosting is less evident—a situation in which the shift to a brownish-orange color should be taken as the limit. In summary, a safe and reproducible technique results from the integration of a homogeneous solution, segmented and uniform application, careful assessment of the endpoint, and judicious choice of occlusion—always modulating depth primarily by the operator's hand and by adjusting the concentration of croton oil. In practical terms, the recommended technique involves proper skin preparation, use of a phenol and croton oil solution at adjusted concentrations, application by units with controlled strokes and pressure, visual monitoring of frosting/endpoints, and systematic documentation of clinical experience to refine concentration adjustments and application techniques over time (Tables 8.18 and 8.19).

Table 8.18 Technical parameters for full-face phenol–croton peel

Aspect	Practical recommendations
Applicator	Firm cotton bud, wooden-handled swab, or folded gauze; standardize to avoid differences in depth
Movements	Initial pass should be wetter, followed by continuous circular and back-and-forth movements; uniform friction
Anatomical sequence	Start with the forehead → sides of the face/nose → periorbital and perioral regions
Time per unit	Each unit: 10–15 min; interval of 10–15 min between areas
Emulsion control	Keep the bottle closed and shake before and during use to prevent phase separation
Endpoint assessment	Initial white frost indicates epidermal coagulation; endpoint: homogeneous grey-blue in the papillary dermis
Common errors	Excessive layers/friction, changing applicator, undertreatment of transitions, overdose in higher phototypes

Main technical parameters of full-face phenol–croton peel, including applicators, anatomical sequence, time per unit, endpoint criteria, and most common technical errors. *Notes. Clinical endpoint = visual reference that defines the depth of penetration. Table prepared by the author*

Table 8.19 Occlusion methods after deep phenol–croton peel

Type of occlusion	Advantages	Limitations/risks	Indications
No occlusion (open technique)	Allows continuous inspection of the skin	Greater microenvironmental variation; more active exudate management	Selected cases, lower systemic risk
Vaseline (reapplied ointment)	Moist environment, fewer crusts, protects against irritants, painless	Requires frequent reapplication (every 2–6 h)	Routine use; patient comfort
Impermeable plastic tape/mask	Deepens and evens out the effect; useful for deep static rhytids	Does not allow skin inspection; increases edema; traumatic removal	Deep rhytids; complex contours
Others (hydrocolloids, biosynthetics)	Improve comfort and exudate control	May deepen the effect if used too early	Special cases; careful assessment

Occlusion methods after deep phenol–croton peel: characteristics, advantages, limitations, and indications. *Table prepared by the author*

8.8.3.2 Segmental Peeling

Segmental phenol–croton oil peel is indicated for the focal treatment of deep static rhytids, localized scars, or areas with disproportionate aging between cosmetic units, allowing preservation of untreated areas, reduced overall aggressiveness, and shorter recovery time. It is also an alternative for patients at higher risk of systemic complications, such as those with cardiovascular or respiratory comorbidities and low physiological reserve. In such cases, the procedure may be planned in stages, treating one cosmetic unit at a time in pre-scheduled sessions, thereby minimizing the systemic phenol load. Re-epithelialization generally occurs between 7 and 9 days, followed by residual erythema (Fig. 8.24).

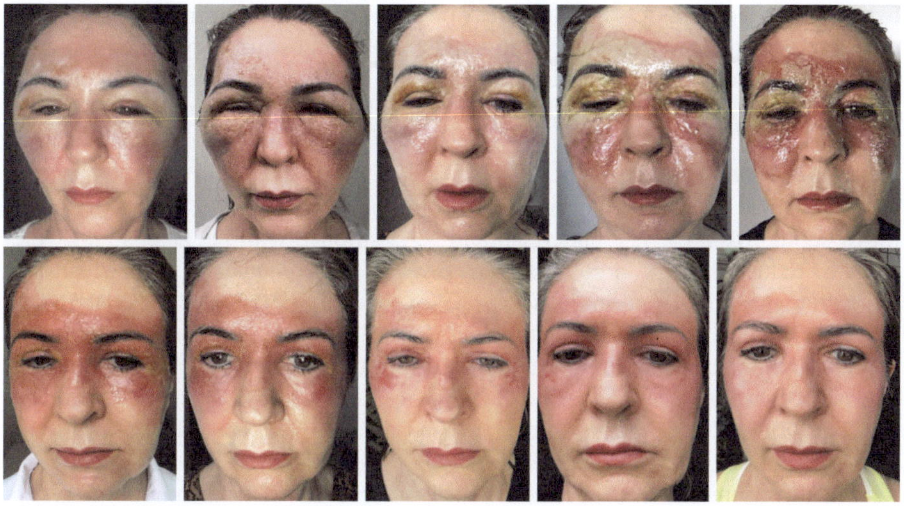

Fig. 8.24 Clinical progression after segmental phenol–croton oil peel (Hetter 0.8%), performed for focal treatment of static rhytids in the periorbital region. Marked edema is observed, peaking at approximately 36 h, accompanied by intense erythema and initial exudation. Between the third and fifth day, yellowish crusts and the onset of irregular desquamation are noted, with progressive reduction of edema. From the sixth to the ninth day, crust detachment and near-complete re-epithelialization of the treated area are observed. By the tenth day, the skin is re-epithelialized, with uniform residual erythema, marking the transition to subsequent dermal remodeling. (*Source: Author's personal archive, Dr Carolina Marçon)*

The ideal selection falls on patients with lower phototypes, with lower concentrations of croton oil being modulated when it is necessary to reduce the risk of demarcation. Solution preparation must strictly follow the principles of homogeneous emulsion under intermittent agitation, and application, regardless of the area, requires precise control of the volume in the applicator, number of passes, pressure applied, and contact time in each zone. Before starting, the treatment area is carefully delineated, establishing a transition zone (feathering) to soften the junction between treated and untreated skin and avoid abrupt demarcation lines. Each cosmetic unit is treated in its entirety before moving on to the next, allowing detailed assessment of tissue response and control of manipulation time.

For segmental peels, the most commonly used concentrations are phenol 35%–50%, and it is possible to work with croton oil within a range from 0.1% to 1.6%, adjusted according to skin thickness and the severity of rhytids. In cases where the rest of the face requires global photorejuvenation, a medium-depth peel (for example, Jessner + TCA or dry CO_2 + TCA) may be applied to the remaining units to ensure a uniform result.

Application is performed using a "semi-dry" cotton applicator, with small volumes and minimal pressure, aiming to achieve a solid, uniform grey-white frost. In thinner areas, application begins laterally, where the skin is thicker, progressing towards the medial region. At the border between treated and untreated skin, a fanning motion is used to soften the depth gradient. Post-inflammatory hyperpigmentation is an expected complication and should be managed with strict physical photoprotection and, as tolerated, low-irritation depigmenting agents.

8.8.3.3 Periorbital Segment

The periorbital segment is often the starting point, given the aesthetic impact of rejuvenating this area. The patient should be positioned with the head slightly elevated to reduce the risk of solution flow towards the conjunctiva. After cleansing, the cotton swab is dipped in the solution, squeezed at the edge of the container to prevent dripping, and the initial strokes are made along the infraorbital rim, while the non-dominant hand stretches the skin. As the cotton dries, the application approaches the lash line, feathering the edge over untreated skin to avoid a demarcation line. Either 0.2% croton oil can be used in multiple passes or 0.8% in fewer passes, depending on skin thickness and the desired endpoint. On the upper eyelid, treatment is limited to the upper tarsal border (Fig. 8.25). This technique is safer in patients with lower phototypes, especially Fitzpatrick I and II. Immediate occlusion of the lower eyelid can be performed with impermeable tape for 24 h to achieve greater depth, or with petrolatum ointment as a protective measure (Fig. 8.26); if tape is used, it is essential to wait for the solution to dry completely to avoid accidental contact with the ocular surface.

8.8.3.4 Perioral Segment and Lips

The *lip peel* with phenol–croton oil is indicated to promote eversion and augmentation of the vermilion without the need for injectables, as well as to treat actinic cheilitis. Phenol 35% combined with croton oil between 0.4% and 1.6% is used, with the concentration selected according to skin thickness and the desired volumizing effect. In cases of focal dysplasia in actinic cheilitis, higher concentrations, such as 4% croton oil in 84.5% phenol, may be applied locally to achieve a deeper effect. The field must remain dry, with protection of the mucosa and teeth, and the patient is positioned to facilitate lip traction (Fig. 8.27). Application is performed with a moist cotton swab—without dripping—covering the entire vermilion uniformly, from the outer border to the *wet–dry line*, with gentle traction to expose all grooves and columns and avoid untreated areas. After application, occlusion with petrolatum is performed and maintained throughout the healing period to preserve moisture and promote re-epithelialization. The degree of volumization achieved depends on the baseline lip size and the concentration used. Improvement in contour and increased volume result from neocollagenesis and tissue contraction, with long-lasting effects, often exceeding 2 years.

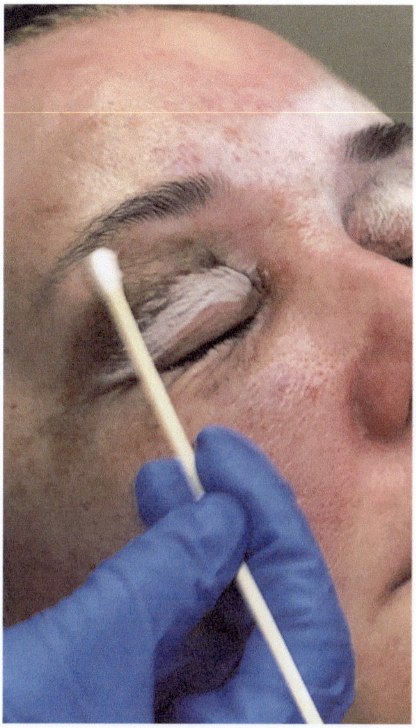

Fig. 8.25 Application technique for phenol-croton oil peel in the periorbital region (blepharopeeling). The cotton applicator is used with minimal, semi-dry volume, avoiding dripping and inadvertent contact with the conjunctiva. Application begins at the infraorbital rim, in areas of thicker skin, carefully progressing to the medial region. Manual traction of the skin with the non-dominant hand assists in controlling the application and achieving a homogeneous frost, respecting anatomical boundaries and the transition zone to prevent demarcation lines. In the blepharopeeling technique, the lower eyelid is treated up to the lash margin and the upper eyelid up to the upper tarsal border, avoiding extension beyond the palpebral fold. This segmental approach allows for safe, focal rejuvenation of the periocular region, with significant aesthetic impact. (*Source: Author's personal archive (Dr Carolina Marçon)*)

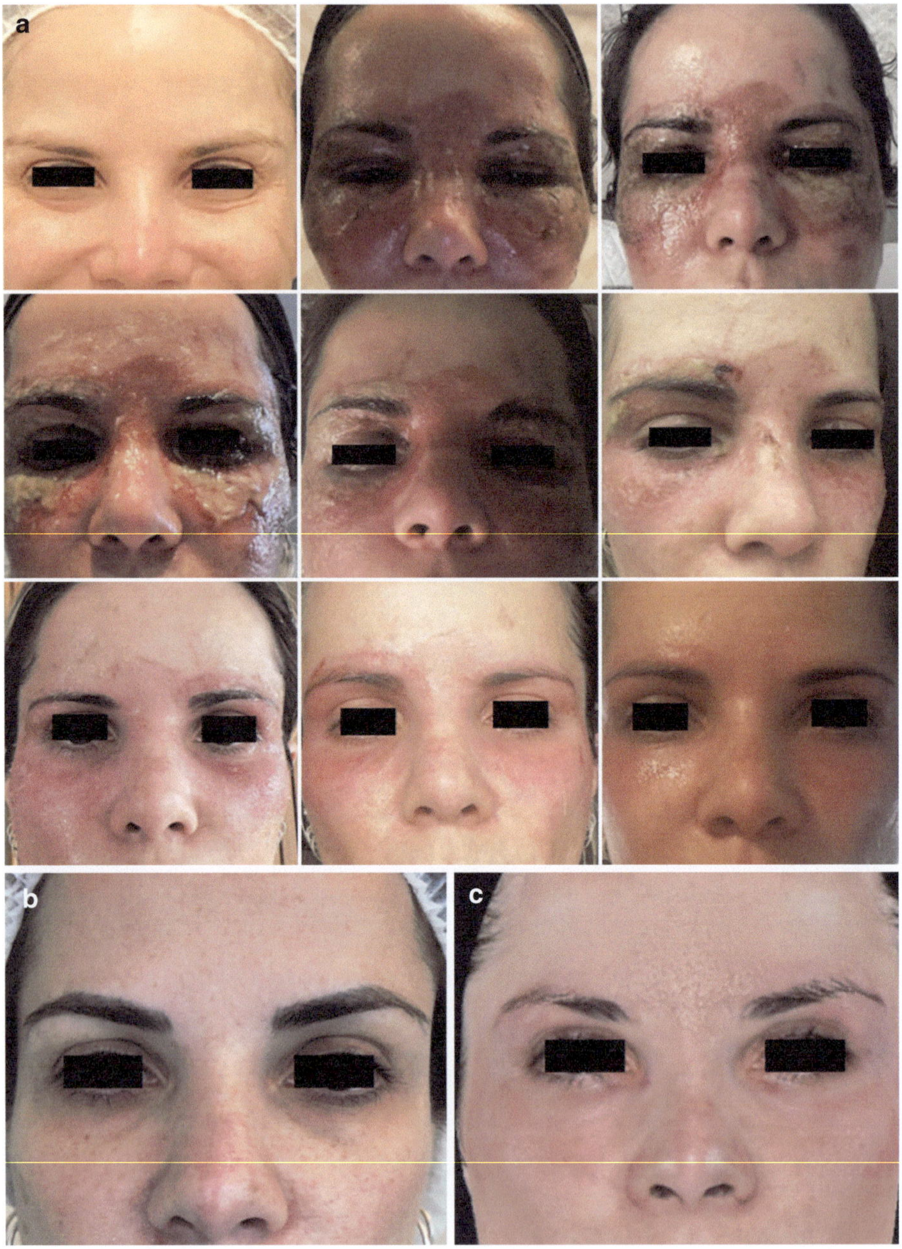

Fig. 8.26 Clinical evolution after segmental periorbital phenol-croton oil peel (Hetter 0.8%). (**a**) Top row (days 1–3): marked edema and initial serous exudation, with irregular crusts and predominantly brown-orange coloring. Second row (days 4–6): progressive detachment of crusts, onset of re-epithelialization in central areas, and gradual reduction of edema. Third row (days 7–9): complete re-epithelialization, residual homogeneous erythema, and mild peripheral desquamation. Bottom row (**b**) preoperative appearance, with pronounced static rhytids, eyelid laxity, and hyperpigmentation; (**c**) 3 months post-procedure, showing significant reduction of fine and medium rhytids, improvement in pigmentation and dermal density, with more even skin tone and overall rejuvenation of the periorbital region. (*Source: Personal archive, Dr Carolina Marçon)*

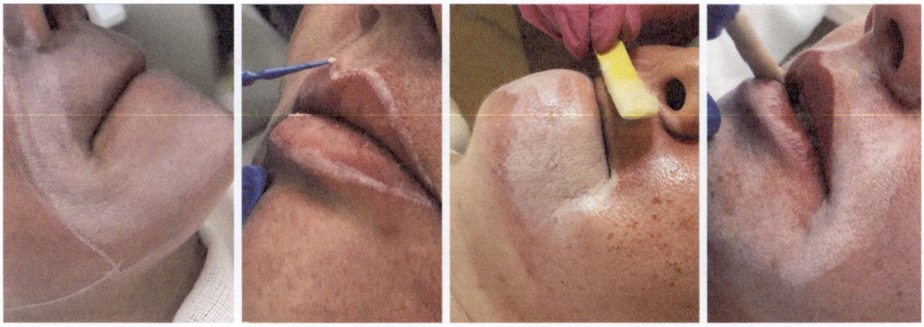

Fig. 8.27 Examples of perioral peel application with phenol–croton oil. Recommended for the treatment of static wrinkles around the mouth and for rejuvenation of the perioral region. A 35% phenol solution is used in combination with croton oil at concentrations ranging from 0.4% to 1.6%, selected according to skin thickness and therapeutic objective. The area must remain dry, with appropriate protection of the mucous membranes and teeth, and the patient should be positioned to allow skin traction and uniform application. (Source: Author's personal archive (Dr Carolina Marçon))

8.9 Post-procedure Care

The postoperative period following phenol–croton oil peeling requires strict monitoring and detailed guidance, as it involves intense inflammatory changes and a potential risk of local and systemic complications. Pain and edema are expected within the first 12 h, followed by exudation and crust formation during the first week. Edema typically peaks around 36 h, with progressive resolution (Fig. 8.28). Analgesia should be administered according to individual tolerance, following the pre-established protocol. In most cases, pain decreases significantly after 8–12 h, leaving only mild discomfort. Complete re-epithelialization of the skin occurs in approximately 10–15 days, and residual erythema may persist for up to 6 months, being most intense in the first month (Fig. 8.29). The deeper the peel, the longer the duration of erythema, which gradually evolves from bright red to pink, until returning to the normal skin tone.

Clinical follow-up should be structured to enable early detection and management of complications. Assessment is recommended within the first 24–48 h, especially in patients with risk factors, to identify signs of infection, necrosis, delayed healing, or systemic toxicity. A second review should take place between 7 and 10 days, a phase when complications such as infection, delayed re-epithelialization, and pigmentary changes are more likely. Between 3 and 6 weeks, follow-up focuses on the progression of healing, prevention of hypertrophic or keloid scarring, and management of persistent pigmentary alterations. Patients and their families should be instructed to report immediately any severe pain, fever, purulent exudate, areas of necrosis, or systemic symptoms such as nausea, palpitations, and dizziness.

In the immediate postoperative period, the choice of occlusion method and maintenance of wound moisture are crucial for comfort and quality of healing. In cases where vaseline is chosen as the occlusive agent, after 12 h post-peel the patient may perform soaks with mildly acidic solutions, such as boric acid combined with

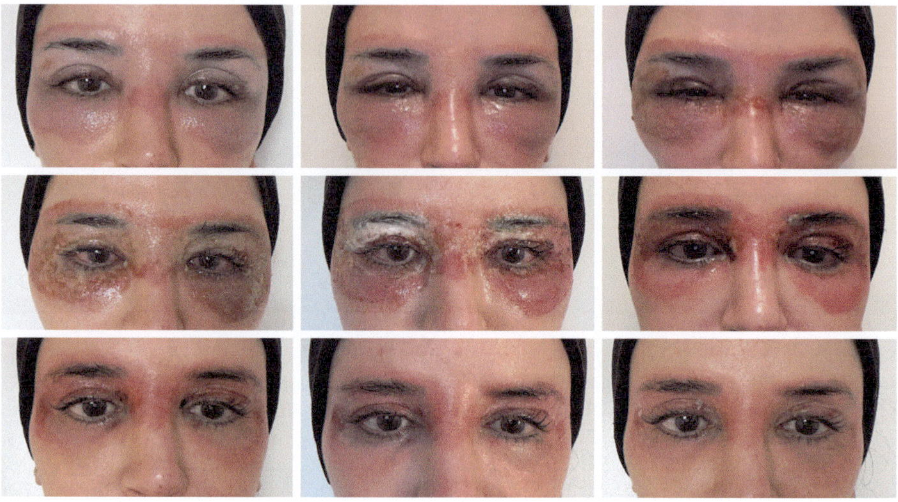

Fig. 8.28 Clinical progression from day 1 to day 9 after deep phenol–croton oil peel (Hetter 0.8%) performed in a "Zorro mask" pattern, covering the periorbital and malar regions. Initial edema and erythema are observed, followed by the formation of sero-hematic crusts and exudate between days 2 and 4. The phase of crust detachment and onset of re-epithelialization occurs between days 5 and 7, with progressive resolution by day 9, when the surface is already epithelialized, though with characteristic residual erythema. (*Source: Author's personal archive (Dr Carolina Marçon)*)

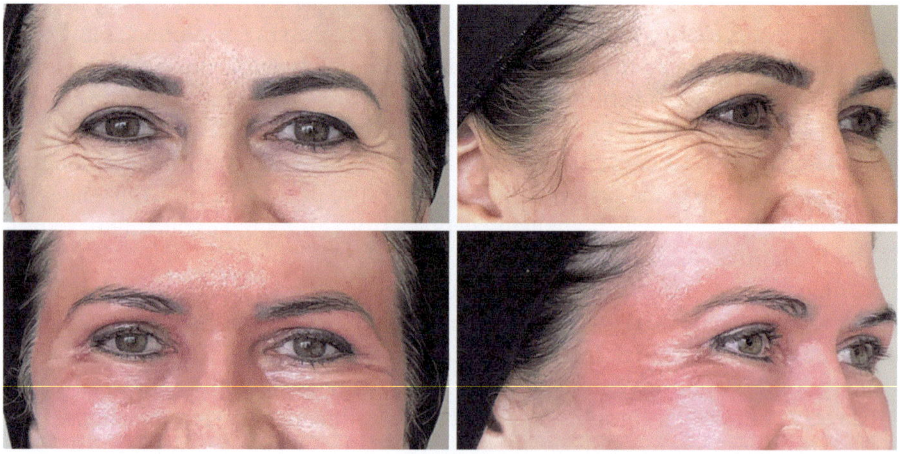

Fig. 8.29 Residual erythema 15 days after phenol–croton peel (Hetter 0.8%) performed in the periorbital region. Complete re-epithelialization is observed, with persistent intense erythema, a finding expected at this early stage. Residual erythema may persist for weeks to months, being more pronounced in the first month and gradually evolving from bright red to a pinkish hue until the normal skin color is restored. There is also a noticeable improvement in skin density and reduction in eyelid laxity, already evident even at this initial stage of recovery. (*Source: Author's personal archive (Dr Carolina Marçon)*)

sodium hyaluronate and 0.9% benzyl alcohol, or apple cider vinegar solution (2 teaspoons diluted in 240 mL of water), followed by reapplication of vaseline. The skin should remain constantly moist. After 24 h, gentle cleansing with hypoallergenic products may be initiated, and hair may be washed with baby shampoo or a mild, fragrance-free formula. The use of products containing lanolin should be avoided due to their allergenic potential. Patients should avoid excessive mouth opening, opting for a soft diet in the first few days (Fig. 8.30).

Pruritus, which may arise around the fifth day and persist during the first month, is controlled with oral antihistamines. To aid sleep and reduce anxiety, especially in the initial days, melatonin 10 mg, zolpidem hemitartrate 2.5–10 mg, or clonazepam (3–5 drops) may be prescribed for up to five nights, with melatonin preferred over benzodiazepines due to its lower risk of motor impairment.

After removal of the adhesive tape occlusion (when used), between 24 and 48 h, the skin should be gently cleansed to remove debris, and thymol-iodine powder, which has a drying and bacteriostatic effect, or bismuth subgallate, may be applied. Two days after tape removal, petroleum jelly should be used to keep the eschar pliable, avoiding mechanical removal of crusts, which can impair healing.

Strict photoprotection must be instituted from the onset of re-epithelialization (10–15 days), initially with broad-spectrum physical sunscreens, reapplied throughout the day, and the use of barrier repair creams such as Cicalfate+ (Avene) or Cicaplast Baume B5+ (La Roche Posay). In patients with Fitzpatrick skin types III–IV, it is recommended to start non-irritating lightening agents prophylactically to reduce the risk of post-inflammatory hyperpigmentation. Make-up may be used from 2 weeks onwards, and actives such as hydroquinone or tretinoin are gradually reintroduced between 3 and 4 weeks, according to skin tolerance (Table 8.20).

In addition to physical care, post-peel follow-up should include psychological support, as the intensity of visual changes and temporary discomfort may cause anxiety. Close and supportive follow-up contributes to greater adherence, safety, and patient satisfaction.

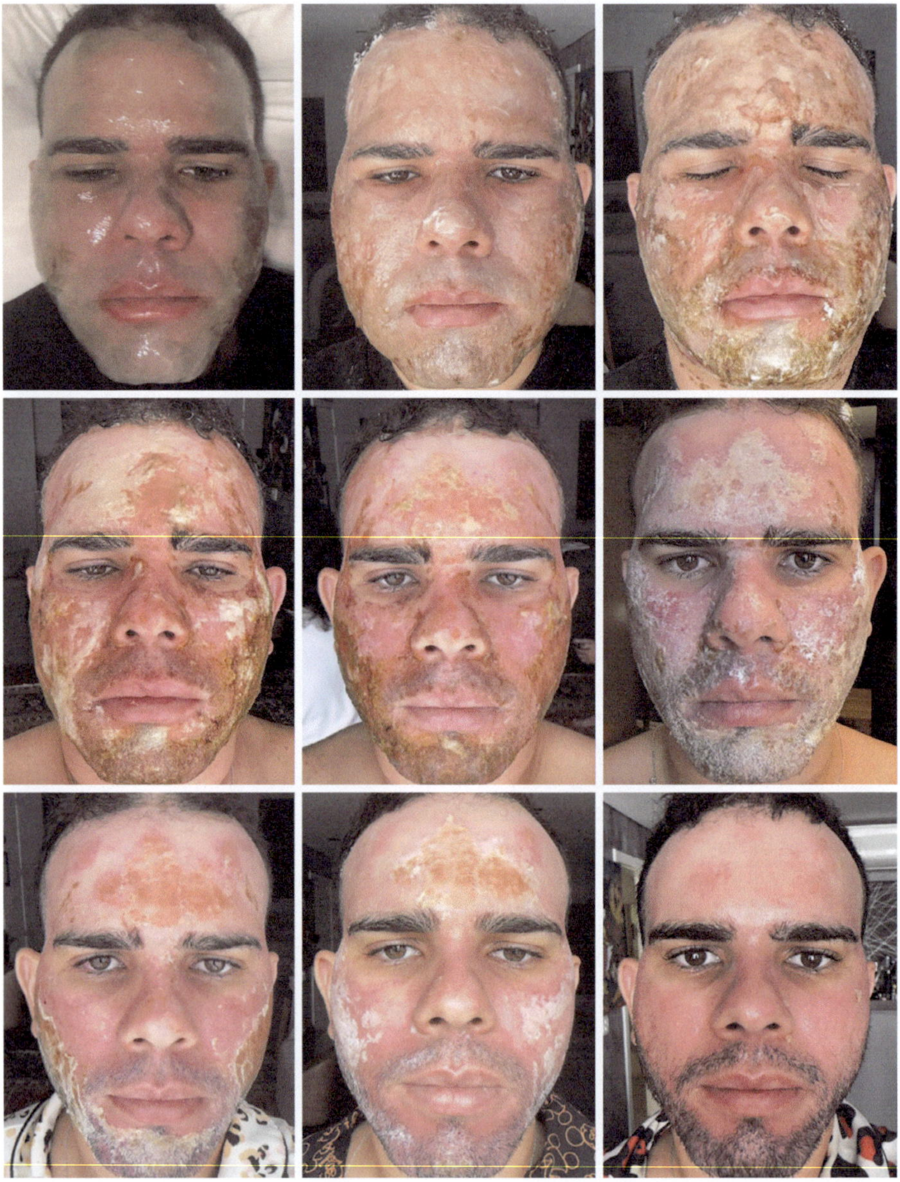

Fig. 8.30 Daily progression after full-face deep peel with Hetter's solution (phenol 35% + croton oil 1.2%) for acne scars, sparing the eyelids. An initial inflammatory response with edema and exudate is observed, with progressive detachment of crusts until days 7–9 and complete re-epithelialization accompanied by residual erythema. The use of vaseline as an occlusive, combined with mildly acidic solutions, keeps the wound moist and promotes more comfortable and uniform healing. (*Source: Author's personal archive (Dr Carolina Marçon)*)

Table 8.20 Post-procedure care following phenol–croton peel: main recommended measures and warning signs

Period	Recommended measures	Warning signs
First 12–48 h	Analgesia as tolerated; maintain chosen occlusion; continuous wound hydration; gentle soaking after 12 h (mild acidic solutions); soft diet	Severe pain, palpitations, nausea, fever, mental confusion
1st week (up to 7 days)	Reapply petroleum jelly; gentle cleansing; avoid crust removal; avoid lanolin; antihistamines for pruritus	Purulent exudate, necrosis, delayed healing
7–15 days	Complete re-epithelialization expected; light make-up permitted after 2 weeks; strict photoprotection with physical barriers	Persistent intense erythema, signs of infection
3–6 weeks	Gradual introduction of non-irritating lightening agents (darker skin types); reintroduction of hydroquinone/tretinoin if tolerated	Significant pigmentary changes, keloids, delayed healing
1–6 months	Ongoing photoprotection; barrier repair creams; psychological support to encourage adherence	Hypertrophic scars, persistent dyschromia

Post-procedure care following phenol–croton peel, organized by recovery period, main recommended measures, and warning signs requiring medical reassessment. (*Source: Table prepared by the author (Dra. Carolina Marçon)*)

Sources

1. Dargan D, Mandal A, Shokrollahi K. Hand burns surface area: a rule of thumb. Burns. 2018;44(5):1346–51.
2. Wambier CG, King BA. Rule of thumb: a simple tool to estimate 1% scalp surface area. J Am Acad Dermatol. 2019;81(2):630–1.
3. Rajan BM, Bhardwaj A. Comment on "Rule of thumb: a simple tool to estimate 1% scalp surface area": whose thumb is it anyway? J Am Acad Dermatol. 2019;81(6):e183.
4. Darouiche RO, Wall MJ Jr, Itani KM, Otterson MF, Webb AL, Carrick MM, Miller HJ, Awad SS, Crosby CT, Mosier MC, Alsharif A, Berger DH. Chlorhexidine-alcohol versus povidone-iodine for surgical-site antisepsis. N Engl J Med. 2010;362(1):18–26.
5. Sterling JB, Lee KC, Wambier CG, Soon SL, Landau M, Rullan PP, Brody HJ. Depth map for face and neck deep chemical peel resurfacing. Dermatol Surg. 2020;46(9):1204–9. https://doi.org/10.1097/DSS.0000000000002268.
6. Bensimon RH. Croton oil peels. Aesthet Surg J. 2008;28(1):33–45. Erratum in: Aesthet Surg J. 2008;28(2):221.
7. Wambier CG, Lee KC, Soon SL, et al. Advanced chemical peels: phenol-croton oil peel. J Am Acad Dermatol. 2019;81(2):327–36.
8. Wambier C. Safety of deep chemical peels. In: Steiner D, Ribeiro F, editors. Peeling químico: manual prático do dia a dia. 1st ed. Rio de Janeiro: Di Livros; 2021. p. 28–38.
9. Binstock JH. Safety of chemical face peels. J Am Acad Dermatol. 1982;7(1):137–8.
10. Koopmann CF Jr. Phenol toxicity during facial peels. Otolaryngol Head Neck Surg. 1982;90(4):383–4.
11. Hetter GP. An examination of the phenol-croton oil peel: Part III. The plastic surgeon's role. Plast Reconstr Surg. 2000;105(2):752–63.
12. Hetter GP. An examination of the phenol-croton oil peel: Part IV. Facial peel outcomes with varying concentrations of phenol and croton oil. Plast Reconstr Surg. 2000;105(3):1061–83.

13. Wambier CG, Brody HJ, Hetter GP. Comments: Hemiface comparative study of two phenol peels (Baker-Gordon and Hetter formulas) for the correction of facial rhytids. Surg Cosmet Dermatol. 2017;9(2):190–1.
14. Sorkin MJ. Cardiac arrhythmias during phenol facial peel. J Dermatol Surg Oncol. 1988;14(5):477.
15. Botta SA, Straith RE, Goodwin HH. Cardiac arrhythmias in phenol facial peeling: a suggested protocol for prevention. Aesthet Plast Surg. 1988;12(2):115–7.
16. Wambier CG, Beltrame FL. Air safety and personal protective equipment for phenol–croton oil peels. Dermatol Surg. 2018;44(7):1035–7.
17. Wambier CG, Wambier SPF, Pilatti LEP, Grabicoski JA, Wambier LF, Schmidt A. Prolongation of rate-corrected QT interval during phenol-croton oil peels. J Am Acad Dermatol. 2018;78(4):810–2.
18. Truppman ES, Ellenby JD. Major electrocardiographic changes during chemical facial peeling. Plast Reconstr Surg. 1979;63(1):44–8.
19. Marçon CR. Phenol in dermatology: updated evidence on efficacy and safety. An Bras Dermatol. 2025;100(5):501200.
20. Gross BG. Cardiac arrhythmias during phenol facial peeling. Plast Reconstr Surg. 1984;73(4):590–4.
21. Wexler MR, Halon DA, Teitelbaum A, Tadjer G, Peled IJ. The prevention of cardiac arrhythmias produced in an animal model by the topical application of a phenol preparation commonly used for facial peeling. Plast Reconstr Surg. 1984;73(4):595–8.
22. Schmidt RJ. "Chemical peel recipe": caution—phenol is not safe for use in chemo-exfoliation. J Cosmet Dermatol. 2023;22(10):2744–5.
23. Bensimon RH. Phenol-croton oil peels. In: Obagi S, editor. Procedures in cosmetic dermatology: chemical peels. 3rd ed. London: Elsevier; 2020. p. 81–99.
24. Frankel EB. Baker's phenol chemical peel. J Dermatol Surg Oncol. 1990;16(6):581–2.
25. Wambier CG, Brody HJ. Introduction: classification of peels. In: Costa A, editor. Minimally invasive aesthetic procedures. Cham: Springer International Publishing; 2020. p. 3–13.
26. Lee KC, Sterling JB, Wambier CG, et al. Segmental phenol–croton oil chemical peels for treatment of periorbital or perioral rhytids. J Am Acad Dermatol. 2019;81(6):e165–6.
27. Sun C, Lim D. Chemical peels for atrophic acne scarring: evolution of peel types and methods. Australas J Dermatol. 2023;64(1):18–27.
28. Cox SV, Zachary CB, Cohen JL. Skin preparation for photodynamic therapy, chemexfoliation, and ablative laser resurfacing: a systematic literature review. Dermatol Surg. 2021;47(7):938–41.
29. ChloraPrep One-Step [package insert]. U.S. Food and Drug Administration; 2025 Jul 2 [cited 2025 Aug 9]. https://dailymed.nlm.nih.gov/dailymed/drugInfo.cfm?setid=3e7b2d1c-1c6f-4f6f-b3b1-0a56d4e7a0d0.
30. Prevantics Maxi Swabstick [package insert]. U.S. Food and Drug Administration; 2023 Jun 30 [cited 2025 Aug 9]. https://dailymed.nlm.nih.gov/dailymed/drugInfo.cfm?setid=7d3b2c3e-8f07-4c47-bb67-7a8f9d1a2b3e.
31. Widgerow AD, Cohen SR, Fagien S. Preoperative skin conditioning: extracellular matrix clearance and skin bed preparation, a new paradigm. Aesthet Surg J. 2019;39(Suppl 3):S103–11.
32. Cavallini M, Montanaro F, Papagni M. A topical depigmentation programme against hyperpigmentation enhances the benefits of previously performed chemical peeling procedures of the face. J Cosmet Sci. 2020;71(6):385–97.
33. Moghadamyeghaneh Z, Phelan MJ, Carmichael JC, Mills SD, Pigazzi A, Nguyen NT, Stamos MJ. Preoperative dehydration increases risk of postoperative acute renal failure in colon and rectal surgery. J Gastrointest Surg. 2014;18(12):2178–85.
34. Engel D, Löffel LM, Wuethrich PY, Hahn RG. Preoperative concentrated urine increases the incidence of plasma creatinine elevation after major surgery. Front Med (Lausanne). 2021;8:699969.
35. Rahm D. A guide to perioperative nutrition. Aesthet Surg J. 2004;24(4):385–90.

36. Bauer JD, Isenring E, Waterhouse M. The effectiveness of a specialized oral nutrition supplement on outcomes in patients with chronic wounds: a pragmatic randomized study. J Hum Nutr Diet. 2013;26(5):452–8.
37. Niimi N, Yuki K, Zaleski K. Long QT syndrome and perioperative torsades de pointes: what the anaesthetist should know. J Cardiothorac Vasc Anesth. 2022;36(1):286–302.
38. D'Souza RS, Warner NS. Phenol nerve block. In: StatPearls. Treasure Island, FL: StatPearls Publishing; 2025. Jan– [cited 2025 Aug 9].
39. Sung DH, Han TR, Park WH, Je Bang H, Kim JM, Chung SH, Woo EJ. Phenol block of peripheral nerve conduction: titrating for optimum effect. Arch Phys Med Rehabil. 2001;82(5):671–6.
40. Aroke EN, Nkemazeh RZ. Perianaesthesia implications and considerations for drug-induced QT interval prolongation. J Perianesth Nurs. 2020;35(2):104–11.
41. Spevak C, Hamsher C, Brown CQ, Wedam EF, Haigney MC. The clinical significance of QT interval prolongation in anesthesia and pain management: what you should and should not worry about. Pain Med. 2012;13(8):1072–80.
42. Ruiz-Maldonado R. Saturated phenol as a local anesthetic for manual dermabrasion. Dermatol Surg. 1997;23(3):187–9.
43. Staikou C, Stamelos M, Stavroulakis E. Impact of anesthetic drugs and adjuvants on ECG markers of torsadogenicity. Br J Anaesth. 2014;112(2):217–30.
44. Mędrzycka-Dąbrowska W, Lange S, Dąbrowski S, Długoborska K, Piotrkowska R. Vitamin C as an adjuvant analgesic therapy in postoperative pain management. J Clin Med. 2025;14(11):3994.
45. Suter M, Bollen Pinto B, Belletti A, Putzu A. Efficacy and safety of perioperative vitamin C in patients undergoing non-cardiac surgery: a systematic review and meta-analysis of randomized trials. Br J Anaesth. 2022;128(4):664–78.
46. Occupational Safety and Health Administration (US). Phenol. Washington, DC: OSHA; 2025 [cited 2025 Aug 9]. https://www.osha.gov/chemicaldata/94.
47. National Institute for Occupational Safety and Health (US). NIOSH pocket guide to chemical hazards: phenol. Washington, DC: Centers for Disease Control and Prevention; 2016 [cited 2025 Aug 9]. https://www.cdc.gov/niosh/npg/npgd0495.html.
48. National Institute for Occupational Safety and Health (US). Immediately dangerous to life or health concentrations (IDLH): phenol. Washington, DC: Centers for Disease Control and Prevention; 1994 [cited 2025 Aug 9]. https://www.cdc.gov/niosh/idlh/108952.html.
49. Brazil. National Health Surveillance Agency. Resolution RDC No. 222, of 28 March 2018. Provides regulations for the management of healthcare service waste and other provisions. Brasília, DF: ANVISA; 2018 [cited 2025 Aug 9]. https://bvsms.saude.gov.br/bvs/saudelegis/anvisa/2018/rdc0222_28_03_2018.pdf.
50. National Health Surveillance Agency (BR). Questions and answers: Resolution RDC No. 222/2018—Management of Healthcare Service Waste. Brasília, DF: ANVISA; 2018 [cited 2025 Aug 9]. https://www.gov.br/anvisa/pt-br/assuntos/servicosdesaude/gerenciamento-de-residuos/PerguntaseRespostasRDCn.2222018.pdf.
51. Brazilian Association of Technical Standards. ABNT NBR 13853: container for sharp healthcare service waste—requirements and test methods. Rio de Janeiro: ABNT; 1997.
52. United States Pharmacopeia. USP <795> pharmaceutical compounding—nonsterile preparations. Rockville, MD: The United States Pharmacopeia Convention; 2023.
53. Marçon CR, Coppinger AJ, Salomão C, Alves Dos Reis V, Alves Dos Reis VN, de Menezes Gomes JL, Gianvecchio VAP, Medeiros de Aquino E, de Seixas Alves MT, Canzian M, Coelho Frenkelis Brandão SA, Fusel de Ue RR, Ribeiro F, Bageorgou F, Wambier CG, International Peeling Society (IPS) and São Paulo's Legal Medical Institute (IML-SP). Fatal phenol peel by an unlicensed social media practitioner: a forensic medical analysis. J Am Acad Dermatol. 2025;93(6):e211–3.
54. Hewett Brumberg EK, Douma MJ, Alibertis K, et al. 2024 American Heart Association and American Red Cross Guidelines for First Aid. Circulation. 2024;150(24):e519–79.
55. Rullan P, Lin EM, Schaut E, Wambier CG. Cardiac safety in full-face phenol-croton oil peels: a 22-year retrospective study. J Am Acad Dermatol. 2024;91:762–3.

56. Wambier C. Brown dermatology phenol–croton oil peeling: standard operating procedure v1.1. 2023 [cited 2024 Oct 15]. https://www.peelingsociety.com/fileadmin/user_upload/pdf/press/2024/Brown_SOP_Phenol-croton_oil_2023.pdf.
57. Murari A. A modified Lund and Browder chart. Indian J Plast Surg. 2017;50(2):220–1.
58. Agency for Toxic Substances and Disease Registry (US). Toxicological profile for phenol. Atlanta, GA: ATSDR; 2008. https://www.ncbi.nlm.nih.gov/books/NBK599443/.
59. Kadunc BV, Vanti AA. Evaluation of the systemic toxicity of phenol in facial peels. Surg Cosmet Dermatol. 2009;1:10–4.
60. Capote ACMO, Campos PM, Perera W, Strangman WK, Williamson RT, Beltrame FL. Authentication of commercial *Croton tiglium* L. oils used as raw material for peeling formulations. In: Proceedings of the ICSB & ISE joint meeting; 2025; [location]. Abstract PA-7.
61. Capote ACMO, Justo AS, Wambier CG, Beltrame FL. Effects of *Croton tiglium* oil as a deep chemical peel in skin rejuvenation [poster presentation]. In: Proceedings of the XXII international congress of pharmaceuticals, cosmetics and natural products (CIFARP); 2023 Oct; Ribeirão Preto, Brazil.
62. Capote ACMO, Justo AS, Wambier CG, Beltrame FL. Shelf-life evaluation of *Croton tiglium* L. oil solution used in the Hetter formula for deep chemical peeling [poster presentation]. In: Proceedings of the XXII international congress of pharmaceuticals, cosmetics and natural products (CIFARP); 2023 Oct; Ribeirão Preto, Brazil.
63. Wambier CG, da Costa Filha ARC, Koga AY, Beltrame FL, Döll-Boscardin PM. Emulsifiers maximize the safety and efficacy of deep chemical peels. J Am Acad Dermatol. 2025;92(1):e23–4.
64. Justo AS, Lemes BM, Nunes B, Antunes KA, Carletto B, Koga AY, Lipinski LC, Montemor Netto MR, Campagnoli EB, Beltrame FL, Wambier CG. Depth of injury of Hetter's phenol-croton oil chemical peel formula using two different emulsifying agents. J Am Acad Dermatol. 2020;82(6):1544–6.
65. National Institute for Occupational Safety and Health (NIOSH). Phenol—NIOSH pocket guide to chemical hazards. Atlanta, GA: Centers for Disease Control and Prevention; 2019 [cited 2025 Aug 10]. https://www.cdc.gov/niosh/npg/npgd0493.html.
66. Kampf G, Kramer A. Epidemiological background of hand hygiene and evaluation of the most important agents for scrubs and rubs. Clin Microbiol Rev. 2004;17(4):863–93, table of contents.
67. Boyce JM, Pittet D; Healthcare Infection Control Practices Advisory Committee; HICPAC/SHEA/APIC/IDSA Hand Hygiene Task Force. Guideline for hand hygiene in health-care settings. Recommendations of the Healthcare Infection Control Practices Advisory Committee and the HICPAC/SHEA/APIC/IDSA Hand Hygiene Task Force. Society for Healthcare Epidemiology of America/Association for Professionals in Infection Control/Infectious Diseases Society of America. MMWR Recomm Rep. 2002;51(RR-16):1–45, quiz CE1–4.
68. Maiwald M, Chan ES. The forgotten role of alcohol: a systematic review and meta-analysis of the clinical efficacy and perceived role of chlorhexidine in skin antisepsis. PLoS One. 2012;7(9):e44277.
69. Evidence review for the effectiveness of skin antiseptics in the prevention of surgical site infection: surgical site infections: prevention and treatment: evidence review B. London: National Institute for Health and Care Excellence (NICE); 2019 Apr. (NICE Guideline, No. 125). https://www.ncbi.nlm.nih.gov/books/NBK569835/.
70. Stone PA, Lefer LG. Modified phenol chemical face peels: recognizing the role of application technique. Clin Plast Surg. 2001;28(1):13–36.
71. Brown AM, Kaplan LM, Brown ME. Phenol-induced histological skin changes: hazards, technique, and uses. Br J Plast Surg. 1960;13:158–69.
72. Soon SL, Wambier CG, Rullan PR, Sterling JB, Brody HJ, Lee KC, Kreyden OP, Landau M, International Peeling Society. Phenol-croton oil chemical peeling induces durable improvement of constitutional periorbital dark circles. Dermatol Surg. 2023;49(4):368–73.

73. Lee KC, Sterling JB, Wambier CG, Soon SL, Landau M, Rullan P, Brody HJ, International Peeling Society. Segmental phenol-croton oil chemical peels for treatment of periorbital or perioral rhytids. J Am Acad Dermatol. 2019;81(6):e165–6.
74. Larson DL. Phenol-croton oil peel: an update. Aesthet Surg J. 2005;25(2):197–200.
75. Kass LG, Kass K. The lost art of chemical peeling: my fifteen year experience with phenol-croton oil peel. Adv Ophthalmol Optom. 2017;2(1):391–407.
76. Gross BG, Maschek F. Phenol chemosurgery for removal of deep facial wrinkles. Int J Dermatol. 1980;19(3):159–64.
77. Litton C, Szachowicz EH II, Trinidad GP. Present day status of the chemical face peel. Aesthet Plast Surg. 1986;10(1):1–7.
78. Stone PA. The use of modified phenol for chemical face peeling. Clin Plast Surg. 1998;25(1):21–44.
79. Baker TJ, Gordon HL. Chemical peeling as a practical method for removing rhytids of the upper lip. Ann Plast Surg. 1979;2(3):209–12.
80. Beeson WH, McCollough EG. Chemical face peeling without taping. J Dermatol Surg Oncol. 1985;11(10):985–90.
81. Wambier CG, Neitzke IC, Lee KC, Soon SL, Rullan PP, Landau M, Simão JCL, Sterling JB, Brody HJ, International Peeling Society. Augmentation and eversion of lips without injections: the lip peel. J Am Acad Dermatol. 2019;80(5):e119–20.

9 Combined Treatments with Phenol-Croton Oil Peel

9.1 Introduction

The phenol–croton peel is the non-surgical intervention with the greatest capacity for deep dermal remodeling, providing significant improvement in elastosis, rhytids, and skin texture. However, facial aging is a multifactorial phenomenon, resulting from simultaneous changes in the skin, subcutaneous tissue, musculature, and osteoligamentous support. In this context, contemporary practice has moved away from isolated procedures and adopted a multimodal approach, with the phenol–croton peel as the central axis of skin quality.

This strategy is based on the rational integration of complementary techniques: neuromodulators (botulinum toxin) to modulate movement, fillers and biostimulators to restore or reposition structure, adjunctive technologies to refine and sustain results, and, when indicated, plastic surgery for specific anatomical corrections. Thus, the phenol–croton peel is positioned as the foundational intervention, around which integrated, safe, and individualized protocols are constructed.

In the context of acne scarring, the procedure plays a fundamental role by inducing diffuse dermal remodeling, and may be combined, according to scar morphology, with focal approaches such as CROSS with phenol–croton, subcision, and punch techniques. Such combinations must respect safe temporal windows to avoid undesirable summation of depth or overlapping inflammatory insults within the same field.

Still within the scope of multimodality, segmental treatment is highlighted, in which the phenol–croton peel is applied in a targeted manner to specific regions—such as the perioral or periocular area—and, in the same session, may be combined with medium-depth peels or technologies in adjacent areas. This practice requires technical rigor, with attention to avoiding field overlap and protecting the borders of transition, ensuring aesthetic uniformity, optimized recovery, and greater predictability of outcomes.

C. Marçon, C. Wambier, *Phenol-Croton Oil Peel*,
https://doi.org/10.1007/978-3-032-25993-6_9

The essence of this approach lies in personalization. Although phenol-croton oil peel is the most potent chemical resurfacing technique for the treatment of static rhytids, elastosis, and deep scars, many patients present with concomitant concerns such as lipoatrophy or muscular hyperkinesis. In such cases, adjunctive interventions, scheduled sequentially and/or in different areas, enhance overall results. Clinical reasoning should consider the biology of wound healing, the pharmacology of phenol and croton oil, and the need to respect the inflammatory window, so that procedures do not result in excessive tissue injury.

In general, medium and deep procedures should be indicated judiciously over time, while home care regimens — with retinoids, antioxidants, depigmenting agents, and alpha- or beta-hydroxy acids—serve to maintain results. The planned sequencing of techniques promotes clinical synergy: the peel addresses static rhytids and skin quality; botulinum toxin controls residual hyperkinesis; and fillers restore volumetric support when necessary. This combination, when applied judiciously, has been shown to significantly increase patient satisfaction.

The aim of this chapter, therefore, is to detail the rationale, order of execution, appropriate intervals, and precautions involved in combining phenol-croton oil peel with other dermatological interventions. The intention is to highlight the clinical scenarios in which such strategies maximize aesthetic and functional outcomes, always preserving patient safety.

9.2 General Principles of Sequencing

The planning of combinations must respect the biology of wound healing induced by phenol-croton oil peel. After application, an inflammatory phase is observed with re-epithelialization occurring in approximately 7 to 14 days, followed by an initial remodeling phase between the fourth and eighth weeks, and an expansive remodeling phase extending from 3 to 6 months, potentially evolving up to 12 months. Interventions that depend on stable tissue planes, such as fillers and biostimulators, are more predictable when performed after the inflammatory peak and tissue consolidation. Modulation of movement with botulinum toxin may be performed prior to phenol-croton oil peel to reduce traction during healing, or alternatively, after complete re-epithelialization when the aim is merely to refine residual facial expression. Technologies work best as remote tissue preparation—in mild sessions performed weeks beforehand—or as late maintenance, months later, when new collagen is already organized. In all scenarios, overlapping deep interventions in the same field during early inflammatory windows should be avoided, and extra caution is required in areas with compromised vascularization, especially where recent surgical undermining has occurred (Table 9.1).

Table 9.1 Temporal sequencing and safe windows for combination with phenol-croton oil peel

Modality	Main objective	Timing in relation to phenol-croton oil peel	Field/plane	Safety notes
Botulinum toxin (A)	Reduce facial expression/traction during healing; refine dynamic wrinkles	Preferably 2–3 weeks before; alternatively: ≥3–4 weeks after re-epithelialization	Areas of strong expression (forehead, glabella, periocular); conservative doses	Avoid on the same day as deep peel; reassess at 2–4 weeks for adjustments; possible reduced duration post-peel
Hyaluronic acid (HA)	Volumetric restoration/contouring	≥8–12 weeks after	Deep planes; prefer cannula; avoid superficial deposition	Early inflammation may accelerate degradation; particular caution in lips
Calcium hydroxyapatite (CaHA)	Structural support/skin quality (when hyperdiluted)	≥12–16 weeks after (may extend to 4–6 months)	Deep planes; hyperdilution when the focus is skin quality	Reduce risk of nodules in still-reactive tissue; advise on possible reduced initial longevity
Biostimulators (PLLA, PCL, hyperdiluted CaHA)	Sustained neocollagenesis; maintenance of firmness	Ideal between 3–6 months after	Plans appropriate to the technique; avoid areas with active nodules	Biological synergy (PLLA ~6 months peak); avoid early use on eyelids/perioral area
Technologies—Preparation	Standardize epidermis/texture before the peel	4–8 weeks prior; mild/sub-ablative protocols	Areas planned for phenol or adjacent (without deep injury)	Avoid disrupting the barrier so as not to combine depths during the phenol session
Technologies—Post-peeling (maintenance/refinement)	Fine texture/residual pigment; late tightening	On different fields: 14–30 days; coincident: NA/Q-switched ≥30–60 days; ablative ≥4–6 months; RFM/CO_2/Er:YAG fractional 6–12 months for refinement	Adjust according to phototype/skin thickness	Avoid simultaneous overlap in the same field; conservative parameters in higher phototypes
Other peels (Jessner + TCA; glycolic/salicylic)	Modulate depth by subunit; homogenize transitions	Same timing on distinct fields (no overlap); second peel only after full re-epithelialization (14–30 days)	Delimit zones; protect transition borders	"Retouch" if no sustained erythema at 7–10 days; consider new session in 2–6 months

(continued)

Table 9.1 (continued)

Modality	Main objective	Timing in relation to phenol-croton oil peel	Field/plane	Safety notes
Surgeries (rhytidectomy, blepharoplasty)	Vectors, skin excess and deep support	Option 1 (same procedure): TCA 20–40% on flaps; phenol-croton oil only on intact areasoption 2 (staged): Peeling 6–12 months after surgery	Respect perfusion; do not apply phenol to undermined flaps	Cardiology screening when indicated; document fields to avoid overlap
Acne scars (CROSS, subcision, microneedling)	Treat specific morphologies and diffuse remodeling	Alternate in separate sessions with 6–8 weeks between techniques; avoid microneedling/dermabrasion in the same phenol procedure	Focal CROSS with minimal volumes; subcision for fibrous bands; microneedling for diffuse areas	Strict photoprotection/depigmenting preparation in higher phototypes; monitor PIH

Summary of safe windows for combining botulinum toxin, fillers, biostimulators, technologies and surgeries with phenol-croton oil peel, based on the phases of wound healing (inflammatory, early remodeling and late remodeling). *Note: HA = hyaluronic acid; CaHA = calcium hydroxyapatite; PLLA = poly-L-lactic acid; PCL = polycaprolactone; NA = non-ablative; PIH = post-inflammatory hyperpigmentation. Source: Table prepared by the author (Dr Carolina Marçon)*

9.3 Combination with Botulinum Toxin

Type A botulinum toxin is one of the most frequent and effective combinations with phenol-croton oil peel, both in the overall management of photoaging and in specific segmental indications. Its main role is to reduce the muscular hyperactivity responsible for dynamic wrinkles, thereby lessening traction forces on the dermis during the healing process. This reduction in facial mimicry during the inflammatory and remodeling phases promotes more organized neocollagenesis, improves the quality of tissue regeneration, and contributes to more stable and long-lasting results. In addition to controlling dynamic wrinkles, the muscle relaxation induced by the toxin results in less mechanical tension on the regenerating dermis, which reduces repetitive microtrauma, optimizes collagen fiber alignment, and leads to more uniform scar remodeling. Clinical and experimental evidence further supports that botulinum toxin acts as an adjunct in wound healing by reducing tension at the margins, modulating fibroblast activity, and decreasing the expression of profibrotic cytokines such as TGF-β1, resulting in finer and aesthetically superior scars in various clinical trials. Although there are no specific studies evaluating this effect in the context of phenol-croton oil peel, the pathophysiological rationale suggests potential benefit in this setting as well. Additionally, there is evidence that muscle paralysis contributes to reduced peripheral nociceptive activation, attenuating the release of pain-related inflammatory mediators. Thus, the toxin may reduce intra- and post-operative discomfort, adding to the transient hypomimetic effect induced by phenol itself—due to its neurotoxicity—and the initial edema.

The most widely recommended sequence involves administering botulinum toxin 2–3 weeks prior to phenol-croton oil peel. This interval ensures that, during the critical period of re-epithelialization and inflammation—typically between 10 and 14 days—facial mimicry is already attenuated, reducing tension on healing wound edges and promoting more homogeneous remodeling. (Fig. 9.1) When pre-treatment is not feasible, toxin may be administered after complete re-epithelialization, from 3 to 4 weeks onwards, when the skin is stable and receptive. This approach is particularly useful for the forehead, glabella, and periocular region, always using conservative doses to avoid undesirable ptosis during edema. Reassessments between 2 and 4 weeks after the peel allow for minimal dose adjustments, preserving a natural appearance. Administration on the same day as deep peeling is not recommended, due to the risk of excessive diffusion caused by intense inflammation and immediate edema.

In the literature, Landau (2006) reviewed the clinical practice of combining chemical peels, including phenol-croton oil peel, botulinum toxin, and fillers. The author emphasized that muscle relaxation improves post-peel regeneration by reducing mechanical tension during dermal remodeling, recommending toxin administration two weeks before deep peeling, or three weeks after re-epithelialization, thus avoiding the most intense inflammatory phase that could disperse the toxin. Clinical cases presented demonstrated benefit in periocular rhytids treated with toxin after phenol-croton oil peel, without functional

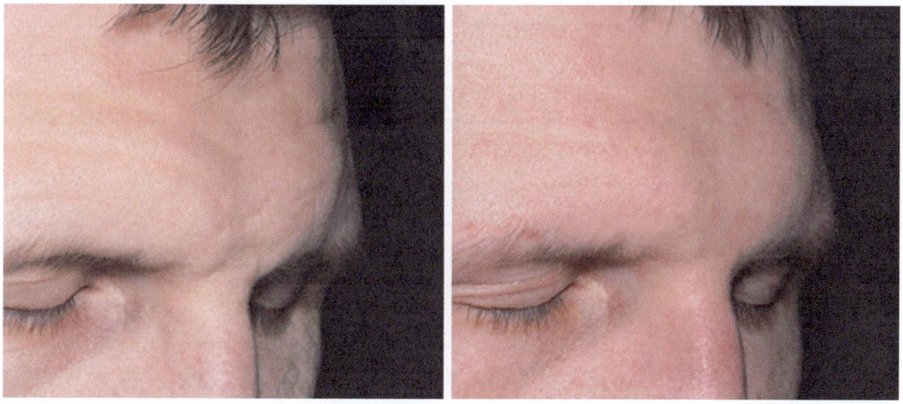

Fig. 9.1 Combination of pre-treatment with botulinum toxin type A and phenol-croton oil peel. Pre-treatment reduced pain perception and inhibited facial mimicry during the healing phase, resulting in improved outcomes. However, remodeling reduced the duration of neuromuscular blockade, necessitating reinjection at 3–4 months (earlier than the usual 5–6 month interval). *Left: pre-treatment. Right: 4 months after the peel, on the day of reinjection. Source: Personal archive of Dr Carlos Wambier*

distortions. Additionally, Tung et al. (2016) conducted a randomized, evaluator-blinded clinical trial comparing medium-depth peel (Jessner + TCA 35%) with and without pre-treatment with botulinum toxin A for lateral periocular rhytids. Twenty-six patients (Fitzpatrick I–III) were included, of whom 25 completed 10 weeks of follow-up. The combined group showed superior results, with a mean reduction in wrinkle score (FWSS—Fitzpatrick Wrinkle Severity Score) of 1.91 versus 0.93 in the peel-only group ($p = 0.001$). All patients in the combined group improved, while in the peel-only group, 12 out of 14 benefited. Although limited to medium-depth peels and short-term outcomes, this study provides randomized-level evidence that prior immobilization of facial mimicry enhances resurfacing results, which translates into a practical message for phenol-croton oil peel: schedule toxin administration 1–2 weeks before the procedure, preferably with a two-week interval, to reduce tension during healing. It is important to note that the study assessed only the aesthetic outcome (reduction in wrinkle severity via FWSS) and not healing parameters, re-epithelialization time, or complications. Thus, while the results indicate that prior immobilization of facial mimicry enhances the clinical effects of resurfacing, there is no evidence that toxin accelerates healing or reduces adverse events.

More recent reviews on periorbital rejuvenation also reinforce the importance of neuromodulators in attenuating dynamic wrinkles and optimizing multimodal protocols, highlighting even longer-acting formulations such as daxibotulinumtoxinA. In clinical practice, therefore, the combination of phenol-croton oil peel with botulinum toxin should follow certain principles: prioritize pre-treatment 2–3 weeks before the peel in areas of strong facial mimicry; consider administration from 3 weeks after re-epithelialization when the aim is only to refine residual wrinkles; avoid administration on the same day as deep peeling; and accept administration in different areas within the same therapeutic plan, as in the example of perioral phenol-croton oil peel combined with frontal toxin. Patients accustomed to toxin should also be advised that its duration may be reduced after phenol-croton oil peel, and early reinjection may be required, around 3–4 months.

In summary, the combination of botulinum toxin and phenol-croton oil peel has a solid clinical and biological rationale: in addition to standardizing healing by reducing mechanical tension and muscle mimicry, it is supported by external evidence that toxin improves scar quality in various settings. Although specific studies with phenol-croton oil peel are lacking, the sum of experimental and clinical evidence justifies its strategic use in combined protocols, provided safe intervals, rational planning, and therapeutic individualization are observed (Table 9.2).

Table 9.2 Clinical evidence for the combination of phenol-croton oil peel with other modalities

Author/year	Design	Combined interventions	N (phototypes)	Main findings	Limitations
Landau, 2006	Narrative review	Botulinum toxin + peels (including phenol-croton oil)	–	Recommends toxin 2 weeks before or ≥ 3 weeks after re-epithelialization; reduced traction favors regeneration	No specific RCTs with phenol-croton oil
Tung et al., 2016	Assessor-blinded RCT	Prior botulinum toxin A + medium-depth peel (Jessner +35% TCA) periocular	25 (I–III)	FWSS better in the combined group (1.91 vs 0.93; $p = 0.001$); 100% of combined group improved	Short-term; did not assess healing/ complications
Langsdon, Milburn & Yarber, 2000	Hemifacial comparative	Non-fractional CO_2 vs phenol (baker-Gordon)	4 (61–73 years)	Peel more comfortable and effective on thin skin; laser initially better on thick areas; hypopigmentation more frequent with laser	Small sample; outdated laser
Kaye et al., 2016 (PAVE)	Retrospective (6 years)	Rhytidectomy +20–40% TCA on undermined flaps + phenol-croton oil on intact areas	159	High satisfaction; social downtime 14–16 days; safe when perfusion maintained; 1 arrhythmia	Retrospective; no control
Ozturk et al., 2013	Case series	Rhytidectomy + perioral phenol-croton oil	–	Marked improvement in perioral rhytids; no increase in necrosis when vascularization preserved.	No control group; N not specified
Gatti, 2008	Clinical cohort	Lower blepharoplasty + periocular phenol (~50%; traces of croton oil when needed)	>700	Lightening and smoothing of rhytids; re-epithelialization 7–10 days; mild/ moderate complications	No standardized scores
Sterling, 2014	Pilot series	Micropunch blepharopeeling +89% phenol	8	Palpebral retraction without linear scar; re-epithelialization 7–10 days; erythema up to 4 months.	Small sample
Asilian et al., 2018	Prospective randomized trial	Surgical blepharoplasty vs micropunch blepharopeeling	22 (I–III)	Fewer scars (0% vs 36.4%) and higher satisfaction with micropunch; comparable aesthetics	Short follow-up; no histology
Lee & Rullan, 2019	Retrospective series	CROSS (88% phenol) + subcision (Nokor/biplanar cannula) + microneedling	139 (includes IV–VI)	Uniform improvement; low PIH with preparation; biplanar technique safer (fewer bruises)	No control; no universal scores

(continued)

Table 9.2 (continued)

Author/year	Design	Combined interventions	N (phototypes)	Main findings	Limitations
Lopez, 2024	Observational series	Serial microneedling + CROSS (60% phenol +0.2% croton oil)	21 (IV–V)	GAIS 50–75%; improvement of 1–2 grades (Goodman & Baron); 6–8 week intervals guided by TGF-β; minimal events	Without systemic monitoring; co-intervention; small N
Ayhan et al., 1998	Historical series	Phenol ≈50% + dermabrasion	>300	Long-lasting results (6–10 years) vs isolated dermabrasion (2–4); less bleeding	Outdated methodology; risk of cumulative tissue injury

Main publications evaluating the combination of phenol-croton oil peel or related techniques with botulinum toxin, fillers, technologies, surgeries, and approaches for acne scars. Authors, study design, number of patients, main findings, and limitations are presented, providing a critical overview of the available body of evidence. *Note: FWSS = Fitzpatrick Wrinkle Severity Score; TCA = trichloroacetic acid; PIH = post-inflammatory hyperpigmentation; GAIS = Global Aesthetic Improvement Scale; TGF-β = transforming growth factor beta. Source: Table prepared by the author (Dr Carolina Marçon)*

9.4 Combination with Fillers

The phenol-croton oil peel profoundly transforms skin quality, but does not, by itself, restore the volume lost with aging. Therefore, combining it with fillers represents an important complementary strategy to restore facial contours and proportions. The most common indications involve the use of hyaluronic acid and, in specific situations, calcium hydroxyapatite, both applied in deep planes for structural replacement.

Planning the combination must respect the time required for tissue recovery and consolidation. For hyaluronic acid, it is recommended to wait 8–12 weeks after the peel, by which time the initial inflammatory process has resolved, offering greater predictability of integration. For calcium hydroxyapatite, the ideal interval is usually even longer, from 12 to 16 weeks or more, reducing the risk of nodules and complications in still-reactive tissue.

Skin subjected to peeling is temporarily thinner, with increased vascularization and intense inflammatory activity, making it essential to prefer deep planes and cannulas, avoiding superficial deposits that may result in irregularities or visibility of the material. The most frequently treated areas after peeling include the nasolabial fold, marionette lines, jawline contour, and malar area. The lip region, in turn, requires particular caution due to residual inflammation, which increases the risk of complications when treatment is performed too early. Clinical reports describe good outcomes in elderly patients with malar lipoatrophy treated with hyaluronic acid after deep peeling, as well as in depressed scars, with adequate integration and persistence of effects for up to 1 year. There is also a case report of lip augmentation performed 6 weeks after peeling, with a satisfactory aesthetic result, although this interval is considered borderline.

A critical point is understanding how the robust inflammation triggered by the phenol-croton oil peel may impact the longevity of fillers. The activation of hyaluronidases and metalloproteinases, together with the dermal remodeling process, may accelerate the degradation of hyaluronic acid, reducing its duration. Although specific clinical studies are lacking, this biological plausibility explains the practical observation of shorter filler duration when injected in the early phases of healing. For this reason, it is recommended that filling in overlapping areas be postponed for at least 8–12 weeks for hyaluronic acid and 12–16 weeks for calcium hydroxyapatite, with the interval extended to 4–6 months in situations requiring greater safety.

In distinct areas, the combination may be performed on the same day, provided there is no overlap of treated fields. Nevertheless, it should be considered that the systemic inflammation and remodeling triggered by deep peeling may theoretically accelerate the degradation of fillers in adjacent or even distant regions, which justifies advising the patient about the possibility of reduced longevity.

Another relevant aspect is the presence of previous fillers. In the case of permanent fillers, such as polymethylmethacrylate (PMMA), although there are no studies directly evaluating its interaction with peeling, it is known that intense

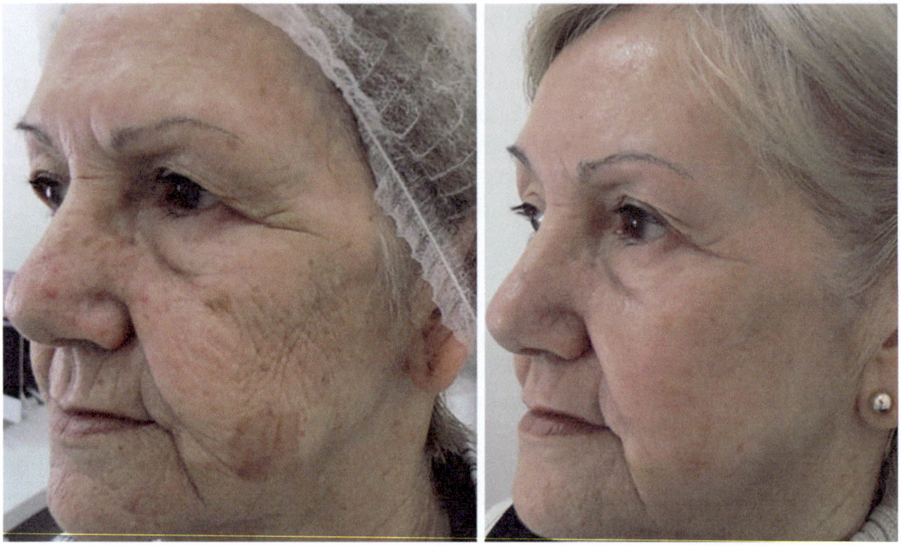

Fig. 9.2 Combination of multiple treatments with phenol-croton oil peel. Left: before. Right: one year after full facial phenol-croton oil peel (Hetter 1.2%) and periocular phenol-croton oil peel (Hetter 1.6%), followed by deep-plane malar filling with 30% polymethylmethacrylate (PMMA) using a 21G microcannula, with persistent and satisfactory results. Two months after the initial chemical peel, additional treatment was performed with Q-switched 532 nm laser for residual seborrheic keratosis lesions. Macular on the mandibular line. Source: *Personal archive of Dr Carlos Wambier*

inflammatory processes may serve as a trigger for late complications, such as granulomatous reactions, nodules, or irregularities. Therefore, performing the peel is not contraindicated, but requires careful assessment and transparent discussion with the patient. (Fig. 9.2) For temporary fillers, the recommendation is similar: the peel does not contraindicate their presence, but it should be clarified that resorption may be accelerated, and expectations regarding maintenance of results should be adjusted.

In summary, the combination of phenol-croton oil peel and fillers is synergistic and enhances the overall outcomes of facial rejuvenation, provided that the appropriate timing for each technique is respected and an individualized risk assessment is maintained. Understanding that the inflammatory process is the main modulator of this interaction is essential to safely guide the patient, align expectations, and achieve stable and harmonious results.

9.5 Combination with Collagen Biostimulators

Collagen biostimulators—notably poly-L-lactic acid, calcium hydroxyapatite in induction dilutions, and polycaprolactone—can prolong and amplify the remodeling initiated by phenol-croton oil peel by inducing sustained neocollagenesis, predominantly of collagen types I and III, and to a lesser extent neoelastogenesis, through a controlled inflammatory response around the particles, with macrophage polarization and subsequent fibroblast stimulation. In the case of poly-L-lactic acid, histotemporal studies show that, after approximately 1 month, microparticles become encapsulated by inflammatory cells, followed by intensified fibroblastic activity around 3 months, reaching a peak of collagen deposition at about 6 months, with prolonged clinical maintenance. This behavior explains the rationale for using it as matrix reinforcement once the healing process of the phenol-croton oil peel has passed the initial phases and entered mature remodeling.

Hyper-diluted calcium hydroxyapatite, used without volumizing intent, has demonstrated in clinical and histological studies an improvement in skin quality, including firmness, thickness, and mechanical properties, attributed to the stimulation of neocollagenesis and neoelastogenesis around the microspheres after dilution. Results have been documented in serial protocols, and although there is no direct evidence following phenol-croton oil peel, they support its role as an "active maintenance" strategy for the quality achieved. Polycaprolactone, in turn, also acts as a long-lasting collagen stimulator; recent reviews and experimental studies in animal and human models have demonstrated an increase in collagen types I and III, supporting its use as a late matrix reinforcement after scar stabilization of the treated area.

Regarding timing, there are no clinical trials that definitively establish a single window after phenol-croton oil peel. The recommendation to introduce biostimulators between three and 6 months is based on the biology of deep wound healing and the histotemporal data of the biostimulators themselves: after a deep peel, re-epithelialization occurs in approximately 8 to 14 days, erythema may persist for several weeks, and dermal remodeling continues for months, with progressive fiber maturation. Thus, from 3 months onwards, the tissue tends to be more stable to receive a new collagen-inducing stimulus, and around 6 months, there is even a synergy of biological peaks, as poly-L-lactic acid reaches its peak fibroblastic activity during this period. In other words, this interval minimizes cumulative inflammation and maximizes the predictability of integration.

From a pathophysiological perspective, biostimulators can enhance the results of phenol-croton oil peel through three main mechanisms: they reduce the "gap" in fibrillar support that may persist after the initial reorganization induced by the peel, promoting secondary deposition of collagen I and III; they increase dermal density and the mechanical resistance of the tissue, with effects documented in studies of the neck and décolletage with hyper-diluted calcium hydroxyapatite; and they provide maintenance between the sixth and twelfth months, a period in which the clinical curve of the peel tends to stabilize or decline, thereby prolonging skin firmness and texture.

Regarding the potential interference of prior use of biostimulators with phenol-croton oil peel, there are no direct studies demonstrating impairment of the peel in the presence of previously implanted particles. The clinical reasoning is one of caution: the robust and diffuse inflammation induced by a deep peel could, in theory, modulate the response to the biostimulator, transiently altering the dynamics of degradation or encapsulation. However, unlike permanent implants, biostimulators have a programmable integration and degradation profile, as in the case of poly-L-lactic acid and polycaprolactone, or controlled bioactivity, as with calcium hydroxyapatite. Thus, the practical approach is to avoid peeling directly over areas with active nodules and to respect intervals that prevent overlapping inflammatory windows. Beyond this, the prior presence of a biostimulator is not an absolute contraindication, and the patient should simply be informed that the overall clinical response may vary.

In areas of greater sensitivity, such as the eyelids and perioral region in the immediate post-phenol-croton oil peel period, the risk of nodulation or hyperreactivity with poly-L-lactic acid is higher for two reasons: the thin skin and superficial planes favor suboptimal deposits, which is already described in product leaflets as a risk factor for papules and nodules in the periorbital area, and the exacerbated inflammatory state of the first weeks after the peel increases the likelihood of a granulomatous response or irregular organization. Therefore, in these regions, early use should be avoided and, when indicated, appropriate application depth should be prioritized.

In summary, biostimulators may potentially prolong the quality curve initiated by phenol-croton oil peel when introduced late, around 3–6 months after the procedure, in already stabilized tissue. Poly-L-lactic acid acts as a medium-term fibrillar reinforcement, hyper-diluted calcium hydroxyapatite improves mechanical properties and skin quality in serial protocols, and polycaprolactone provides long-lasting collagen stimulation. All share a histological basis and indirect clinical evidence consistent with the strategy of maintaining and enhancing results.

9.6 Combination with Technologies

The combination of phenol-croton oil peel with technologies has been explored both as a preparatory strategy and for the maintenance of medium- and long-term results. Fractional lasers and microneedling radiofrequency can be employed prior to the peel, in mild and sub-ablative protocols performed 4–8 weeks beforehand, with the aim of evening out the epidermis, reducing pore size, controlling oiliness, and improving the homogeneity of the cutaneous field to be treated. Subsequently, between 6–12 months after deep peeling, these technologies serve to refine residual texture and persistent pigmentation, provided that conservative parameters and wide intervals between sessions are observed. Additional interventions are not recommended in the first 8–12 weeks after peeling, a period during which the inflammatory response remains intense and the risk of aberrant scarring and post-inflammatory dyschromia is higher. The choice of device and energy calibration should always consider phototype, skin thickness, and individual history of hyperpigmentation.

Although phenol-croton oil peel and laser resurfacing are distinct techniques, there are consistent reports of sequential and combined use, especially in cases of deep rhytids and scarring. CO_2 laser, in particular, is described as a modern alternative to deep peeling, but the literature does not establish a consensus regarding the superiority of one technique over the other. Comparative studies suggest that the results may be complementary and that integration should respect the principle of field separation, avoiding the overlap of chemical and thermal injuries in the same region. The work of Langsdon, Milburn, and Yarber (2000) illustrates this discussion by comparing, in a hemifacial model, CO_2 laser resurfacing (Silktouch Flashscanner, non-fractional) and deep phenol-croton oil chemical peel. Four women aged between 61 and 73 years were treated with phenol peel on one hemiface, using a formulation containing phenol, croton oil drops, antimicrobial soap, and distilled water (Baker-Gordon formula), applied according to the traditional technique, while the opposite hemiface received laser with two passes (differentiated parameters for the periocular and central facial regions). In one patient, subsequent rhytidoplasty allowed direct histological analysis of the treated areas. The authors observed that, clinically, discomfort was shorter on the peel side, whereas the laser side produced more intense erythema, more pronounced edema, and prolonged hypersensitivity. In thin skin (eyelids and lateral malar region), both techniques were equivalent for rhytid reduction, with results maintained at 1 year. In thicker and more glandular areas (nasolabial fold and chin), the laser showed an initial advantage in texture and smoothing, a difference that diminished after 6 months but persisted slightly at 1 year. Regarding pigmentary changes, hypopigmentation was more frequent and pronounced on the laser side, with only one case of mild hyperpigmentation, which resolved with topical therapy. Histology confirmed that the peel reached the reticular dermis, while the laser was limited to the papillary dermis, both eliminating solar elastosis and promoting subsequent remodeling. Thus, the study reinforces that deep peeling maintains superior efficacy in areas of thin skin, while the laser offers better initial performance in thicker regions, at the cost of a higher risk of hypopigmentation and prolonged downtime.

The physical-biological differences between platforms help to design combined regimens. Er:YAG (2940 nm), due to its very high absorption in water, causes minimal thermal damage, faster re-epithelialization, and shallower penetration—useful for fine lines and superficial resurfacing; CO_2 (10,600 nm), with greater thermal effect, penetrates deeper and promotes tightening, but with a higher risk of persistent erythema and dyschromia. Classic comparative and clinical series support these distinctions, although techniques, parameters, and devices vary between studies. In parallel, fractional photothermolysis (non-ablative and ablative) introduced the concept of "microscopic treatment zones" (MTZ), preserving islands of intact skin to accelerate healing; this reduces downtime and risk in higher phototypes, at the cost of more sessions to achieve results equivalent to full ablative protocols.

In clinical practice, integration with laser can serve different functions. Q-switched systems (532/1064 nm) are used for residual pigmentary disorders, including freckles, melanoses, and post-inflammatory hyperpigmentation, and may be applied even in areas not treated with phenol. Ablative lasers, such as Er:YAG (2940 nm) and fractional CO_2 (10,600 nm), are reserved for mild residual rhytids, generally between 6 and 12 months after peeling, when the initial remodeling process has stabilized. The ideal timing varies according to the type of energy and the area: in different fields, lasers can be used between 14 and 30 days after peeling; in overlapping areas, caution is advised—Q-switched or non-ablative systems only after 30–60 days, and ablative lasers not before 4–6 months.

Regarding "simultaneous" and "same area" application, the literature specific to phenol-croton oil is scarce, but data on the facilitation of chemical penetration after ablation highlight the risk of unpredictable summation of depth. There is evidence that removal epidermal/fractional approaches may enhance the delivery of trichloroacetic acid (TCA) and potentiate the effect of chemical peeling; by prudent extrapolation, combining laser and phenol in the same field and session—especially with ablative platforms—may exceed the safety threshold, increasing the risk of complications. Therefore, it is recommended to segment treatment fields (laser for thick/sebaceous areas; phenol for thin skin) or to stagger the timing between modalities when treating the same area.

Microneedling radiofrequency (RFM) adds a dermal thermal stimulation axis that relatively spares the epidermis, making it an interesting option for maintaining texture after phenol peeling and for higher phototypes when conservative parameters are used. Histological studies have demonstrated neoelastogenesis and neocollagenesis with fractional needles, and recent clinical series confirm texture improvement with minimal interference in daily activities—an approach that aligns well with a late "polishing" strategy following a deep peel.

The combination of microfocused ultrasound (HIFU) and phenol-croton oil peel has not yet been the subject of published scientific studies. Nevertheless, HIFU is widely recognized for its ability to induce tissue contraction and neocollagenesis in deeper layers without significantly affecting the epidermis, which theoretically makes it compatible as a complementary technology to chemical peeling. Clinical studies have demonstrated the safety and efficacy of HIFU when combined with monopolar radiofrequency, with significant improvement in the degree of skin rejuvenation and no serious complications, only transient erythema.

Observational aesthetic protocols and clinical guidelines recommend the sequential use of these technologies—first the peel to restore texture and pigmentation, followed by HIFU a few weeks later to promote lifting and tightening—respecting intervals that preserve healing integrity and minimize risks. This approach, based on physiological principles and practical consensus, appears promising but lacks validation from specific controlled studies; therefore, its use should be cautious, individualized, and preferably conducted within observational protocols.

Another relevant issue is the management of post-peel erythema. Although some authors propose the use of vascular technologies, such as intense pulsed light (IPL) or pulsed dye laser (PDL), to hasten the resolution of persistent erythema, there is controversy regarding the appropriateness of this approach. Post-procedural erythema represents not only vasodilation but also essential inflammatory activity for dermal remodeling and new collagen synthesis. Thus, early intervention on these vessels could theoretically reduce the regenerative stimulus and compromise long-term outcomes. The literature is scarce and inconclusive regarding this interference, and most experts recommend a conservative approach, limiting the treatment of persistent erythema to topical measures and strict photoprotection, reserving vascular technologies only for refractory and prolonged cases where there is significant functional or psychological impact.

Finally, three practical messages underpin the multimodal strategy: (1) avoid simultaneous overlap in the same area of phenol-croton oil with ablative platforms; (2) reserve fractional CO_2/Er:YAG for late maintenance of fine lines/texture or remote preparation in thick/sebaceous fields; (3) use Q-switched 532/1064 nm conservatively for residual pigment, especially in non-phenolised areas or late in phenolised areas. Other technologies, such as LEDs, photodynamic therapy, and IPL/BBL (broadband light), have a role as adjuncts in maintaining results and treating residual pigmentation, at a later stage, with a secondary role in protocols combined with phenol-croton oil.

In summary, the combination of phenol-croton oil peel with technologies should follow principles of caution and segmentation. Sequential use, with appropriate intervals and respect for the characteristics of each facial area, allows for enhanced results and reduced risks, while simultaneous overlap in the same field should be avoided. Careful integration, supported by histological and clinical knowledge, broadens therapeutic possibilities and contributes to safe and long-lasting global rejuvenation.

9.7 Combination with Other Peels in Segmental Treatment

Segmental treatment is a valuable strategy to optimize the efficacy and reduce the risks of phenol-croton oil peeling. This approach allows modulation of depth according to the needs of each anatomical subunit, reserving the phenol-croton oil solution for areas of marked elastosis and deep rhytids—such as the perioral and periocular regions—and employing medium or superficial peels in areas with less damage or higher risk of complications. In this way, harmonious global rejuvenation is achieved, with a reduction in the body surface area exposed to phenol and a consequent decrease in systemic risk (Fig. 9.3).

One of the classic combinations described in the literature by Monheit consists of the application of Jessner's solution followed by trichloroacetic acid (TCA) at concentrations between 20% and 35% to areas such as the forehead, nasal dorsum, and malar regions, while phenol-croton oil is applied segmentally to the perioral and periocular regions, without overlapping fields. Jessner's solution acts as a preparatory agent, removing the epidermal barrier and increasing skin permeability, thereby enhancing TCA penetration and ensuring greater predictability of the depth achieved. The efficacy of this combination has been demonstrated for various indications, including photoaging and pigmentary disorders, with significant improvement in texture and pigmentation. (Fig. 9.4) Alternatively, serial medium-depth peels may be performed 6–8 weeks before or after the phenol-croton oil peel, with the aim of evening out the texture of adjacent areas and softening transitions. This approach requires strict demarcation of treatment zones with a surgical marker, protection of the borders with occlusive barriers, and standardized photographic documentation—essential measures to reduce the risk of solution spillover and minimize demarcation lines.

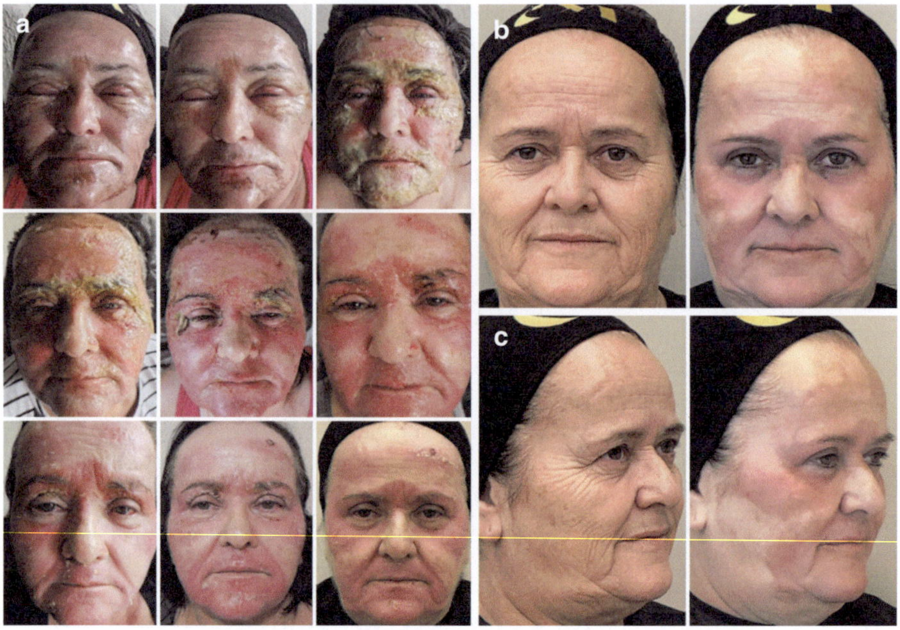

Fig. 9.3 Clinical evolution after phenol-croton oil peel (Hetter 1.2% in the periocular region and 1.6% in the perioral region) combined with Jessner's peel +35% TCA (Monheit) on the forehead. A more intense inflammatory response, with marked erythema and desquamation, is observed in the areas treated with phenol-croton oil compared to TCA. Full-face peeling was avoided due to the patient's cardiovascular risk factors. (**a**) daily progression of the inflammatory process. (**b**) frontal view before and 3 months after treatment. (**c**) oblique views before and 3 months after treatment. *Source: Author's personal archive (Dr Carolina Marçon)*

The "touch-up" may be considered in cases where, after 7–10 days, there is no sustained erythema in the treated area, indicating insufficient injury. In such cases, it is possible to reapply the same formula, opt for a more potent solution, or schedule a new session between 2 and 6 months. When it is necessary to combine another chemical agent, one must always respect the window for complete re-epithelialization—generally between 14 and 30 days—before a second peel, avoiding reapplication to areas already exposed to phenol-croton oil.

Another relevant aspect is the possibility of combining phenol-croton oil peel on the face with TCA on the neck, a strategy already described in classic publications. This combination provides integrated aesthetic improvement while respecting safety limits, since TCA, unlike phenol, does not have cardiotoxic effects. Comparative experimental evidence has shown that phenol may induce arrhythmias and myocardial depression, whereas TCA, even at high concentrations (50%), does not cause significant cardiovascular changes. Thus, in patients at higher systemic risk, segmenting and partially replacing phenol with TCA in adjacent areas is a rational approach to reduce the body surface area exposed to phenol and, consequently, minimize complications.

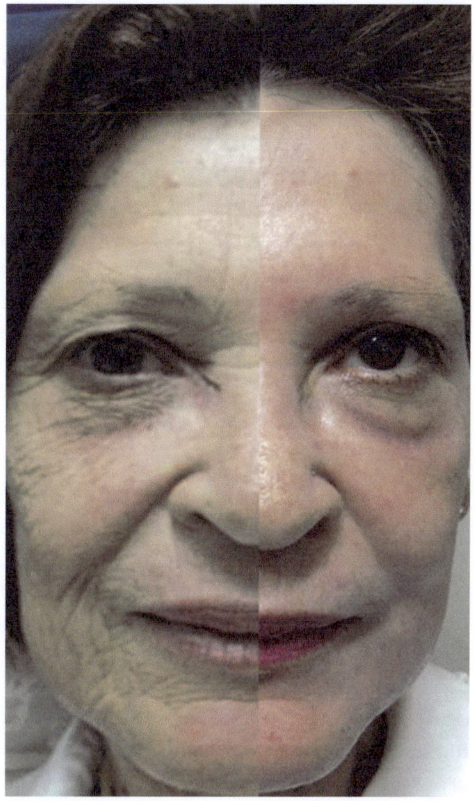

Fig. 9.4 Phenol-croton oil peel to the full face, sparing the lower periocular region due to marked laxity demonstrated by the snap-back test. After 30 days, the lower periocular area was treated with Monheit's medium-depth peel (Jessner's solution followed by 35% trichloroacetic acid). Left and right: same hemiface, identified by a frontal intradermal nevus. Left: before. Right: 2 months after phenol-croton oil peel and 1 month after Monheit's peel to the lower eyelid. *Source: Personal archive of Dr Carlos Wambier*

In summary, the combination of phenol-croton oil peel with other chemical peels—especially Jessner's solution plus TCA, but also glycolic or salicylic acid in preparatory or maintenance superficial peels—is a validated practice of great clinical utility. This strategy allows precise modulation of depth, maintains homogeneity of results, and broadens the safety margin, integrating the unique remodeling potential of phenol-croton oil with the versatility and safety profile of medium and superficial peels.

9.8 Combination with Plastic Surgery

The combination of phenol-croton oil peel with aesthetic surgical procedures, particularly rhytidectomy and blepharoplasty, has been the subject of investigation since the earliest formulations and remains an area of great interest due to its ability to deliver more comprehensive and long-lasting results. Surgery alone corrects skin excess, repositions deep structures, and restores support, but does not significantly improve texture, elastosis, or diffuse fine rhytids. Phenol-croton oil peel, on the other hand, acts on skin quality, inducing extensive and long-lasting dermal remodeling. When combined judiciously, these approaches offer synergistic results, enhancing overall rejuvenation.

In rhytidectomy, phenol-croton oil peel has proven particularly effective for treating areas where surgery has limited impact, such as the perioral region, glabellar rhytids, and peri-nasal folds. Ozturk et al. (2013) described a series of patients undergoing rhytidectomy combined with perioral phenol-croton oil peel, documenting marked improvement in deep vertical wrinkles in this region, which represent a classic surgical challenge. The authors emphasized that the combination enabled more homogeneous rejuvenation with greater impact on perceived age, without a significant increase in the risk of necrosis when the absolute contraindication of applying the peel to undermined flaps was respected. This principle was reinforced by histological studies by Gonser et al. (2017), which demonstrated that phenol-croton oil applied to undermined areas reaches the upper reticular dermis, compromising residual vascularization and increasing the risk of flap ischemia. Thus, the recommendation to limit deep peels to intact skin, applying more superficial agents to flaps, is now a consensus in the literature.

Another important contribution comes from Kaye et al. (2016), who published a six-year retrospective analysis of 159 patients treated with the PAVE protocol (Peeling-Assisted Volume Enhancing Lift), in which rhytidectomy with SMAS plication was combined with fat grafting and selected chemical peels according to the vascularization of the flap: TCA 20–40% in undermined areas and phenol-croton oil peel in non-undermined areas with intact perfusion, especially perioral, nasal, and glabellar regions. In more advanced cases (Glogau IV), the mosaic technique was used, with TCA applied to undermined flaps and phenol-croton oil to non-undermined areas. The average time for social reintegration was 14–16 days. The authors reported high subjective satisfaction, safety comparable to that described in the literature for each isolated procedure, and manageable complications such as transient hyperpigmentation, milia, and prolonged erythema. One case of cardiac arrhythmia underscored the need for preoperative cardiological screening and ECG. The study, with a robust case series, supports the safety and technical rationale of combining both procedures in a single operative stage, provided that phenol-croton oil peel is not applied to areas with compromised vascularization.

In the classic study by Peled, Ullmann, and Ramon (1996), deep chemical peeling with phenol (Baker-Gordon formula) was presented as a non-surgical alternative to rhytidectomy in selected patients, especially those whose main concern was the presence of fine wrinkles, trophic changes, and sun-induced skin damage, situations in which surgical traction alone does not yield satisfactory results. Conversely, in cases of greater skin laxity, the authors highlighted the superiority of combining both modalities, emphasizing that rhytidectomy should be performed first to correct tissue laxity, while phenol peel acts subsequently as an indispensable adjunct to promote skin renewal, improve texture, and treat residual rhytids. Thus, the chemical procedure is not indicated prior to surgery, but rather as an isolated alternative in patients who do not wish to undergo or are not candidates for surgical intervention, or as a postoperative adjunct in combined protocols aiming to rejuvenate both facial contour and skin quality simultaneously. The interval between procedures was not specified in the publication.

Phenol-croton oil peel remains one of the most effective techniques for treating periorbital skin changes, especially in the management of hyperpigmentation and fine rhytids, which respond poorly to blepharoplasty alone. The clinical experience accumulated by John E. Gatti (2008) over more than two decades, in over 700 procedures, demonstrates that combining phenol peel with lower blepharoplasty significantly enhances aesthetic outcomes. This protocol provides skin lightening and smoothing of wrinkles in the lower eyelid and lateral periorbital region, promoting overall rejuvenation of the gaze. The technique used by the author consisted of a modified 50% phenol solution, prepared by diluting 1 mL of phenol in 1 mL of water and adding a drop of liquid soap to facilitate homogenization. In cases of deeper wrinkles, minimal traces of croton oil were added to increase penetration and efficacy. Application was performed with a cotton swab, extending from the lower eyelid to the malar and temporal regions, until initial frosting appeared, followed by erythema. The procedure was usually performed 6–8 weeks after blepharoplasty, although it could also be indicated as a standalone treatment in patients seeking only cutaneous aesthetic improvement.

Postoperative care included immediate occlusion of the treated area with petroleum jelly, cold compresses in the first days, and subsequently the use of moisturizers and makeup after re-epithelialization, which occurred in about 7–10 days. In cases of residual hyperpigmentation, 4% hydroquinone was prescribed from the first month. The results obtained were consistent: most patients showed marked improvement in skin texture, with reduction of fine wrinkles and skin lightening, softening dark circles and periorbital shadows. Even in individuals with thicker skin, deep wrinkles, or in men, where the aesthetic response was less pronounced, the procedure proved valuable as an adjunct. The complications observed were mostly mild and transient, including prolonged erythema and post-inflammatory hyperpigmentation, both managed with topical therapy. Isolated areas of deeper desquamation resulted in mild hypopigmentation, which was nonetheless considered aesthetically acceptable. Severe complications such as necrosis, hypertrophic scarring, or eyelid deformities were not reported. In his critical analysis, Gatti emphasized that, even in the face of the increasing replacement of chemical peels by ablative technologies such as lasers, phenol remains a simple, predictable, safe option with long-lasting results, with mild hypopigmentation often being an aesthetically favorable effect, capable of reducing dark circles and eyelid shadowing.

While lower blepharoplasty greatly benefits from the combination with phenol-croton oil peel to correct skin texture and pigmentation, excess skin of the upper eyelid has historically been treated almost exclusively by surgical blepharoplasty, which involves linear skin excision and scar formation. Although the Baker-Gordon phenol formulation had already been tested as a non-surgical option for eyelid tightening, its limitations—such as prolonged healing time and risk of persistent hypopigmentation—reduced its clinical acceptance. In this context, Sterling (2014) proposed micropunch blepharopeeling, a hybrid technique that combines diffuse application of 89% phenol with multiple non-linear micro-excisions of skin, performed in a random pattern and healing by secondary intention, aiming to reduce skin excess without a linear scar and with less aggressiveness compared to traditional deep peels.

In his pilot study, Sterling treated eight patients with a mean age of 59.6 years, all with thin to medium skin, diffuse rhytids, and mild to moderate upper eyelid skin excess. After application of phenol until uniform frosting was achieved, micro-excisions were performed with curved scissors, ranging from 5 to 20 per eyelid, depending on skin thickness. The areas were left to heal openly, treated only with petrolatum. Re-epithelialization occurred within 7–10 days, although erythema persisted for up to 4 months. No linear scars or severe complications were observed, and the results demonstrated effective upper eyelid skin tightening, improvement of periocular rhytids, and a natural aesthetic appearance, without the inherent risks of traditional blepharoplasty, such as asymmetries, changes in the eyelid crease, or a "hollow eye" appearance due to fat removal (Fig. 9.5).

Subsequently, Asilian and colleagues (2018) conducted a prospective, randomized clinical trial with 22 patients, directly comparing surgical blepharoplasty to micropunch blepharopeeling. The participants, with phototypes I to III, had thin to medium skin, mild to moderate skin excess, and diffuse rhytids. After follow-up at 2 weeks and 2 months, the micropunch group showed a lower incidence of scarring (none, versus 36.4% in the blepharoplasty group), greater satisfaction regarding symmetry, pain, and scarring, as well as more favorable physician assessments in terms of naturalness and absence of surgical stigmata. Complications such as hypopigmentation, hyperpigmentation, dry eye, bruises, and ecchymoses occurred in both groups, with no statistically significant differences, and no serious complications such as diplopia or infections were recorded. From an aesthetic perspective, the results of the micropunch technique were comparable to those of conventional blepharoplasty, but with advantages in the complication profile and in the degree of satisfaction among patients and evaluators, establishing it as a promising, less invasive technique with faster recovery.

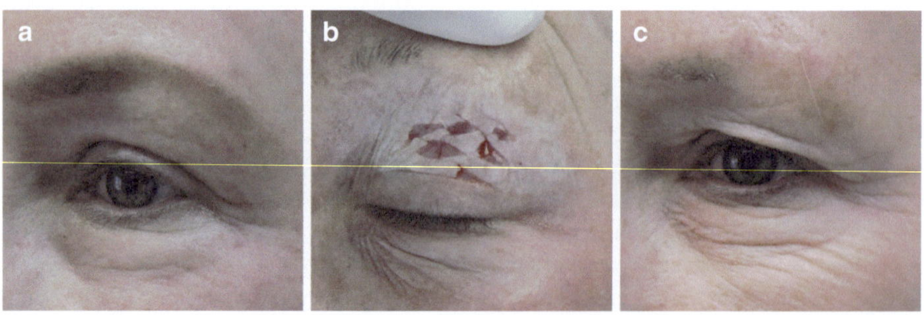

Fig. 9.5 Phenol-croton oil peel (Hetter 1.2%) combined with micropunch on the upper eyelid. (**a**) pre-treatment. (**b**) immediately after the peel and micro-excisions. (**c**) 6 weeks post-procedure, showing effective skin tightening and smoothing of rhytids without linear scarring. *Source: Courtesy of Dr J. Barton Sterling*

The periocular region, therefore, represents one of the most challenging areas in facial rejuvenation, as surgery alone is not always able to satisfactorily correct residual hyperpigmentation, fine rhytids, and irregular eyelid skin texture. In these scenarios, phenol-croton oil peel, when applied segmentally and judiciously, has proven to be a highly valuable tool both as an adjunct and, in certain cases, as an alternative to surgery.

9.9 Combination of Phenol-Croton Oil Peel in the Treatment of Acne Scars

Atrophic acne scars are among the greatest challenges in aesthetic dermatology due to their morphological diversity, involving icepick, boxcar, and rolling patterns, often found in combination. This heterogeneity explains the need for combined therapeutic approaches that act complementarily on the different components of the scar—whether fibrous bands, pinpoint depressions, or collapse of the dermal matrix. Phenol-croton oil peel, due to its recognized potential for deep dermal remodeling and improvement of skin texture, occupies a central role in this context, especially when applied segmentally or focally, in protocols integrated with other techniques that enhance the clinical response (Fig. 9.6).

One of the most recent reports on this approach is the study by Lopez (2024), which evaluated the combination of serial microneedling and CROSS (Chemical Reconstruction of Skin Scars, a technique involving focal chemical application to atrophic scars to induce protein coagulation and localized dermal remodeling) using 60% phenol combined with 0.2% croton oil in 21 patients, predominantly Fitzpatrick skin types IV and V. The protocol involved microneedling with variable depths from 0.5 to 1.75 mm,

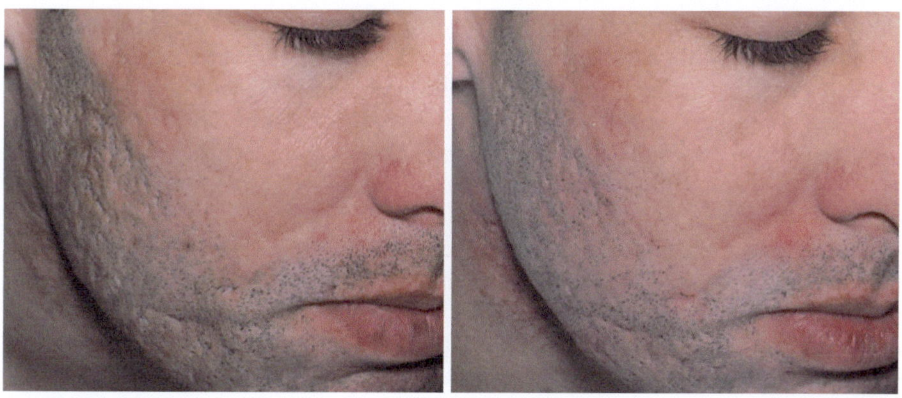

Fig. 9.6 Chemical reconstruction of acne scars (CROSS) performed in three monthly sessions, using phenol solution 88% (full-strength stock solution, diluted with 1 drop of croton oil per mL) combined with full-face treatment using Q-switched Nd:YAG laser (1064 nm) prior to each application, aiming to improve irregular skin pigmentation and melasma. *Source: Personal archive of Dr Carlos Wambier*

including a stamping technique for thicker scars, followed by focal CROSS application to narrow icepick and boxcar scars. Improvements of 1–2 grades on the Goodman & Baron scale and GAIS (Global Aesthetic Improvement Scale) responses of 50–75% were observed in most patients, with rapid recovery and minimal adverse events. The author justifies the 6- to 8-week intervals between sessions based on TGF-β kinetics, suggesting that sessions performed too frequently could accentuate pro-fibrotic stimulation, whereas waiting allows predominance of TGF-β3, which is associated with regenerative healing. Despite the encouraging results, the study has significant limitations: small sample size, absence of a control group, concomitant use of a growth factor serum, and lack of hemodynamic or laboratory monitoring to assess systemic absorption of phenol. Another important aspect concerns safety: by disrupting the epidermal barrier, microneedling theoretically increases the risk of systemic penetration of phenol and croton oil. Although no serious complications were reported in this series, the lack of objective monitoring warrants caution, especially in light of recent clinical reports of fatal events when microneedling and phenol were performed during the same surgical session. Thus, although the combination appears promising, the practical recommendation is to alternate the techniques in separate sessions, maintaining a 6- to 8-week interval, and not to combine them in the same procedure.

Another multimodal protocol was described by Lee and Rullan (2019), who retrospectively evaluated 139 patients, including a significant proportion of higher Fitzpatrick skin types, treated with CROSS using 88% phenol, subcision, and microneedling. CROSS was applied to icepick and boxcar scars, followed by subcision—performed with both an 18G Nokor needle and an 18G blunt cannula using a biplanar approach, which proved safer and carried a lower risk of hematoma. Subsequently, microneedling was performed to the endpoint of pinpoint bleeding, aiming for diffuse collagen induction. Photographic results demonstrated uniform improvement, accompanied by high patient satisfaction and a low incidence of post-inflammatory hyperpigmentation, even in skin types IV to VI, provided that skin preparation and photoprotection protocols were followed. Although this was a retrospective study without a control group or standardized objective scores, the robust sample size and detailed technical description confer significant clinical applicability, supporting the rationale for a sequential approach: focal CROSS for pinpoint defects, subcision for fibrotic bands, and microneedling for diffuse dermal remodeling. This rationale can be extended to the use of phenol-croton oil, provided that minimal volumes are used and strict monitoring is maintained.

In the field of combinations with mechanical procedures, the classic work of Ayhan and colleagues (1998) deserves mention. They described the combination of chemical peeling with phenol (≈ 50%) and dermabrasion in over 300 patients treated over two decades. The proposed rationale was to use phenol as a coagulating agent and "biological marker" of depth, followed by high-speed mechanical dermabrasion to level the surface. The authors reported greater durability of results—up to 6–10 years for facial rejuvenation, compared to 2–4 years with dermabrasion alone—less intraoperative bleeding, and a more comfortable postoperative period. The figures presented showed significant improvement in acne scars, post-traumatic scars, and wrinkles, although standardized scoring systems were not used. Despite the accumulated experience, this is a historical series with limited methodology, no measurement of systemic toxicity parameters, no precise sample description, and technical elements that are outdated by current standards. Nevertheless, the study is valuable for documenting the inherent risk of increased penetration and cumulative injury when chemical and mechanical techniques are applied to the same skin field, reinforcing the need for caution. The concomitant use of dermabrasion and phenol-croton oil peel, although theoretically possible, should be restricted to well-validated protocols, preferably with sessions spaced over time or performed on different areas, in order to reduce the risk of systemic toxicity and permanent scarring.

Overall, the literature demonstrates that phenol-croton oil peel can be integrated into combined strategies for acne scars, enhancing the results achieved with monotherapy. However, safety must remain the guiding principle. The simultaneous use of techniques that disrupt the skin barrier, such as microneedling or dermabrasion, together with phenol-croton oil application increases the risk of systemic absorption and should not be recommended outside controlled protocols. The safest clinical practice involves alternating the procedures over time, with intervals of 6–8 weeks, rigorous prophylaxis against post-inflammatory hyperpigmentation in higher skin types, careful selection of scar morphology, and minimal volumes of phenol for focal CROSS. At the same time, patients should be informed that scars may initially appear larger after CROSS, due to breakdown of the borders, before collagen remodeling leads to elevation of the surface. Thus, phenol-croton oil retains its role as a powerful tool in the arsenal against atrophic acne scars, provided it is used within scientifically grounded combination protocols, adhering to principles of safety and individualized treatment.

9.10 Final Considerations

The combination of phenol-croton oil peel with other therapeutic modalities should be planned according to skin phenotype, degree of aging, scar morphology, and the individual goals of the patient. In individuals with predominantly dynamic wrinkles associated with advanced photoaging, a sequence involving botulinum toxin 2–3 weeks prior to deep peeling, followed by refinement fillers at 3–6 months and, if necessary, light-based technologies between the sixth and twelfth month, promotes natural results and durability. In candidates for rhytidoplasty, surgery corrects laxity and gravitational vectors, while phenol-croton oil peel performed later—between 6 months and 1 year—restores skin texture and uniformity; if mild regional laxity persists, biostimulators may be considered between 9 months and 1 year after the peel. For higher phototypes, preparation with depigmenting agents for 4–6 weeks, strict photoprotection, and a preference for segmented application are essential safety measures, with serial medium-depth peels reserved for areas not treated with phenol-croton oil. In the context of acne scars, the approach remains morphology-driven: icepick and narrow boxcar scars respond best to focal CROSS; rolling and broad boxcar scars require subcision and serial microneedling; phenol-croton oil peel acts as a surface harmonizer and inducer of diffuse remodeling, provided adequate intervals are maintained between procedures to avoid overlap of scarring phases and risk of toxicity.

Integrative models help visualize these strategies. The "relax-resurface-refine" protocol applies toxin pre-procedure, uses phenol-croton oil peel as the central step, and after 3–6 months incorporates hyaluronic acid for contour adjustments, reserving light-based technologies for late maintenance. In patients with more pronounced volume loss, the "contour + skin quality" approach begins with phenol-croton oil peel, followed by structural fillers at 3–6 months, and may include biostimulators between 9 months and 1 year, sometimes combined with segmented medium-depth peels in adjacent areas. In the "lift & finish" protocol, aimed at surgical candidates, rhytidoplasty addresses ptosis and skin excess, and late phenol-croton oil peel, between 6 months and 1 year, evens out the skin; when indicated, biostimulators and light-based energies consolidate the result. For acne scars with actinic damage, the "release-harmonize" sequence organizes management in stages: subcision, punch techniques or CROSS according to morphology, scar stabilization, and then segmented phenol-croton oil peel to equalize texture and stimulate diffuse remodeling, complemented by microneedling and appropriate brighteners for the phototype during maintenance.

Phenol-croton oil peel should be understood as a central component of a deep rejuvenation strategy, but its full potential is realized when methodically integrated with other modalities. Respecting the chronobiology of healing, selecting the correct order of interventions, and allowing generous intervals are principles that transform the sum of techniques into clinical synergy—with more natural results, greater durability, and safety. Personalization, guided by phenotype, phototype, degree of tissue damage, and patient expectations, is essential, as is execution by experienced professionals capable of recognizing risks and managing potential complications.

Overall, the benefits of the combination include enhanced rejuvenating effects, improved skin texture and uniformity, more effective treatment of scars and deep wrinkles, greater patient satisfaction, and, in some cases, faster and more comfortable recovery. However, combinations should only be performed judiciously: techniques that disrupt the epidermal barrier, such as microneedling or dermabrasion, should not be combined with phenol-croton oil in the same session due to the risk of systemic absorption; when necessary, they should be performed at different times or in separate areas. The literature shows that, in higher phototypes, depigmenting preparation and spacing between procedures are crucial to reduce the incidence of post-inflammatory hyperpigmentation.

Finally, several key messages should be emphasized: phenol-croton oil peel is extremely potent and versatile, but does not, on its own, address all aspects of aging; combinations may be planned before, during, or after the peel, provided complete healing of the area is awaited before further intervention; when the goal is tone uniformity in a single session, controlled variation of the phenol-croton oil peel's own potency is preferable to simultaneous use of classic medium-depth peels. Throughout this chapter, the guiding principle remains the same: sequence methodically, stratify by aesthetic units, and respect biological windows, transforming phenol-croton oil-centered combination into a contemporary, safe, and effective standard of rejuvenation (Table 9.3).

Table 9.3 Recommended sequencing of combinations with phenol-croton oil peel

Modality	Recommended time window	Objective/benefit	Key notes
Botulinum toxin A	Pre: 2–3 weeks prior. Post: ≥3–4 weeks (after re-epithelialization)	Reduces mimicry/traction; promotes organized neocollagenesis; postoperative comfort	Avoid on the same day as phenol; possible reduced duration after peeling
Fillers—HA	Post: 8–12 weeks	Structural restoration; contour improvement	Deep planes and cannula; avoid early lip treatment; reduced longevity if applied too soon
Fillers—CaHA	Post: 12–16 weeks (or longer)	Support/skin quality (when indicated)	Deep planes; avoid superficial deposits to reduce risk of nodules
Biostimulators (PLLA, hyper-diluted CaHA, PCL)	Post: 3–6 months	Sustained neocollagenesis; maintenance of firmness/texture	Avoid overlapping inflammation; do not use over active nodules; select appropriate depth
Technologies—Mild/sub-ablative preparation	Pre: 4–8 weeks prior (distinct fields)	Evens epidermis; reduces pores/oiliness; improves field homogeneity	Conservative parameters; consider phototype and thickness
Technologies—Maintenance (NA/Q-switched; fractional ablative)	Same area: NA/Q--switched ≥30–60 days; fractional ablative 4–6 months. Distinct fields: 14–30 days	Refinement of texture and residual pigment	Avoid simultaneous overlap in the same area; PIH prophylaxis in higher phototypes
Other peels (Jessner + TCA; superficial)	Same session in distinct fields or 6–8 weeks before/after.Reapplication in the same field: After full re-epithelialization (14–30 days)	Precise depth modulation; smooths transitions and evens adjacent areas	Delimit zones; protect borders; document with photographs; avoid spillage
Surgery (rhytidoplasty /blepharoplasty)	Same session: TCA on undermined areas; phenol-croton oil only on intact skin.Staging as needed	Synergy between surgical support and skin quality	Never apply phenol-croton oil to flaps; cardiological/ECG screening; mosaic technique when indicated
Acne scars (CROSS, subcision, microneedling, dermabrasion`)	Alternate techniques every 6–8 weeks; avoid combining in the same surgical session when there is barrier disruption	Multimodal approach to icepick/boxcar/rolling scars with improved overall response	Use minimal volumes of phenol in CROSS; strict PIH prophylaxis; monitoring and documentation

Practical timeline (pre- and post-) for safe application across different modalities. Focus on time windows and clinical objectives. Management should consider phototype, skin thickness, and history of PIH. *Notes: PIH = post-inflammatory hyperpigmentation; NA = non-ablative; TCA = trichloroacetic acid. Source: Table prepared by the author (Dr Carolina Marçon)*

Sources

1. Ozturk CN, Huettner F, Ozturk C, Bartz-Kurycki MA, Zins JE. Outcomes assessment of combination face lift and perioral phenol-croton oil peel. Plast Reconstr Surg. 2013;132(5):743e–53e.
2. Peled IJ, Ullmann Y, Ramon I. Chemical peeling: an alternative to rhytidoplasty. Aesth Plast Surg. 1996;20(4):333–6.
3. Lopez Q. Treatment of acne scars with microneedling and chemical reconstruction of scarred skin therapy (CROSS) using phenol/croton oil combination. J Drugs Dermatol. 2024;23(6):418–22.
4. Ayhan S, Baran CN, Yavuzer R, Latifoglu O, Cenetoglu S, Baran NK. Combined chemical peeling and dermabrasion for deep acne and post-traumatic scars as well as facial ageing. Plast Reconstr Surg. 1998;102(4):1238–46.
5. Ersek RA. Comparative study of dermabrasion, phenol peel, and acetic acid peel. Aesth Plast Surg. 1991;15(3):241–3.
6. Logsdon PR, Milburn M, Yarber R. Comparison of laser and phenol chemical peel in facial skin resurfacing. Arch Otolaryngol Head Neck Surg. 2000;126(10):1195–9.
7. Gatti JE. Eyelid phenol peel: an important adjunct to blepharoplasty. Ann Plast Surg. 2008;60(1):14–8. discussion 19-20
8. Hetter GP. An examination of the phenol-croton oil peel: Part I. Dissecting the formula. Plast Reconstr Surg. 2000;105(1):227–39. discussion 249-251
9. Hetter GP. An examination of the phenol-croton oil peel: Part IV. Face peel results with different concentrations of phenol and croton oil. Plast Reconstr Surg. 2000;105(3):1061–83. discussion 1084-1087
10. Wambier CG, Lee KC, Soon SL, Sterling JB, Rullan PP, Landau M, Brody HJ, International Peeling Society. Advanced chemical peels: phenol-croton oil peel. J Am Acad Dermatol. 2019;81(2):327–36.
11. Justo AS, Lemes BM, Nunes B, Antunes KA, Carletto B, Koga AY, Lipinski LC, Montemor Netto MR, Campagnoli EB, Beltrame FL, Wambier CG. Depth of injury of Hetter's phenol-croton oil chemical peel formula using two different emulsifying agents. J Am Acad Dermatol. 2020;82(6):1544–6.
12. Lee KC, Sterling JB, Wambier CG, Soon SL, Landau M, Rullan P, Brody HJ, International Peeling Society. Segmental phenol-croton oil chemical peels for the treatment of periorbital or perioral rhytids. J Am Acad Dermatol. 2019;81(6):e165–6.
13. Gonser P, Kaestner S, Jaminet P, Kaye K. Histological case-control study of skin changes induced by different peeling agents in surgically subcutaneous undermined skin flaps in face-lift patients. J Plast Reconstr Aesthet Surg. 2017;70(11):1660–5.
14. Tung R, Mahoney AM, Novice K, Kamalpour L, Dubina M, Hancock M, Krol C. Treatment of lateral canthal rhytids with a medium-depth chemical peel with or without pretreatment with onabotulinum toxin type A: a randomized controlled trial. Int J Womens Dermatol. 2016;2(1):31–4.
15. Yamauchi PS, Lask G, Lowe NJ. Botulinum toxin type a provides adjunctive benefit to periorbital laser resurfacing. J Cosmet Laser Ther. 2004;6(3):145–8.
16. Landau M. Combination of chemical peels with botulinum toxin injections and dermal fillers. J Cosmet Dermatol. 2006;5(2):121–6.
17. Russell SM, Clark JM. Periorbital rejuvenation in the clinic: a state-of-the-art review. World J Otorhinolaryngol Head Neck Surg. 2023;9(3):242–8.
18. Rendon MI, Berson DS, Cohen JL, Roberts WE, Starker I, Wang B. Evidence and considerations in the application of chemical peels in skin disorders and aesthetic resurfacing. J Clin Aesthet Dermatol. 2010;3(7):32–43.
19. Landau M, Bageorgeou F. Update on chemical peels. Dermatol Clin. 2024;42(1):13–20.
20. Monheit GD. The Jessner's + TCA peel: a medium-depth chemical peel. J Dermatol Surg Oncol. 1989;15(9):945–50.
21. Monheit GD. Medium-depth chemical peels. Dermatol Clin. 2001;19(3):413–25.

22. Aoki KR. Evidence for the antinociceptive activity of botulinum toxin type A in pain management. Headache. 2003;43(Suppl 1):S9–15.
23. Matak I, Lacković Z. Botulinum toxin A, the brain and pain. Prog Neurobiol. 2014;119–120:39–59.
24. Aoki KR, Francis J. Updates on the antinociceptive mechanism hypothesis of botulinum toxin A. Parkinsonism Relat Disord. 2011;17(Suppl 1):S28–33.
25. Fu Z, Huang H, Huang J. Efficacy and safety of botulinum toxin type A for postoperative scar prevention and improvement of wound healing: a systematic review and meta-analysis. J Cosmet Dermatol. 2022;21(1):176–90.
26. Al-Qattan MM, Al-Shanawani BN, Alshomer F. Botulinum toxin type A: implications in wound healing, facial cutaneous scarring, and cleft lip repair. Ann Saudi Med. 2013;33(5):482–8.
27. Li YH, Liu JQ, Xiao D, Zhang W, Hu DH. Advances in research on the mechanisms of prevention and treatment of scars with botulinum toxin type A and its clinical application. Zhonghua Shao Shang Za Zhi. 2017;33(4):254–6.
28. Vengalil N, Council LM, Michalski BM. Foreign body granulomas to polymethylmethacrylate soft tissue filler following COVID-19 infection. JAAD Case Rep. 2023;41:1–3.
29. Quirino MR, Neves AC, Campos MS, Brandão AA, Anbinder AL. Oral granuloma formation after injection of cosmetic filler. J Craniomaxillofac Surg. 2012;40(7):e194–7.
30. Almeida AT, Figueredo V, Cunha T, Casabona G, Costa DL, Lago EA. The risks of polymethylmethacrylate: an integrative review of 587 complication reports. Rev Bras Cir Plast. 2012;27(1):81–7.
31. Wu W, Chayavichitsilp P, Hata T. Extremely delayed granulomatous reaction to soft-tissue injectables (polymethyl methacrylate). J Am Acad Dermatol. 2012;67(5):e206–7.
32. Kroumpouzos G, Treacy P. Hyaluronidase for dermal filler complications: review of applications and dosage recommendations. JMIR Dermatol. 2024;7:e50403.
33. Ao YJ, Yi Y, Wu GH. Application of PLLA (poly-l-lactic acid) for rejuvenation and regeneration of facial cutaneous tissue in aesthetics: a review. Medicine (Baltimore). 2024;103(11):e37506.
34. Bauer U, Graivier MH. Optimising injectable poly-L-lactic acid administration for soft tissue augmentation: the rationale for three treatment sessions. Can J Plast Surg. 2011;19(3):e22–7.
35. Yutskovskaya YA, Kogan EA. Improved neocollagenesis and skin mechanical properties after injection of diluted calcium hydroxyapatite in the neck and décolletage: a pilot study. J Drugs Dermatol. 2017;16(1):68–74.
36. Pavicic T, Kerscher M, Kuhne U, Heide I, Dersch H, Odena G, Graul V. A prospective, multicenter, evaluator-blinded, randomized study of diluted calcium hydroxyapatite to treat décolletage wrinkles. J Drugs Dermatol. 2024;23(7):551–6.
37. Berlin AL, Hussain M, Goldberg DJ. Calcium hydroxyapatite filler for facial rejuvenation: a histological and immunohistochemical analysis. Dermatologic Surg. 2008;34(Suppl 1):S64–7.
38. Fitzgerald R, Vleggaar D. Facial volume restoration of the ageing face with poly-L-lactic acid. Dermatol Ther. 2011;24(1):2–27.
39. Kim JA, Van Abel D. Neocollagenesis in human tissue injected with a polycaprolactone-based dermal filler. J Cosmet Laser Ther. 2015;17(2):99–101.
40. de Melo F, Nicolau P, Piovano L, Lin SL, Baptista-Fernandes T, King MI, Camporese A, Hong K, Khattar MM, Christen MO. Recommendations for volume augmentation and rejuvenation of the face and hands with the new generation polycaprolactone-based collagen stimulator (Ellansé®). Clin Cosmet Investig Dermatol. 2017;10:431–40.
41. Beasley KL, Weiss MA, Weiss RA. Hyaluronic acid fillers: a comprehensive review. Facial Plast Surg. 2009;25(2):86–94.
42. Khatri KA, Ross V, Grevelink JM, Magro CM, Anderson RR. Comparison of erbium:YAG and carbon dioxide lasers in resurfacing of facial rhytids. Arch Dermatol. 1999;135(4):391–7.
43. Oh BH, Hwang YJ, Lee YW, Choe YB, Ahn KJ. Skin characteristics after fractional photothermolysis. Ann Dermatol. 2011;23(4):448–54.

44. Piccolo D, Fusco I, Crisman G, Zingoni T, Conforti C. Efficacy and safety of Q-switched 1064/532 nm Nd:YAG lasers on benign hypermelanosis in dark-skinned individuals—a preliminary study. J Clin Med. 2024;13(6):1615.
45. Elmorsy E, Aboukhadr N, Tayyeb M, Taha AAA. Low-power fractional carbon dioxide laser followed by Jessner's peel versus Jessner's peel alone for the treatment of melasma. J Clin Aesthet Dermatol. 2021;14(2):61–7.
46. Kauvar ANB, Gershonowitz A. Clinical and histologic evaluation of a fractional radiofrequency treatment of wrinkles and skin texture with novel 1-mm long ultra-thin electrode pins. Lasers Surg Med. 2022;54(1):54–61.
47. Park H, Kim E, Kim J, Ro Y, Ko J. High-intensity focused ultrasound for the treatment of wrinkles and skin laxity in seven different facial areas. Ann Dermatol. 2015;27(6):688–93.
48. Ayatollahi A, Gholami J, Saberi M, Hosseini H, Firooz A. Systematic review and meta-analysis of safety and efficacy of high-intensity focused ultrasound (HIFU) for face and neck rejuvenation. Lasers Med Sci. 2020;35(5):1007–24.
49. Yoon HJ, Lee DH, Kim SO, Park KC, Youn SW. Acne erythema improvement by long-pulsed 595-nm pulsed-dye laser treatment: a pilot study. J Dermatolog Treat. 2008;19(1):38–44.
50. Huang YC, Tseng CF, Lee SS, Chan HL. Intense pulsed light therapy for the treatment of facial erythema and hypertrophic scar after phenol peeling. Dermatologic Surg. 2004;30(1):88–92.
51. Yepuri V, Patil AD, Fritz K, Salavastru C, Kroumpouzos G, Nisticò SP, Piccolo D, Sadek A, Badawi A, Kassir M, Gold MH, Große-Büning S, Grabbe S, Goldust M. Light-based devices for the treatment of facial erythema and telangiectasia. Dermatol Ther (Heidelb). 2021;11(6):1879–87.
52. Stagnone GJ, Orgel MG, Stagnone JJ. Cardiovascular effects of topical 50% trichloroacetic acid and Baker's phenol solution. J Dermatol Surg Oncol. 1987;13(9):999–1002.
53. Herbig K, Trussler AP, Khosla RK, Rohrich RJ. Combination Jessner's solution and trichloroacetic acid chemical peel: technique and outcomes. Plast Reconstr Surg. 2009;124(3):955–64.
54. Sterling JB, Lee KC, Wambier CG, Soon SL, Landau M, Rullan PP, Brody HJ. Depth map for face and neck deep chemical peel resurfacing. Dermatologic Surg. 2020;46(9):1204–9.
55. Wambier CG, de Freitas FP. Combining phenol-croton oil peel. In: Issa MCA, Tamura B, editors. Chemical and physical procedures. Cham: Springer; 2018. p. 101–13.
56. Kadunc BV. Combining trichloroacetic acid peel. In: Issa MCA, Tamura B, editors. Chemical and physical procedures. Cham: Springer; 2018. p. 63–71.
57. Marçon CR, Coppinger AJ, Salomão C, Alves Dos Reis V, Alves Dos Reis VN, de Menezes Gomes JL, Gianvecchio VAP, Medeiros de Aquino E, de Seixas Alves MT, Canzian M, Coelho Frenkelis Brandão SA, Fusel de Ue RR, Ribeiro F, Bageorgou F, Wambier CG. International Peeling Society (IPS) and São Paulo's Legal Medical Institute (IML-SP). Fatal phenol peel by an unlicensed social media practitioner: a forensic medical analysis. J Am Acad Dermatol. 2025;93(6):e211–3.
58. Marçon CR. Phenol in dermatology: updated evidence on efficacy and safety. An Bras Dermatol 2025; 100(5): 501200.8

10 Risks and Management of Complications

10.1 Introduction

Phenol–croton oil peel is among the most effective and long-lasting tools for the treatment of advanced photoaging and various dermatological indications. However, as a deep ablative procedure with significant dermal penetration and potential systemic impact, its execution requires not only proficiency in the technique but also a thorough understanding of the pathophysiology of possible complications, preventive measures, and immediate management protocols.

Historically, complications arising from phenol peel have been underestimated or reported in a fragmented manner, often limited to isolated case series. With the consolidation of medical practice and systematic outcome analysis, it has become clear that, although rare in experienced hands, both local and systemic complications can occur and must be anticipated. These include: cardiac arrhythmias, airway edema, hepatic and renal toxicity, permanent scarring, dyschromia, bacterial and viral infections, as well as complications related to individual patient characteristics, such as inflammatory skin diseases.

The distinction between expected effects (erythema, edema, crusting, desquamation, and transient post-inflammatory hyperpigmentation) and true complications is essential for the correct interpretation of clinical progression. Delayed re-epithelialization, persistent erythema beyond six months, or exacerbated pain should serve as warning signs for infectious or scarring complications.

Another crucial point is targeted prevention. Although general safety guidelines have already been discussed in previous chapters, this chapter will take a practical and specific approach: each complication will be presented along three axes—risk and pathophysiology, targeted prevention, and management—enabling the dermatologist to adopt an objective and evidence-based clinical reasoning.

The management of complications requires promptness and precision: minor superficial infections, when treated promptly, do not progress to permanent sequelae; the

C. Marçon, C. Wambier, *Phenol-Croton Oil Peel*,
https://doi.org/10.1007/978-3-032-25993-6_10

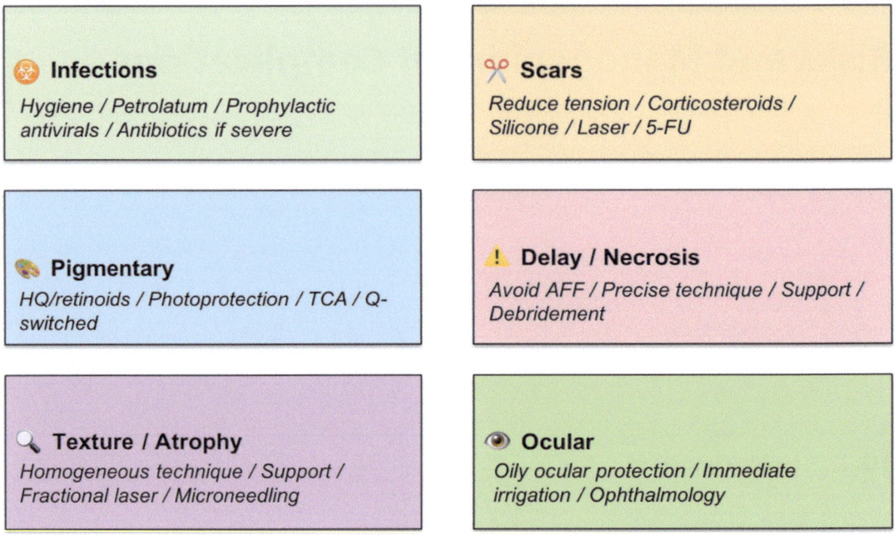

Fig. 10.1 Local complications of phenol-croton oil peel. Summary table of the main local complications of phenol-croton oil peel, organized into six practical axes (infections, scarring, pigmentary changes, delayed re-epithelialization/necrosis, textural changes/atrophy, and ocular alterations), with respective risk factors, preventive measures, and initial therapeutic approaches. Notes. ATB = antibiotic; HQ = hydroquinone; ATX = tranexamic acid; 5-FU = 5-fluorouracil; CO_2 = carbon dioxide; Er:YAG = erbium:yttrium-aluminim-garnet; AFF = frontal fibrosing alopecia; BSS = *balanced salt solution*; SF = saline solution; CMC = carboxymethylcellulose; PEG = polyethylene glycol. *Source: Figure prepared by the author (Dr Carolina Marçon)*

same applies to post-inflammatory dyschromia and early scarring, whose prognosis depends directly on early intervention. On the other hand, systemic complications, such as arrhythmias or hepatorenal toxicity, although extremely rare with modern formulations containing diluted croton oil, remain within the risk spectrum and require the physician to be adequately prepared and supported by appropriate infrastructure.

Finally, it is essential to emphasize that the occurrence of complications, in addition to compromising aesthetic outcomes, can severely impact the patient's self-esteem and the credibility of the procedure. Thus, recognizing, preventing, and treating complications is not merely a technical skill, but an ethical and professional responsibility that underpins the safe and responsible practice of phenol-croton oil peel in modern dermatology (Fig. 10.1).

10.2 Local Complications

10.2.1 Infections

Cutaneous infections following deep chemical peels, although uncommon, are clinically significant complications as they may impair healing and result in permanent aesthetic sequelae. Phenol solutions are bactericidal, although this effect is not relevant after application. In phenol-croton oil peels, the skin remains incompletely epithelialized for 7–10 days, a critical period of vulnerability during which the cutaneous barrier is weakened and susceptible to microbial colonization. Opportunistic agents from the microbiota, such as *Staphylococcus aureus* and β-hemolytic streptococci—especially *Streptococcus pyogenes*—may trigger impetiginized, folliculitis, or cellulitis. Bacterial colonization is favored by the presence of crusts and serous exudate, which act as a culture medium, particularly in the context of inadequate hygiene or excessive manipulation of the treated area. As preventive measures, strict local hygiene is recommended, with gentle and regular cleansing of the skin during the initial healing phase, avoiding the formation of thick crusts. Although specific literature for phenol is scarce, evidence from analogous ablative procedures, such as CO_2 laser resurfacing, demonstrates bacterial infection rates between 1% and 7%, depending on the care protocol adopted.

The risk is increased by predisposing conditions such as immunosuppression, advanced age, diabetes mellitus, a history of herpes simplex, and the use of occlusive dressings. Occlusion, while reducing pain and accelerating initial epithelialization, hinders direct inspection and creates a moist environment conducive to bacterial proliferation, and has been associated, in rare cases, with toxic shock syndrome due to toxigenic S. aureus. Toxic shock syndrome (TSS) is an exceedingly rare but potentially fatal complication described after deep chemical peels. The first reports appeared in 1983, when Dmytryshyn et al. described a case of TSS following facial peeling in a transgender patient with staphylococcal pyoderma, which evolved favorably with intensive support and targeted antibiotic therapy. In 1987, LoVerme et al. published two additional cases of TSS after phenol peel, one associated with an occlusive dressing and the other without occlusion, both in previously healthy patients. In all cases, the clinical picture was characterized by high fever, hypotension, scarlatiniform rash followed by desquamation, and multisystem involvement, with positive cultures for toxigenic *Staphylococcus aureus*. Importantly, none of the patients described in these reports died, but the severity of the condition required immediate hospitalization, aggressive fluid replacement, and antibiotic therapy with beta-lactamase-resistant agents, such as oxacillin and first-generation cephalosporins, in combination with clindamycin to inhibit toxin production. Since then, no new cases have been documented in the literature, which underscores the rarity of this complication, although its risk should always be considered, especially when occlusive dressings are used post-peeling. Another relevant risk factor is improper handling of ointments, particularly the practice known as "double-dipping," which involves re-immersing the same applicator into ointment jars used after the procedure. This seemingly harmless behavior turns the product into a potential culture medium, facilitating cross-contamination by bacteria, fungi, or viruses originating from the patient's own skin, the environment, or even the practitioner. Once contaminated, the ointment may act as a microbial reservoir, increasing the risk of infection in areas of incomplete epithelialization. To prevent this complication, it is recommended that application always be performed using strict aseptic technique, with sterile disposable applicators, needleless syringes, or individual spatulas, as well as pre-portioning the product into single-use units for each patient. Instructing the patient never to insert their fingers into ointment jars for home use and to apply the product only with clean hands or applicators is equally essential to reduce the risk of microbial colonization and ensure greater safety during the healing process. Furthermore, immunocompromised individuals are at increased risk not only of bacterial infections but also of viral and fungal complications, such as infection by atypical mycobacteria, which have been described in settings with inadequate asepsis.

In a classic study on facial resurfacing with CO_2 laser and the use of occlusive dressings, Christian et al. evaluated 354 patients who received prophylactic antibiotics with cephalexin for 10 days, as well as antiviral prophylaxis, with polyurethane foam dressings removed on the third postoperative day. The infection rate was 1.13%, all bacterial and confirmed by culture, with three of the four cases occurring late, between the third and fifth week after the procedure, in contrast to the pattern described in the literature of early infections, usually within the first 10 days. The isolated agents included *Staphylococcus aureus*, *Pseudomonas aeruginosa*, *Escherichia coli*, *Klebsiella pneumoniae*, and *Hafnia alvei*, with one case directly linked to contamination of an emollient used by the patient. The late onset suggested that exogenous factors, such as improper handling of ointments and home care products, are decisive. Thus, this study reinforces the need to instruct patients on strict hygiene throughout the healing period and to maintain close follow-up, as infections may present weeks after the procedure, posing a risk of permanent scarring.

Prevention is based on rigorous hygiene protocols during and after the procedure, gentle and frequent cleansing to prevent thick crust formation, and maintenance of a controlled moist environment. Robust evidence from dermatological surgery and CO_2 resurfacing demonstrates that plain petrolatum is as effective as topical antibiotics for wound healing, but with a lower risk of contact dermatitis and reduced cost, as shown in the randomized study by Smack et al.. Subsequent trials, such as those by Draelos et al. confirm that antibiotic ointments offer no additional benefit and may increase the risk of allergy and bacterial resistance. Therefore, 100% petrolatum remains the recommended standard, while formulations such as Aquaphor® may be associated with a higher incidence of allergic dermatitis due to lanolin. When initial occlusion is chosen, its duration should be limited to 48–72 h, followed by direct inspection of the skin and transition to a generous layer of petrolatum. In the viral context, herpes simplex reactivation is a frequent and potentially serious complication, justifying universal prophylaxis with oral antivirals—such as valaciclovir 500 mg twice daily for 7–10 days—a measure supported by international consensus in ablative facial resurfacing. Universal systemic antibiotic prophylaxis, on the other hand, remains controversial; the current recommendation is to individualize its use in high-risk patients, prioritizing hygiene, antiviral prophylaxis, and strict clinical surveillance.

Intensive monitoring in the first 48–72 h is essential. Local signs suggestive of infection include progressive erythema, exacerbated or disproportionate pain, marked edema, local warmth, purulent discharge, and suspicious-looking crusts (Fig. 10.2). It is crucial to distinguish the serous exudate characteristic of the post-phenol period from true pus (Fig. 10.3), which is associated with a foul odor and

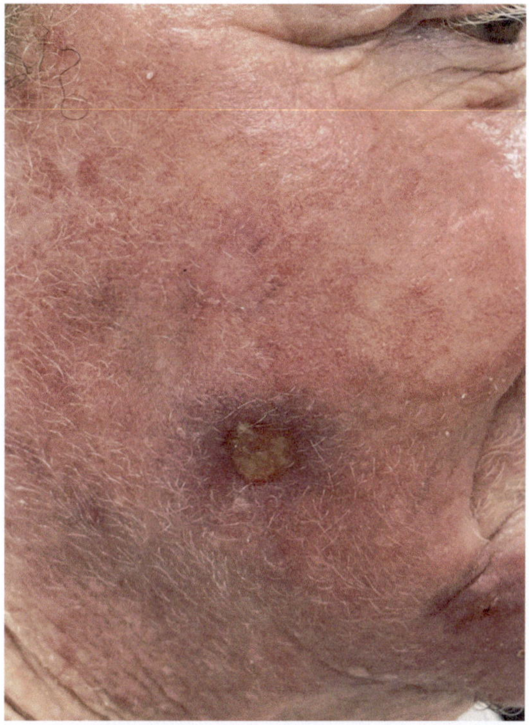

Fig. 10.2 Localized bacterial skin infection in the malar region following re-epithelialization after deep phenol-croton oil peeling, characterized by a yellowish crust over an erythematous base, accompanied by persistent pain beyond 48 h, purulent exudate, and altered local odor. Patient with well-controlled diabetes mellitus. Favorable resolution was achieved after topical antibiotic treatment. *Source: Author's personal archive (Dr Carolina Marçon)*

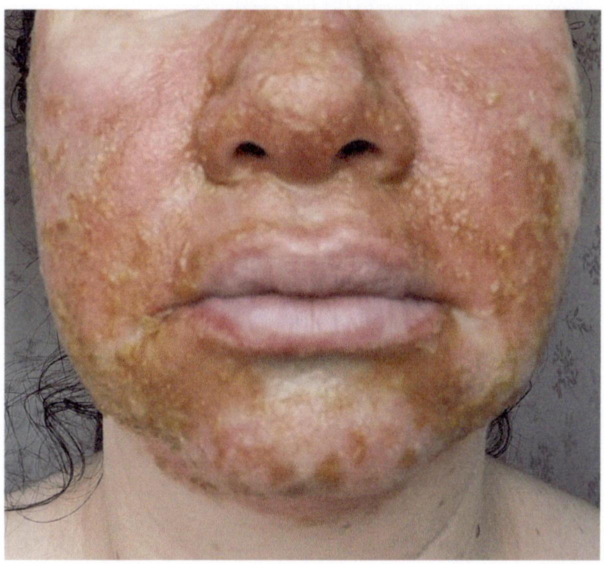

Fig. 10.3 Characteristic serous exudate in the initial period following deep phenol-croton oil peeling, with formation of yellowish crusts over a diffusely erythematous base. This finding should be distinguished from true pus, which is associated with foul odor, disproportionate pain, and progressive clinical deterioration. Recognizing this distinction is essential to avoid misdiagnosis of infection and unnecessary interventions. *Source: Author's personal archive (Dr Carolina Marçon)*

worsening discomfort. Excessive secretion and persistent pain beyond the first 12 h, or any deterioration after 48 h, are warning signs that require immediate attention. Among systemic signs, fever, malaise, chills, and lymphadenopathy are noteworthy, although they may result from intense inflammatory response to peeling. Severe manifestations such as hypotension, tachycardia, diffuse erythema, and altered mental status should raise suspicion of systemic infection. In the viral context, the appearance of grouped vesicles accompanied by itching or burning suggests herpetic reactivation. Fungal or mycobacterial infections, although rare, may present insidiously, with persistent lesions that are difficult to resolve. Daily monitoring allows differentiation between normal scarring progression and signs of infection, thereby reducing the risk of major complications.

Once infection is confirmed or strongly suspected, management must be immediate, based on the triad of culture collection, initiation of appropriate empirical therapy, and intensive clinical monitoring. Samples should be collected before starting antibiotics whenever possible, allowing for targeted treatment. In cases of necrosis, abscess, or devitalized tissue, early debridement is mandatory. The choice of antibiotic should be guided by the likely pathogen, clinical severity, and local epidemiology. For uncomplicated skin infections, cephalexin 500 mg orally every 6 h for 7–10 days is the first-line option, covering sensitive S. aureus and streptococci; clindamycin (300–450 mg orally every 6–8 h) is an effective alternative for penicillin-allergic patients. Amoxicillin-clavulanate (875/125 mg orally every 12 h) broadens coverage in cases of polymicrobial risk, such as infections associated with prolonged occlusion. In areas with high MRSA prevalence or in individual at-risk patients, options such as trimethoprim-sulfamethoxazole (800/160 mg orally every 12 h) or doxycycline (100 mg orally every 12 h) may be used, sometimes in combination with amoxicillin for streptococcal coverage. Severe cases, with extensive cellulitis or systemic signs, require intravenous antibiotics: oxacillin or cefazolin (1–2 g IV every 6–8 h) are first-line, while vancomycin should be used in cases of suspected or confirmed MRSA. For viral complications, antivirals should be started immediately upon symptom onset: acyclovir (400 mg orally every 8 h), valaciclovir (1000 mg orally every 12 h), or famciclovir (250 mg orally every 8 h), for 7–10 days, to reduce lesion extent and risk of scarring. Toxic shock syndrome requires urgent intervention, with hemodynamic support, targeted systemic antibiotic therapy, and hospital admission.

Infection by *Pseudomonas aeruginosa* is a rare but documented complication in the post-deep chemical peel period and should be considered in cases of abrupt and severe wound progression. This opportunistic microorganism thrives in areas of incomplete epithelialization, especially when there is contact with contaminated water, animals, hospital exposure, or prolonged use of moist dressings. Clinically, it is characterized by pain disproportionate to the expected course, greenish exudate, characteristic odor, and, in advanced cases, rapidly progressive cellulitis that may progress to necrosis. Management must be immediate, with culture collection and initiation of empirical antibiotic therapy targeting Gram-negative bacilli, with oral ciprofloxacin (500–750 mg every 12 h for 7–14 days) considered first-line for localized skin infections. In severe or disseminated cases, intravenous antibiotics with antipseudomonal agents are recommended, such as ceftazidime (1–2 g every 8 h), piperacillin-tazobactam (4.5 g IV every 6–8 h), meropenem (1 g IV every 8 h), or combination with aminoglycosides (amikacin 15 mg/kg/day), according to clinical severity and local epidemiological profile. Prevention involves strict aseptic measures throughout the healing process, avoiding the use of tap water or homemade solutions for soaks, and preferring sterile or safe antiseptic solutions, such as diluted chlorhexidine or povidone-iodine, which have been shown to reduce microbial colonization during the period of cutaneous vulnerability.

Fungal and atypical mycobacterial infections, although rare in the context of phenol-croton oil peeling, should be considered in cases of persistent or atypical lesion progression. Fungal infections, usually caused by Candida spp. or dermatophytes, may present as persistent erythema, pustules, or whitish plaques over the healing area, and are favored by prolonged use of occlusive dressings and immunosuppression. Treatment should include topical antifungals, such as nystatin or clotrimazole, combined with systemic therapy in more extensive or refractory cases. Fluconazole (100 mg PO/day for 7–14 days, or 150 mg weekly) is the first-line option, with alternatives such as itraconazole or terbinafine, depending on the causative agent. Infections caused by rapidly growing mycobacteria, such as *Mycobacterium chelonae*, *M. abscessus* and *M. fortuitum*, have a more insidious course, characterized by nodules, abscesses or erythematous plaques that are difficult to resolve and do not respond to conventional antibiotic therapy. Management always requires the collection of material for culture and sensitivity testing, with empirical initiation of clarithromycin (500 mg PO every 12 h), and may require combination with agents such as amikacin, linezolid, imipenem or cefoxitin in severe or disseminated cases, with prolonged treatment duration, generally between three and six months, combined with surgical debridement when indicated. In these situations, joint follow-up with infectious disease specialists is recommended, given the therapeutic complexity and risk of chronic infection.

In summary, the safety of phenol-croton oil peel depends on a clear understanding of infectious risks, the implementation of evidence-based preventive measures, intensive clinical monitoring, and prompt, individualized therapeutic management (Table 10.1). This systematic approach reduces complications, ensures the quality of aesthetic outcomes, and reinforces the need for the procedure to be performed in a qualified medical setting, with strict protocols for prevention, surveillance, and intervention.

10.2.2 Scarring

The development of hypertrophic and keloid scars after deep phenol-croton oil peel is an infrequent complication, but one with significant aesthetic and functional impact. Although phenol-croton oil is known to induce intense dermal remodeling and generally favorable healing, individual and contextual factors may trigger an exaggerated reparative response, resulting in disordered collagen deposition and scar thickening (Fig. 10.4). The anatomical regions most prone include the

Table 10.1 Infections after phenol-croton oil peel

Agent/type of infection	Typical clinical presentation	Risk factors	Prevention	Initial management	Escalation/remarks
Bacterial (*S. aureus*, *S. pyogenes*)	Impetiginization, folliculitis, cellulitis; progressive erythema, disproportionate pain, purulent discharge	Inadequate hygiene, thick crusts, prolonged occlusive dressings, immunosuppression, diabetes	Gentle and frequent cleansing; avoid prolonged occlusion; use of plain petrolatum	Cultures; oral antibiotics (cefalexin 500 mg every 6 h for 7–10 days; clindamycin if allergic)	Severe cases → intravenous antibiotics (oxacillin, cefazolin, vancomycin if MRSA)
Toxic shock syndrome (*S. aureus* toxigenic)	High fever, hypotension, scarlatiniform rash, desquamation, multisystem involvement	Occlusive dressings, poor hygiene, previous staphylococcal infection	Avoid rigid/prolonged occlusion; strict aseptic technique	Immediate hospitalization; intensive support; intravenous antibiotics (oxacillin/first-generation cephalosporin + clindamycin)	Rare but potentially fatal complication; reported in deep chemical peels
Viral (*Herpes simplex*)	Clustered vesicles, pruritus/burning, local pain; risk of extensive scarring	History of HSV; immunosuppression; absence of antiviral prophylaxis	Universal prophylaxis with valaciclovir 500 mg PO every 12 h for 7–10 days	Immediate initiation of antivirals (acyclovir 400 mg every 8 h; valaciclovir 1 g every 12 h)	Prophylaxis is international consensus; reactivations require prompt treatment
Pseudomonas aeruginosa	Disproportionate pain, greenish exudate, characteristic odor; severe cellulitis, necrosis	Prolonged moist dressings, contact with contaminated water, hospitalization	Avoid tap water; use safe sterile/antiseptic solutions	Oral ciprofloxacin (500–750 mg every 12 h for 7–14 days)	Severe cases → IV antibiotics (ceftazidime, piperacillin-tazobactam, meropenem ± amikacin)

Fungal (*Candida spp.*, dermatophytes)	Persistent erythema, pustules, whitish plaques; worsening under occlusion	Prolonged occlusive dressings; immunosuppression	Avoid excessive occlusion; proper hygiene	Topical antifungals (nystatin, clotrimazole)	Extensive cases → oral fluconazole (100 mg/day for 7–14 days); itraconazole/terbinafine according to the agent
Atypical mycobacteria (*M. chelonae, M. abscessus, M. fortuitum*)	Nodules, abscesses, persistent erythematous plaques, refractory to common antibiotics	Poor aseptic environments; immunosuppression	Strict aseptic technique; use of sterile materials; avoid double-dipping	Culture collection; empirical initiation of clarithromycin (500 mg orally every 12 h)	Severe cases → combination therapy (amikacin, linezolid, imipenem, cefoxitin) + debridement; prolonged treatment

Infections following phenol-croton oil peel, with main etiological agents, clinical manifestations, risk factors, preventive measures, initial management, and therapeutic escalation strategies. Notes: TSS = toxic shock syndrome; MRSA = Methicillin-resistant Staphylococcus aureus; PO = oral route; IV = intravenous.
Source: Table prepared by the author (Dr Carolina Marçon)

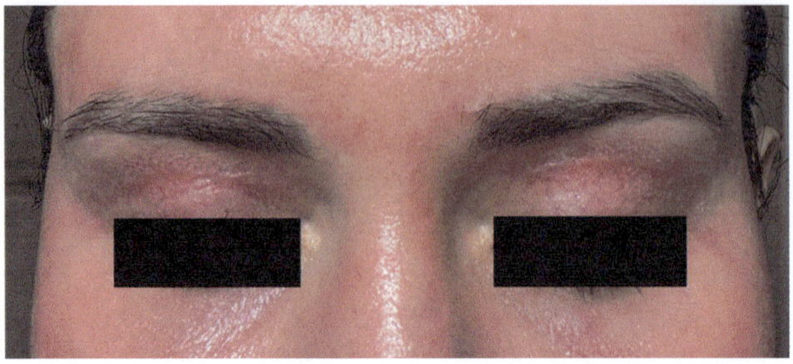

Fig. 10.4 Mild hypertrophic scar on the upper eyelid one month after blepharopeel, located in the area subjected to the greatest number of passes. Complete resolution was achieved after two injections of triamcinolone acetonide 10 mg/mL (Kenalog®) combined with continuous use of a silicone sheet for two months. *Source: Author's personal archive (Dr Carolina Marçon)*

zygomatic arch, preauricular area, medial upper eyelids, lateral lower eyelids, and neck—areas that should be treated with lower intensity, smaller solution volumes, and less friction, especially in cases of lax lower eyelids, compromised snap-back test, history of blepharoplasty or previous ectropion, where a lower croton concentration and drier applicator are recommended. Areas of greater dynamic movement, such as the lips, chin, and perioral region, are also more susceptible to abnormal scarring. Temporary ectropion resulting from the peel may occur as an expected side effect, usually self-limiting and resolving with local massage. In general, hypertrophic scars tend to appear within the first three months after the procedure, and when recognized and treated early, show a good therapeutic response.

The most well-established risk factors for abnormal scarring include genetic predisposition, previous history of hypertrophic or keloid scars, higher phototypes, young age with increased fibroblastic activity, presence of infection at the wound bed, local mechanical tension, and systemic conditions that impair healing, such as diabetes mellitus and nutritional deficiencies. Excessive facial mobility, constrictive tapes, previous rhytidectomy, and intense mastication or speech have been identified as associated factors, although scar formation is not always explained by a single element. Individuals with darker skin are at higher risk, and family and personal history should be assessed. There are reports of necrosis and scarring related to the combination of deep peel and rhytidectomy when performed simultaneously, with compromise of cutaneous circulation. For this reason, an interval between procedures is recommended, avoiding overlapping trauma. Additionally, previous procedures such as dermabrasion and recent use of isotretinoin may increase the risk of scarring complications, and a minimum interval of six months is advisable. Some authors suggest that a propensity for pathological scarring may also be related to mild forms of Ehlers-Danlos syndrome, underdiagnosed in up to 9% of the population, which would justify investigating signs of joint hypermobility, increased skin extensibility, atrophic scars, and frequent bruising during pre-procedure assessment.

Prevention of scarring requires careful patient screening, avoiding deep peels in individuals with a consistent history of severe keloids and proceeding with heightened caution in cases of isolated hypertrophic scars. Careful selection of the treatment area is also essential, avoiding regions known to be predisposed, such as the sternum, shoulders, and earlobes, and reserving phenol-croton oil for the face, which has a lower incidence of exuberant scarring. The procedure must be performed in a controlled medical environment, with infection prevention measures in place, as bacterial colonization promotes inflammation and pathological healing. During the repair process, primary prevention should include reducing mechanical tension on the treated skin, a measure that decreases traction forces and reduces scar hypertrophy. After deep phenol-croton oil peeling, the reduction of mechanical tension should be understood as the attenuation of dynamic forces exerted by facial musculature on the healing skin. In the first weeks, patients should be advised to avoid vigorous chewing, prolonged speaking, exaggerated facial expressions, and activities that increase perioral mobility, as this region is particularly prone to hypertrophic scarring. These measures reduce surface tension and modulate the reparative process, thereby decreasing scar hypertrophy. In high-risk cases or in areas of intense muscular activity, early adjuvant use of botulinum toxin type A may be considered, administered intradermally or into the orbicularis, depressor anguli oris, and mentalis muscles, at intervals of three to four months, in order to temporarily reduce contraction and traction on the healing tissue. Thus, the preventive approach to dynamic tension in the post-peeling period combines behavioral guidance and, in selected cases, pharmacological modulation of muscular activity, working synergistically to reduce the likelihood of hypertrophic scarring. Additional recommendations include avoiding irritating cosmetics, hair dyes, or perm solutions in the week preceding the procedure, as there are reports describing cutaneous necrosis and scarring along the hairline in patients who underwent phenol peeling after using dyes or perm solutions in the previous week; it is believed that caustic agents in these products compromise the epidermal barrier and, upon subsequent contact with phenol, promote cumulative chemical damage and local ischemia, justifying the recommendation to avoid such substances in the immediate preoperative period.

Intensive monitoring is required during the first three months, when there is greater dermal remodeling and risk of fibroblastic hyperplasia. Persistent erythema, more intense localized erythema, progressive skin induration, firm nodules, severe pruritus, and raised areas or those resistant to potent topical corticosteroids such as clobetasol are early warning signs of possible hypertrophic scar formation (Fig. 10.6). Objective monitoring of scars after deep peels can be performed using the POSAS (Patient and Observer Scar Assessment Scale), currently considered one of the most comprehensive and validated tools for this purpose. Unlike classical scales such as the Vancouver Scar Scale, POSAS integrates both the physician's assessment and the patient's subjective perception, providing a comprehensive view of the scar in both functional and aesthetic terms. The current version of the scale consists of two parts: the Observer Scale, in which the medical evaluator examines parameters such as vascularity, pigmentation, thickness, relief, surface irregularity, and extent relative to adjacent skin; and the Patient Scale, in which the patient rates aspects such as pain, pruritus, colour, stiffness, perceived thickness, and overall appearance. Each item is scored from 1 to 10, with higher values reflecting more severe characteristics, and the sum of the domains allows comparison of progress over time and response to different interventions. Systematic use of POSAS, already recommended in international consensus statements on lasers and scar management, enables greater reproducibility between studies, assists therapeutic decision-making, and strengthens the scientific documentation of clinical outcomes following deep phenol-croton oil peels.

Therapeutic management in the face of risk or onset of pathological scarring should always be early, progressive, and individualized. In the initial phase, characterized by persistent erythema, pruritus, or incipient thickening within the first 2–8 weeks after re-epithelialization, the use of potent topical corticosteroids such as clobetasol is recommended to modulate the inflammatory response and reduce fibroblastic hyperproliferation. If there is inadequate response, the introduction of non-invasive adjuvant measures is indicated, such as continuous use of silicone sheets or gels, which help stabilize the scar microenvironment and reduce superficial vascularity. In cases where scar activity persists, therapies with vascular devices such as pulsed dye laser (585–595 nm) or intense pulsed light with specific filters may be instituted to control erythema, vascularization, and associated symptoms. Additionally, non-ablative fractional lasers (1540–1550 nm) or low-density ablative fractional lasers (CO_2 or Er:YAG) may be used to modulate dermal remodeling, reduce scar thickness, and prevent progression to exuberant forms. These treatments may be performed sequentially, for example, PDL followed by fractional laser, and combined with laser-assisted drug delivery, which enhances intradermal penetration of corticosteroids or 5-fluorouracil. All these interventions should be adjusted according to individual skin phototype and reactivity, using conservative parameters in individuals with medium or highly melanized skin, thereby reducing the risk of post-inflammatory hyperpigmentation.

When the hypertrophic scar is already established (≥6–8 weeks) or in cases of early keloid, the treatment of choice involves combined approaches. Intralesional triamcinolone acetonide remains the therapeutic mainstay, used at concentrations of 5–10 mg/mL in the initial phases and up to 40 mg/mL in more refractory scars. The combination of triamcinolone with 5-fluorouracil (50 mg/mL, in a 1:9 ratio to the corticosteroid) has demonstrated superior efficacy, reducing recurrence rates and the adverse effects of monotherapy. Infiltrations should be performed at intervals of two to four weeks, adjusted according to clinical response. Intralesional bleomycin is another option for refractory cases, although it carries a higher risk of adverse effects. Intralesional cryotherapy may be considered for small lesions, but the risk of dyschromia in higher phototypes should be weighed. Lasers also play an important adjunctive role: PDL reduces erythema and vascularity, while fractional CO_2 laser enhances tissue remodeling and increases the penetration of intralesional drugs. Recent studies reinforce that fractional CO_2, although limited as monotherapy, shows superior results when combined with topical or intralesional corticosteroids. In a randomized clinical trial, fractional CO_2 laser followed by topical triamcinolone application demonstrated greater volumetric scar reduction (45.2% versus 28.7% with laser alone), as well as significant improvement in pain and pruritus. More complex multimodal protocols have also been reported, such as the combination of botulinum toxin type A, fractional CO_2 laser, and topical growth factors, with sustained results for up to 15 months. In more recent hybrid systems, which combine fractional CO_2 with a 1570 nm laser, significant improvement in scar texture, thickness, and coloration was observed in two to four sessions, with a favorable safety profile.

Botulinum toxin type A has emerged as a promising adjunct in the prevention and treatment of facial and neck scars, acting by reducing muscular traction and modulating profibrotic signaling. Studies and meta-analyses show that its early application, within the first few postoperative weeks, can reduce scar width, erythema, and improve overall aesthetic appearance. The technique involves intradermal injection at points distributed along the scar or in adjacent muscles with greater mobility, at doses ranging from 2 to 2.5 units per point, in multiple points spaced 0.5 to 1 cm apart, generally totaling 20 to 40 units, adjusted to the treated area. The combination with intralesional triamcinolone enhances outcomes and is recommended at intervals of four to six weeks between applications. This approach is especially useful in highly dynamic regions, such as the perioral area, where temporary reduction in mobility can mitigate mechanical tension and prevent hypertrophic scarring.

Katz et al. reported a notable case of severe hypertrophic scarring with perioral contracture following deep phenol peel (Baker & Gordon formula) in a 75-year-old patient, phototype II, refractory to topical and intralesional corticosteroids, treated with an integrated multimodal protocol in the same session. Each of the ten sessions included sequential application of pulsed dye laser (PDL 595 nm, 7–9 J/cm^2, 7–10 mm spot, 3–10 ms pulse duration, with dynamic cooling) followed by 1450 nm diode laser (12–14 J/cm^2, 6 mm spot, 40 ms cooling), immediately followed by intralesional infiltration of a solution of triamcinolone acetonide 10 mg/mL and 5-fluorouracil 50 mg/mL in a 1:9 ratio, in volumes ranging from 0.02 to 0.35 mL per area. This strategy aimed to harness the synergistic effect of the technologies: PDL to reduce scar vascularity and erythema via selective photothermolysis, diode laser to modulate fibroblast activity and dermal remodeling, and the increased tissue permeability induced by the lasers to optimize intradermal drug diffusion. Functional improvement was noted after the second session, with increased oral opening; after five sessions, overall improvement was 90%, and after ten sessions, it exceeded 95%, remaining stable at 2.5 years' follow-up, with no recurrence. Matsuura et al. reported the case of a 52-year-old patient, phototype II, who developed persistent erythema and bilateral hypertrophic scarring in the mandibular region after deep peel with Hetter 1.2% formula. Treatment consisted of three sessions of intense pulsed light (540 nm filter, 13–18 J/cm^2, 15 ms, with dynamic cooling), applied at monthly intervals, combined with two infiltrations of triamcinolone acetonide 10 mg/mL diluted 1:8 in saline (final concentration approximately 1.25 mg/mL), administered fortnightly and always one week before the light sessions. Significant improvement in erythema, telangiectasia, and scar texture was observed, with reduction in pruritus and additional aesthetic benefit in periocular rhytids. This report reinforces the synergistic role of combined therapies and the importance of early intervention and prolonged follow-up in managing scarring complications after deep peel.

In summary, the management of hypertrophic scars and keloids following deep phenol-croton oil peel should follow the sequence of risk assessment, prevention, monitoring, and intervention, always employing a multimodal and individualized approach (Table 10.2). Early identification of clinical signs of abnormal healing, combined with timely implementation of preventive, pharmacological, and technological measures, is crucial to optimize the aesthetic and functional outcome, reducing recurrences and preserving the overall quality of the rejuvenation achieved.

10.2.3 Pigmentary Changes

Pigmentary changes are among the most common local complications following phenol-croton oil peel, with frequency and severity varying according to phototype, the depth reached by the caustic agent, and patient adherence to photoprotection measures. Additionally, factors such as early sun exposure, prolonged inflammation, inappropriate use of topical agents, and individual predisposition may influence the development of these complications. Although often transient, these dyschromias can compromise the final aesthetic outcome and cause significant dissatisfaction, requiring both well-defined preventive and therapeutic strategies. Proper management includes strict photoprotection, use of topical depigmenting

Table 10.2 Scarring after phenol-croton oil peel

Aspect	Risk factors	Prevention	Management
Hypertrophic scar	Genetics; previous history; smoking; higher phototypes; young age; local infection; mechanical tension; DM; poor nutrition	Careful selection; avoid high-risk areas; infection prevention; reduce mechanical tension (guidance and botulinum toxin in selected cases); avoid caustic cosmetics/dyes before peeling	Topical corticosteroids (clobetasol); silicone; PDL/IPL laser; fractional CO_2/Er:YAG + drug delivery; intralesional triamcinolone ± 5-FU; multimodal protocols
Keloid	Personal/family history; higher phototypes; genetic predisposition	Avoid phenol-croton oil in patients with severe keloids; caution in isolated cases	Intralesional triamcinolone (5–40 mg/mL); combined with 5-FU; cryotherapy for small lesions; adjunctive lasers; combined protocols
Cicatricial ectropion	Lax lower eyelids; compromised snap-test; history of blepharoplasty; excess croton/volume	Avoid excess agent in high-risk areas; use lower concentrations; drier applicator	Local massage; silicone sheets; intralesional corticosteroids; in persistent cases, surgical correction

Scar-related complications after phenol-croton oil peel, including risk factors, preventive measures, clinical warning signs, and main therapeutic options, organized in a practical format to support dermatological management. *Notes: DM = Diabetes mellitus; 5-FU = 5-fluorouracil; PDL = Pulsed Dye Laser; IPL = Intense Pulsed Light. Source: Table prepared by the author (Dr Carolina Marçon)* agents, and, in persistent cases, interventions such as laser or additional superficial peels.

After the epithelialization period, the skin remains erythematous for approximately three to six months, with flushing on physical exertion potentially persisting for up to a year. Erythema peaks around the second week, representing a normal part of the healing process and an indirect marker of new reticular dermal collagen formation (Fig. 10.5). During this phase, the skin is typically dry and sensitive, and irregular brown discoloration may appear about one month after the peel, usually resolving spontaneously or with topical regimens prescribed by the dermatologist. Time itself has a therapeutic effect. Patients should be informed that erythema and transient color changes are benign and expected, and that the degree and duration of erythema are directly related to the depth of the peel and the long-term efficacy of the result.

Post-inflammatory hyperpigmentation is the most common pigmentary complication, resulting from melanocytic activation induced by inflammation (Fig. 10.6). It usually lasts up to six months and may progress to pseudo-hypopigmentation, in which the treated skin appears lighter by contrast with untreated, photodamaged skin (Fig. 10.7). In darker skin types, Fitzpatrick III to VI, the risk of hyperpigmentation is higher, reaching up to 74% of cases. In patients with phototypes IV to VI, the risk is significantly increased, which is why the use of peeling is often restricted to localized treatments, such as for dark circles, refractory melasma, or scars, always with lower parameters, rigorous skin preparation, and close follow-up.

Prevention includes prior preparation with lightening agents such as hydroquinone, retinoids, and mild acids, strict photoprotection, use of broad-spectrum tinted sunscreen for at least six months or until the skin returns to its natural color, as well

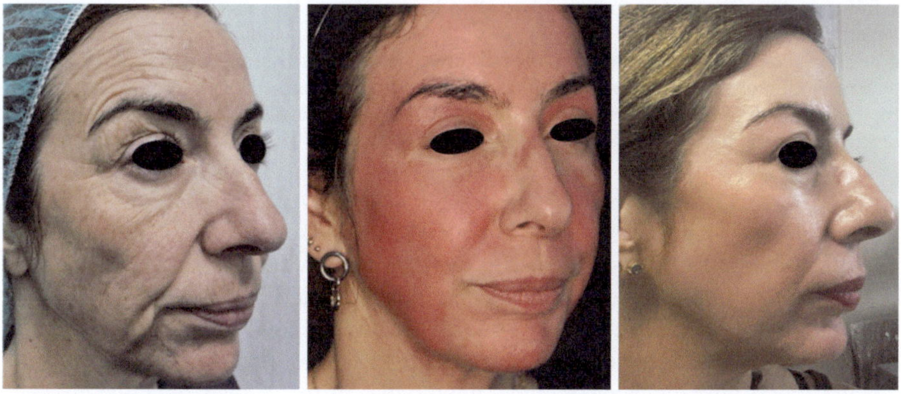

Fig. 10.5 Irregular diffuse erythema observed one month after deep phenol–croton peel. Erythema, which typically peaks around the second week, may persist for three to six months and represents a normal part of the healing process, correlating with new reticular dermal collagen formation. Irregular brown discoloration at this stage is transient, tending to resolve spontaneously or with topical regimens prescribed by the dermatologist. The third image on the right corresponds to the same patient six months after treatment. *Source: Archives of Dr. Carolina Marçon and Dr. María Garcia Baldovi*

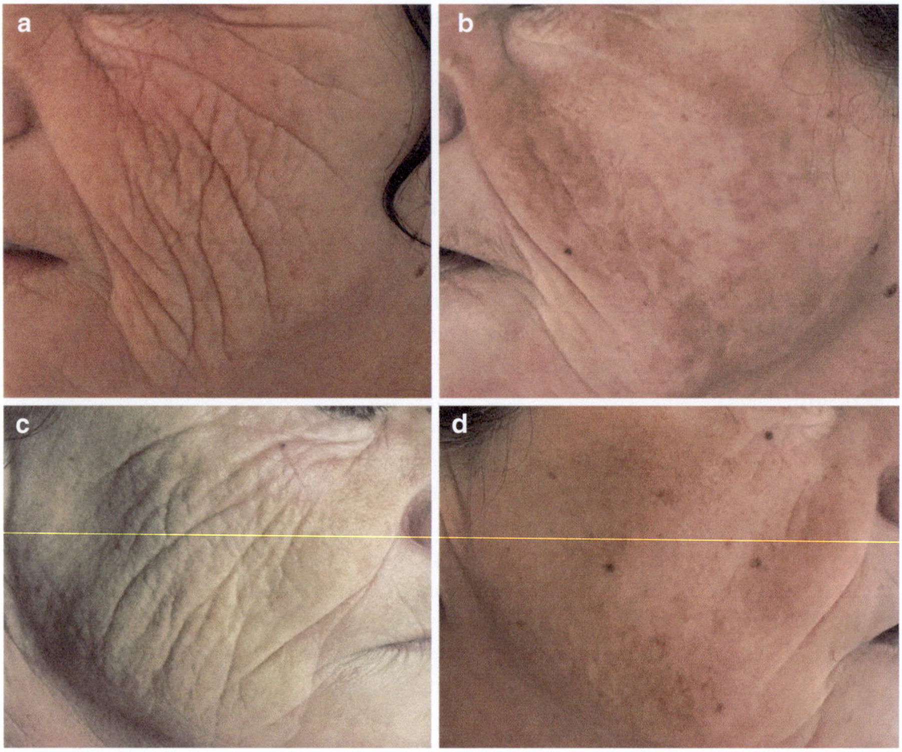

Fig. 10.6 Marked photoaging treated with deep phenol-croton oil peel (Hetter's formula 1.6%), with *degrade* technique applied to the cheeks. There is marked improvement in elastosis, with significant attenuation of rhytids and overall enhancement of skin texture. Post-inflammatory hyperpigmentation (PIH) is evident in the *degrade* areas, the most common pigmentary complication after deep peels, related to melanocyte activation induced by inflammation, especially in patients with higher phototypes (**a**, **c**). Pre-treatment, showing marked elastosis and deep rhytids. (**b**, **d**) Six-month follow-up after the procedure, with overall improvement in elastosis and presence of PIH areas. *Source: Personal archive of Dr Carlos Wambier*

as monthly follow-up visits. Management, when necessary, is based on the reintroduction of depigmenting agents such as hydroquinone, vitamin C, niacinamide, oral or topical tranexamic acid, and classic combinations such as the modified Kligman formula, with the possible use of Q-switched lasers or light-based technologies in refractory cases. Oral tranexamic acid has been incorporated as a preventive strategy in patients with melasma or higher phototypes. Its mechanism of action involves inhibition of the plasmin–keratinocyte–melanocyte interaction, reducing the release of inflammatory mediators that stimulate melanogenesis. The usual dosage ranges from 250 mg to 500 mg/day, starting a few weeks before the procedure and continuing for up to three to six months afterward. However, attention must be paid to the risk of thrombosis, and it is recommended to request preliminary tests such as full blood count, coagulation profile, protein C and S, and investigation of risk factors

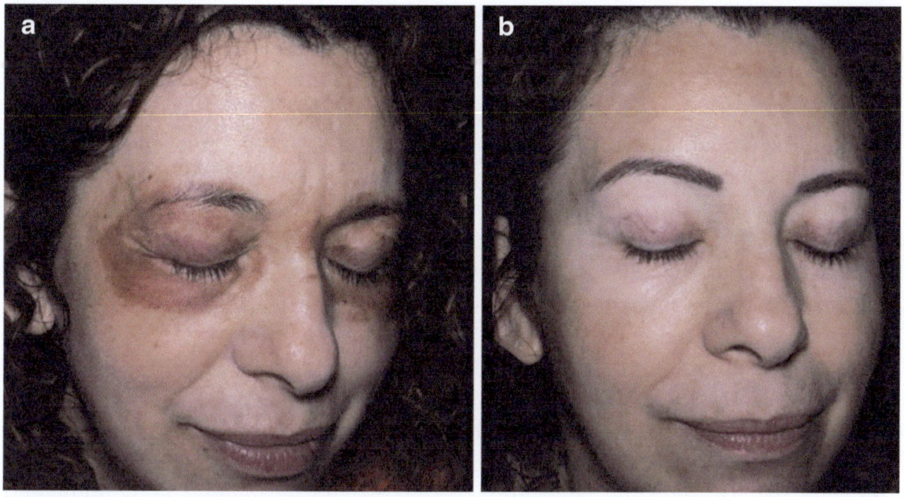

Fig. 10.7 (**a**) Post-inflammatory hyperpigmentation after periocular peel with 35% phenol and 1.2% croton oil. (**b**) After 2 years, pseudo-hypopigmentation is observed in the periocular region, in contrast to the photodamaged skin of the temples and cheeks. *Source: Adapted from Wambier CG, Lee KC, Soon SL, Sterling JB, Rullan PP, Landau M, Brody HJ. Advanced chemical peels: Phenol-croton oil peel. J Am Acad Dermatol. 2019;81(2):327–336. Reproduced with permission from the publisher*

such as personal or family history of thromboembolic events, use of oral contraceptives, and smoking before prescribing.

Localized hypopigmentation, often described as "island" dyschromia or leopard spotting, is characterized by pale areas in contrast to adjacent skin and is associated with deep peels using pure phenol or high concentrations of croton oil, especially when application is uneven. The literature diverges regarding the exact mechanism: while some authors report focal melanocyte destruction, others, such as Kligman, have shown that melanocytes remain present but function irregularly. Prevention depends on uniform technique, respect for anatomical boundaries, and the use of calibrated formulations such as those of Hetter.

Diffuse depigmentation, resulting in porcelain-white skin, is associated with the use of high concentrations of croton oil above 1% (almost universal at concentrations above 2%), with an increased risk of delayed healing and permanent pigment loss, especially outside areas of thicker skin such as the nose and perioral region, or with the use of large amounts of phenol under complete occlusion. Although in fair skin this effect may be considered acceptable, in higher phototypes it is regarded as a significant complication due to the accentuated contrast with adjacent areas. Despite the clinical appearance of depigmentation, histological studies have shown that melanocytes are not destroyed but remain present, producing melanin and distributing it irregularly. Thus, patients may develop freckles after sun exposure, although they do not achieve uniform tanning. Prevention requires careful selection, use of lower concentrations, fewer passes, and prior discussion of aesthetic expectations.

When spontaneous repigmentation is limited, adjuvant therapies with biological rationale and some supporting evidence may be considered: topical immunomodulators such as tacrolimus 0.1% (ointment) or pimecrolimus 1% (cream), applied twice daily for 8–12 weeks (which may be extended up to 24 weeks depending on response/tolerance), act by inhibiting calcineurin (suppressing T-cell-mediated inflammation that perpetuates melanocyte dysfunction) and through experimentally described pro-melanogenic effects (increasing MITF (Microphthalmia-associated Transcription Factor)/tyrosinase and favorable paracrine signaling), with documented efficacy particularly in localized facial vitiligo—a scenario from which their use in well-demarcated post-peel hypochromia is extrapolated. In small, refractory patches, analogues of prostaglandin such as bimatoprost 0.03% (once daily, applied directly to the lesion and slightly beyond its borders, for 8–12 up to 16–24 weeks) may stimulate pigmentation by activating FP receptors (prostaglandin F2α receptor) in melanocytes/keratinocytes, with up-regulation of MITF/tyrosinase and increased melanosome production; clinical series suggest modest to moderate benefit, with the possibility of hypertrichosis/irregular hyperpigmentation, so use should be restricted to small areas under close follow-up. For drug delivery, microneedling (≈0.5–1.5 mm, depending on site/thickness) can enhance the penetration of tacrolimus 0.1% (the main adjuvant) and, in selected and stable protocols, 5-fluorouracil 5%—with studies indicating greater repigmentation with 5-FU than with tacrolimus in certain locations, always weighing the risk of post-inflammatory hyperpigmentation in higher phototypes; typically, one session/month is performed for 3–4 months, with response reassessment. Among light sources, the 308 nm excimer (laser or lamp) is the best-supported technology for focal repigmentation: classic protocols use it twice weekly, starting ≈50 mJ/cm^2 below the lesion's MED (Minimal Erythema Dose) and progressively increasing, with assessment after ≈24 sessions (which may be extended to 36–48 in slow-responding plaques); studies suggest a faster response with 2–3×/week compared to once weekly, and combination with tacrolimus may enhance outcomes. There are also reports of benefit from 308 nm in post-inflammatory/iatrogenic hypopigmentation (e.g., after lichen striatus), reinforcing its role when viable residual melanocytes are present; alternatives such as focused NB-UVB and excimer light show similar performance in selected contexts.

Although hyperpigmentation or hypopigmentation may occur after any chemical peel, lighter phototypes, Fitzpatrick types I to III, are at lower risk. Cellular biology emphasizes that chromatic variation between individuals is less due to the number of melanocytes and more to the size, number, maturation, and distribution of melanosomes and their transfer to keratinocytes. Individuals with dark skin have larger and more dispersed melanosomes; in lighter skin, they are smaller and clustered. Drugs and injuries can alter the clumping and migration of these organelles, modifying the clinical appearance of pigment. Skin type IV can undergo peeling, provided the patient understands that the demarcation line between treated and untreated areas may be more evident. In such cases, the feathering technique under the jawline helps to soften these differences. When performing a peel on an isolated aesthetic unit, it is always recommended to apply the solution approximately 5 mm beyond the natural anatomical boundaries to avoid demarcation lines. In the periorbital region, the peel should be extended to the orbital margins, and in the perioral unit, beyond the nasolabial fold. In skin type V, such as in individuals of East Asian, Latin, or Indian descent, diffuse pigmentation changes are more likely, regardless of the ablative agent, while in skin type VI, diffuse hyperpigmentation is the most common complication, which may take up to 18–24 months to resolve. In these patients, extra caution, specific consent, and more intensive preparation and follow-up protocols are indicated.

An additional aspect to consider is hyperpigmentation or accentuation of melanocytic nevus after phenol-croton oil peel. The literature describes that, after medium and deep peels, pre-existing melanocytic lesions such as nevus and lentigines may become more visible or darkened due to removal of adjacent actinic damage and the contrast difference with the lightened skin, a generally transient phenomenon but one that may cause patient concern. Furthermore, there is the theoretical risk of developing so-called pseudo melanoma or recurrent nevus, characterized by irregular repigmentation of a previously traumatized nevus, which may clinically and histologically mimic melanoma. This phenomenon has already been documented after other methods of chemical and physical injury, such as cryotherapy, laser, and dermabrasion, and although there are no specific series for phenol-croton oil peels, the biological plausibility justifies strict clinical surveillance. Thus, it is recommended not to perform peels over suspicious melanocytic lesions, to carry out prior dermoscopy and, when necessary, excision before the procedure. For clearly benign nevus, physical protective barriers such as thick petroleum jelly or tapes may be used to avoid direct exposure to the caustic agent. During follow-up, any irregular or unexpected repigmentation in treated sites should be assessed with dermoscopy and, if necessary, biopsy, to rule out malignancy.

In addition to technical factors such as concentration, number of passes, and friction, the literature also describes the influence of multiple exogenous and endogenous factors on the risk of dyschromia after phenol-croton oil peel. Among the exogenous factors, phenolic and catecholic substances with depigmenting potential stand out, such as 4-isopropyl catechol, whose experimental action and occupational reports of leukoderma illustrate the ability of these compounds to irreversibly interfere with melanogenesis. This historical observation helps to explain why phenolic derivatives such as hydroquinone, in controlled concentrations, are effective in the prevention and treatment of post-inflammatory hyperpigmentation. Hydroquinone inhibits tyrosinase, reduces melanin formation, and decreases active melanosomes. However, in patients predisposed to post-peel hypopigmentation, or in cases of prolonged use after re-epithelialization, it may potentiate already existing hypochromic areas or accentuate residual hypochromia, resulting in irregular dyschromia. For this reason, its use is recommended with caution, for controlled periods and in an individualized manner, often in combination with other less aggressive lightening agents. Regarding the triple combination, although a mild corticosteroid (such as dexamethasone 0.1% or fluocinolone) helps to reduce inflammation and prevent pigmentary rebound, it should be remembered that the controlled inflammatory process following phenol-croton oil peeling is also one of the main stimuli for dermal neocollagenesis. Thus, prolonged use of topical corticosteroids could theoretically attenuate the remodeling induced by the procedure. For this reason, their use should be restricted, limited to short periods and targeted application, avoiding extensive and prolonged use that could interfere with the desired histological outcome.

Among endogenous factors, hormones such as α- and β-MSH, ACTH, gonadotrophins, and thyroid hormone stand out, as they can stimulate melanogenesis and cause generalized hyperpigmentation. Pregnancy and the use of oral contraceptives, classically associated with melasma, should also be considered, since if the patient becomes pregnant in the months following the peel, this hormonal context may favor the onset or intensification of post-inflammatory hyperpigmentation. Periods of pituitary-hypothalamic stress, such as puberty and pregnancy, are associated with scar hyperplasia and pigment patches after trauma. The influence of the menopause and estrogen therapy should also be considered in risk assessment, as they significantly modulate the pigmentary response. These modulators explain why dyschromias may occur even in appropriately selected patients, including outside periods of sun exposure, with Lotter reporting cases during winter months in Chicago, highlighting the role of hormones, drugs, and inflammation.

Lotter's clinical series, which evaluated 408 patients undergoing phenol-croton oil peeling using the Baker-Gordon formula, demonstrated that pigmentary changes are frequent, multifactorial complications with significant emotional impact. Nine cases of mild irregular pigmentation and one of severe hyperpigmentation were documented, corresponding to approximately 2.4% of the sample, in addition to other non-pigmentary complications, such as five cases of full-thickness skin loss in the context of combined surgeries, one case of prolonged flushing, one of persistent cutaneous hypersensitivity, one of multiple milia, one of hypertrophic scarring, and one death. Management included localized reapplication of the peeling formula to even out residual patches, use of topical hydroquinone, low-current electrocautery for persistent flushing and small post-peel telangiectasias, manual removal of milia, and surgical correction of hypertrophic scars. In one case of severe hyperpigmentation, a second light peel without occlusion led to initial improvement, but pigmentation recurred after four weeks. These findings reinforce that, although some complications can be managed with complementary measures, the most effective way to reduce their occurrence is prevention, based on careful patient selection, detailed investigation of drug and hormone use, strict sun exposure control, meticulous technical execution, and prolonged follow-up. Lotter concludes that, despite the rarity of severe cases, the aesthetic and emotional burden of pigmentary changes demands clear prophylactic and therapeutic strategies. The combination of tretinoin 0.1% + hydroquinone 5% + dexamethasone 0.1% was cited as the standard for minimizing and treating post-peel hyperpigmentation; phenolic/catechol agents with melanocytotoxicity were suggested with caution; and superficial non-occlusive repeels may be useful in selected cases of irregular pigmentation.

In summary, pigmentary changes after phenol-croton oil peeling are common but generally manageable. The biology of pigment and its modulators is complex and extends far beyond sun exposure; dyschromias are frequent but can be prevented and treated with lightening agents, appropriate protocols, and strict photoprotection (Fig. 10.8); and technique, patient selection, and careful follow-up are the main factors determining risk and final aesthetic prognosis (Table 10.3).

10.2.4 Delayed Re-epithelialization and Necrosis

Delayed re-epithelialization is a significant complication following phenol-croton oil peel. Under normal conditions, complete re-epithelialization occurs between 7 and 10 days, but may extend to 12–14 days in more aggressive peels. Delays beyond this period suggest local complications and are associated with multiple factors, such as excessive phenol application, a high number of passes, intense friction, use of high concentrations of croton oil, as well as comorbidities such as diabetes, smoking, malnutrition, and immunosuppression.

A particular scenario warrants attention: frontal fibrosing alopecia (FFA). This is a progressive scarring alopecia, considered a variant of lichen planopilaris, characterized by frontotemporal hairline recession, often accompanied by loss of eyebrows, eyelashes, and facial vellus hair. This condition involves follicular fibrosis and destruction of follicular stem cells, structures crucial for epidermal regeneration after chemical peels or ablative procedures. Thus, patients with FFA may

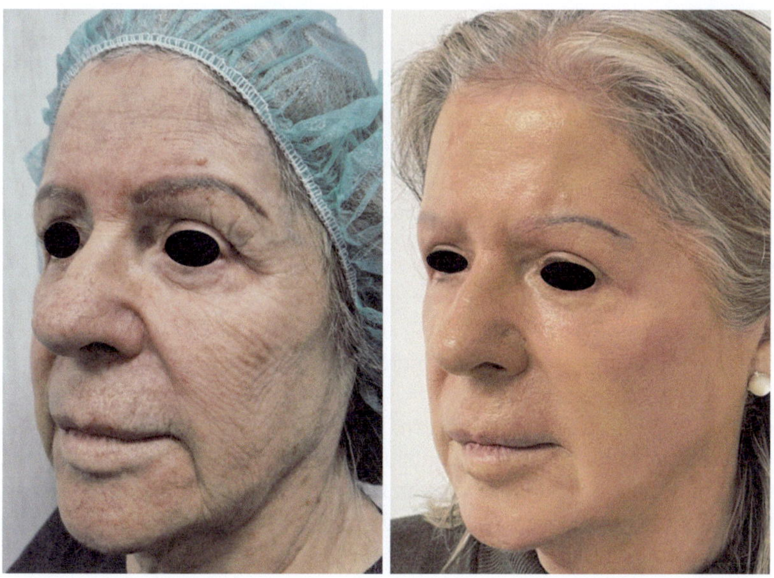

Fig. 10.8 One-month follow-up after deep phenol-croton oil peel (Hetter 1.2%). Persistent diffuse erythema is observed, an expected finding at this stage, during active dermal remodeling. The use of broad-spectrum tinted sunscreen provides not only additional photoprotection but also cosmetic camouflage, helping the patient to better cope with this aesthetically challenging phase and supporting adherence to post-procedure follow-up. *Source: Archives of Dr. Carolina Marçon and Dr. Ramon Pigem*

Table 10.3 Pigmentary changes after phenol-croton oil peeling

Type of change	Risk factors	Prevention	Management
Post-inflammatory hyperpigmentation	Higher phototypes (III–VI); prolonged inflammation; sun exposure; hormone use; aggressive technique	Skin preparation (HQ, retinoids, mild acids); photoprotection rigorous; tinted sunscreen ≥6 months; prophylactic tranexamic acid in selected cases	HQ 4–5%; vitamin C; niacinamide; oral/topical TXA; Kligman's formula; Q-switched lasers; additional superficial peels
Localized hypopigmentation (*leopard spotting*)	Pure phenol or high croton oil; uneven application; excessively deep peels	Calibrated formulations (Hetter); uniform technique; respect for anatomical boundaries	Topical tacrolimus/ pimecrolimus; bimatoprost for small patches; microneedling + drug delivery (tacrolimus/5-FU); excimer 308 nm 2–3x/ week
Diffuse depigmentation (porcelain skin)	Croton oil >1% (universal >2%); phenol under total occlusion; high doses on thin skin	Use of lower concentrations; fewer passes; avoid complete occlusion; careful selection in higher phototypes	Topical tacrolimus; excimer 308 nm on focal patches; microneedling in selected protocols; expectant management if accepted by the patient
Accentuated/ darkening of nevus (pseudo melanoma)	Peels over pre-existing melanocytic lesions; local trauma; removal of adjacent actinic damage	Avoid peeling over suspicious lesions; prior dermoscopy; physical barrier (petroleum jelly/tape) over benign nevus	Dermoscopic follow-up; biopsy if irregular repigmentation or suspicion of malignancy

Pigmentary changes after phenol-croton oil peel, with risk factors, preventive measures, and therapeutic approaches organized for practical use in dermatological practice. *Notes: HQ = hydroquinone; TXA = tranexamic acid; 5-FU = 5-fluorouracil. Source: Table prepared by the author (Dr Carolina Marçon)*

experience significant delays in healing or even areas of incomplete epithelialization after phenol-croton oil peel, with increased risk of dyschromia, persistent ulceration, and atrophic scarring.

Recent reports reinforce this concern. In a series published in 2024 by Landau, Tosti, Kroumpouzos et al. five patients with FFA experienced unusually complicated outcomes after deep phenol-croton oil peels. Presentations included progressive hypopigmentation, persistent erythema, deep ulcerations, and irregular dyschromia, often in areas of hairline recession or previously inflamed skin. Although all procedures were performed using appropriate technical protocols, the absence or compromise of pilosebaceous units appeared to determine the regenerative difficulty and adverse outcomes. These observations are consistent with previous reports of similar complications in ablative procedures in patients with frontal fibrosing alopecia. For example, Sun et al. documented a clinical case of extensive facial scarring after ablative laser resurfacing in a patient with previously undiagnosed FFA. Current literature proposes that the presence of FFA should be considered an absolute contraindication for deep chemical peels, given the incompatibility between the disease's pathophysiology and the dependence of phenol-croton oil peels on follicular integrity for re-epithelialization. The global increase in FFA prevalence makes recognition of this risk even more urgent, especially as the initial presentation may be subtle and easily overlooked during preoperative assessment. Careful clinical screening, including inspection of the hairline, presence of facial papules, eyebrow thinning, and history of lichen planus, should be part of the pre-procedure evaluation, and the procedure should be avoided in these patients.

Cutaneous necrosis, although rare, is described in the literature and constitutes one of the most serious complications. Lotter, in his series of 408 cases, reported five episodes of full-thickness skin loss, always associated with combined surgeries such as blepharoplasties or rhytidectomies, suggesting a cumulative effect of chemical injury with surgical trauma. Hetter also described necrosis as a possible outcome in peels performed with high concentrations of croton oil or excessive volumes of phenol, especially when combined with rigid and complete occlusion. Other publications have reported localized necrosis in areas of thin skin, pre-existing scars with reduced vascularization, and in cases of secondary infection, all of which impair healing and exacerbate tissue loss. Necrotic areas may progress to ulceration, superimposed infection, and permanent atrophic scarring. Experimental histological studies, such as that by Gonser et al. support these findings by demonstrating that, in skin flaps subjected to undermining during rhytidoplasty, phenol-croton oil peels reach an average of 68% of dermal thickness, with necrosis of adnexal structures and a significant risk of vascular compromise. These data highlight that phenol-croton oil peels should not be applied to previously undermined skin flaps due to the risk of necrosis, and should be restricted to areas with intact vascularization.

Another rare but relevant outcome is erosive pustular dermatosis (EPD), a rare condition typically described in elderly patients with atrophic, photoaged scalp, but which may also arise following ablative facial procedures such as laser resurfacing or medium and deep chemical peels (Fig. 10.9). Clinically, it presents as painful or pruritic erythematous plaques, associated with sterile pustules, exudative erosions, and persistent crusting. The etiology remains uncertain, but there is consensus that trauma to actinically damaged skin plays a central role, and studies suggest the involvement of pro-inflammatory cytokines such as IL-1β and TNF-α, as well as matrix metalloproteinases, particularly MMP-3, which is overexpressed in active lesions. Another key histological feature is the absence or destruction of hair follicles, structures that provide essential stem cells for epidermal regeneration, explaining the difficulty in re-epithelialization.

Mervak et al. described three cases of facial EPD in women aged 50–60 years, arising weeks to months after ablative CO_2 resurfacing or medium Jessner + TCA 35% peels, often in association with concomitant blepharoplasty or facelift. All cases progressed with chronic erosions, crusting, and sterile pustules, despite apparently adequate initial healing. Biopsies revealed non-specific changes, such as dermal fibrosis and chronic inflammation, and cultures were negative, reinforcing the sterile nature of the condition. The clinical course was protracted, with slow healing

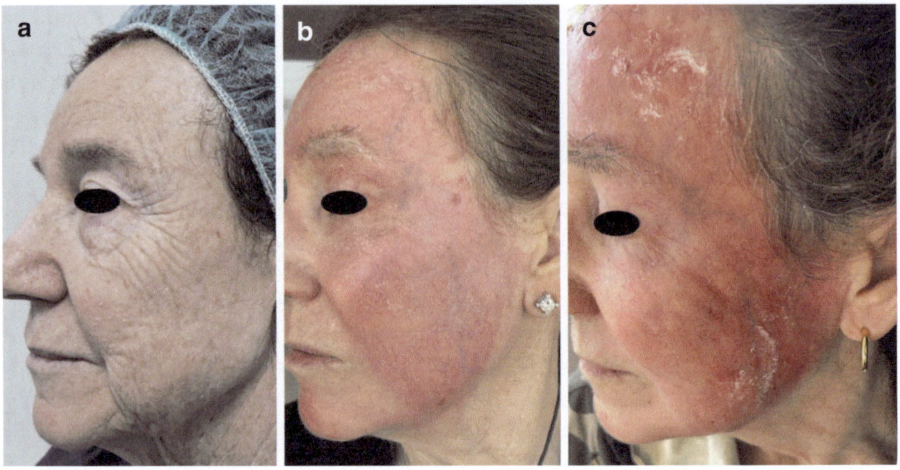

Fig. 10.9 Clinical progression of erosive pustular dermatosis (EPD) following deep phenol-croton oil peel in an elderly patient with atrophic, photoaged skin. (**a**) Pre-procedure. (**b**) Three months post-peel, with recurrent erythematous, erosive, and scaling areas. (**c**) Six months post-procedure, with persistent crusting and erosions, without complete re-epithelialization. EPD is characterized by a chronic sterile inflammatory process, involving pro-inflammatory cytokines (IL-1β, TNF-α) and increased expression of matrix metalloproteinases (MMP-3), and is aggravated by the absence of functional hair follicles, which are fundamental for epidermal regeneration. *Source: Archives of Dr. Carolina Marçon and Dr. Ramon Pigem*

over months to years. Treatment included potent topical corticosteroids, systemic corticosteroids in severe cases, oral and topical antibiotics for secondary infection control, oral dapsone at doses of 100 mg/day (with maintenance at 25–50 mg/day for up to 3.5 years), oral isotretinoin (10–30 mg/day for up to 2.5 years, cumulative dose of 250 mg/kg), topical tacrolimus 0.1%, and emollients. The prognosis was for progressive but slow improvement, requiring years of follow-up, with a risk of secondary bacterial infection and a tendency to relapse.

Additional cases have broadened the understanding of EPD. Van Exel and English reported manifestations both on and off the scalp, always following local trauma or ablative procedures on chronically sun-damaged skin. Histological findings were non-specific but consistent with chronic inflammation and destruction of adnexal structures. Diagnosis is by exclusion and is often confused with folliculitis, impetigo, pustular psoriasis, cicatricial pemphigoid, pyoderma gangrenosum, or even squamous cell carcinoma. Although microorganisms such as *Staphylococcus aureus*, Pseudomonas, and fungi have been isolated, these represent secondary colonization, and antibiotics alone do not resolve the condition. The most effective treatment was with potent topical corticosteroids, which induced rapid improvement, albeit with a risk of further atrophy. In refractory cases, 0.1% tacrolimus proved effective, and there are positive reports with topical calcipotriol, oral isotretinoin, systemic nimesulide, and zinc sulfate.

In addition to the cases described on the face and photoaged scalp, EPD has also been recognized in more complex contexts, such as in areas of extensive thermal burns. Hopley et al. reported three patients previously treated in burns units, with an average of 33% of body surface area affected, who developed late-onset EPD, approximately 18.9 months after the initial trauma and conventional management with skin grafts. Lesions arose in chronically altered areas, characterized by persistent erosions, crusting, and pustules, often mistaken for infection or graft failure. Repeated cultures were negative, reinforcing the sterile nature of the condition. Treatment with potent topical corticosteroids led to complete healing in approximately 32 days, with no recurrences after the gradual withdrawal of medication. These findings broaden the clinical spectrum of EPD beyond atrophic and photoaged skin, demonstrating that it can also occur in previously burned areas, probably due to the loss of pilosebaceous follicles and the consequent limitation of the epidermis's regenerative capacity, associated with a residual chronic inflammatory state.

From a pathophysiological perspective, EPD should be understood as a chronic wound with an intrinsic inability to heal, in which multiple anti-inflammatory, immunomodulatory, and regenerative approaches may be employed. In addition to established therapies, future prospects include the use of biologics such as infliximab, which has been reported as successful in related diseases, the application of silicone gel to modulate the wound microenvironment, fractional CO_2 laser as a healing stimulator, and autologous micrograft's in columns, capable of inducing scarless regeneration at the donor site.

Although EPD was initially described on photoaged scalp and more recently in areas of extensive thermal burns subjected to skin grafts, its pathophysiology can be partially extrapolated to deep chemical peels. In both contexts, intense injury to structurally compromised skin, poor in pilosebaceous units and under a chronic inflammatory microenvironment, favors the development of erosive lesions with delayed healing. Thus, although rare after phenol-croton oil peel, EPD should be considered in the differential diagnosis of cases with delayed or incomplete re-epithelialization, especially in elderly patients with atrophic, scarred, or previously sun-damaged skin.

Prolonged erythema after peeling may also be considered part of the spectrum of complications related to delayed healing. In general, it resolves within 90–180 days, depending on the formulation and technique used, but may be prolonged in patients who have previously received isotretinoin, due to genetic factors, or even the ingestion of small amounts of alcohol. Although rarely permanent, it may occur intermittently for up to two years after peeling, often accompanied by pruritus. Management includes topical application of mild corticosteroid lotions (hydrocortisone), oral antihistamines, and the use of corrective make-up with green pigment. Creams with medium- and high-potency/fluorinated corticosteroids, due to the risk of atrophy or telangiectasia, and chronic use of oral corticosteroids, which may lead to hypercortisolism, are not recommended.

In summary, delayed re-epithelialization and necrosis after phenol-croton oil peel are recognized, multifactorial, and potentially serious complications, resulting from technical factors, individual characteristics, and associated comorbidities.

While delayed healing may be related to conditions such as frontal fibrosing alopecia or the use of excessive concentrations of croton oil, necrosis remains rare but possible, especially in the context of combined surgeries, intense occlusion, or secondary infection. Erosive pustular dermatosis, although rare, should be remembered as a chronic complication in elderly patients with atrophic skin or those subjected to intense chemical trauma. Prevention is based on precise technique, careful assessment of risk factors, appropriate patient selection, and close follow-up, ensuring early intervention when signs of delayed healing, persistent erythema, or necrosis are identified (Table 10.4).

Table 10.4 Delayed re-epithelialization and necrosis after phenol-croton oil peel

Complication	Risk factors	Prevention	Management
Delayed re-epithelialization	Excess phenol/croton; multiple passes; intense friction; diabetes; smoking; malnutrition; immunosuppression; FFA	Precise technique; avoid high concentrations of croton; appropriate patient selection; do not perform peel in FFA	Local support; antibiotics if infection; mild corticosteroids for prolonged erythema; severe cases → hospitalization
Cutaneous necrosis	Combined surgeries (blepharoplasty, rhytidoplasty); high concentrations/volumes of phenol-croton oil; tight occlusion; secondary infection; thin skin or previous scarring	Avoid phenol-croton oil in undermined flaps; respect risk areas; careful technique; avoid intense occlusion	Early debridement; antibiotic therapy; hospital support in severe cases; risk of permanent atrophic scarring
Erosive pustular dermatosis (EPD)	Advanced age; atrophic/photoaged skin; intense chemical trauma; absence of hair follicles; history of burns or previous surgeries	Careful selection; prolonged monitoring in elderly patients and atrophic skin; early differential diagnosis	Potent topical corticosteroids; tacrolimus 0.1%; oral dapsone; oral isotretinoin in chronic cases; extended support
Prolonged erythema	Aggressive peels; genetic predisposition; prior isotretinoin use; alcohol consumption; individual factors	Appropriate selection; adjusted technique; skin preparation; close follow-up	Mild topical corticosteroids (hydrocortisone); oral antihistamines; corrective make-up; avoid potent fluorinated corticosteroids and LIP/PDL

Delayed re-epithelialization and necrosis after phenol-croton oil peel, with risk factors, preventive measures, and recommended management, including associated complications such as erosive pustular dermatosis and prolonged erythema. *Notes: AFF = frontal fibrosing alopecia; EPD = erosive pustular dermatosis. Source: Table prepared by the author (Dr Carolina Marçon)*

10.2.5 Milia

Milia are small epidermal inclusion cysts formed by the entrapment of keratin within the epidermis or superficial dermis. Clinically, they present as firm, whitish or yellowish papules, 1–2 mm in diameter, generally asymptomatic. Although benign and self-limiting, they may cause aesthetic discomfort, particularly in the context of phenol-croton oil peel, when they arise during the skin repair phase.

The occurrence of milia is described as a relatively common complication following resurfacing procedures, reported more frequently after dermabrasion than after deep chemical peels. This difference is related to the nature of tissue trauma. In dermabrasion, mechanical abrasion more extensively removes cutaneous appendages such as hair follicles and sebaceous glands, which play a central role in epidermal regeneration. The loss of these structures compromises the uniformity of healing and favors obstruction of follicular ducts during re-epithelialization, resulting in the formation of milia. In deep chemical peels, although the skin injury is also significant, the chemical action tends to preserve a greater number of pilosebaceous units, allowing for more homogeneous regeneration and, consequently, a lower risk of developing these lesions. When milia do occur in this context, they are usually associated with excessive use of thick ointments or overly occlusive dressings during the initial healing phase.

The most widely accepted mechanism for the development of these lesions involves obstruction of regenerating pilosebaceous ostia, which hinders keratin elimination and leads to microcyst formation. Some authors suggest a higher predisposition in patients with thick skin, although this association has not been objectively confirmed.

Preventive measures include pre-peel skin preparation with topical tretinoin, which helps normalize keratinization, as well as the gradual reintroduction of retinoids after re-epithelialization, reducing the likelihood of milia formation. It is also advisable to avoid occlusion or prolonged use of oily ointments, which may contribute to follicular blockage.

In most cases, milia resolve spontaneously within weeks to months. When persistent or aesthetically concerning, the preferred approach is simple mechanical extraction with a sterile needle or blade. Alternatively, gentle electrodessication may be used, provided care is taken to prevent dyspigmentation or scarring. In multiple or recurrent cases, there are reports of using low-intensity CO_2 or Er:YAG laser technologies, although these are not first-line options in the immediate post-peel period.

In summary, milia represent a benign, low-morbidity complication of resurfacing procedures, including phenol-croton oil peel. Their occurrence is closely related to wound management, being preventable with appropriate care and easily treatable when intervention is required.

10.2.6 Atrophy and Texture Changes

The ideal goal of a deep peel is to use an agent capable of penetrating slightly beyond the depth of the lesion to be treated, as in the case of actinic damage. When the desired depth is not achieved uniformly—whether due to inadequate surfactants in the formulation, high surface tension of the chemical agent, or improper technique—the result may be irregular and manifest clinically as textural changes or even as an atrophic appearance. Such irregularity can be observed, for example, in the inability of medium-depth peels, such as the combination of solid CO_2 and 35% TCA, to penetrate uniformly beneath severe perioral rhytids, producing not scars, but textural irregularities that can only be corrected by repeating the procedure with deeper agents.

So-called cutaneous atrophy, described after deep peels, refers clinically to the loss of normal skin markings without apparent scar formation. This finding is classically described after multiple phenol peels or when deep-acting agents are applied to very thin skin areas, such as the periorbital region. Clinically, the skin may acquire a translucent appearance, with visualization of the underlying musculature when illuminated, which gives the impression of a true atrophy. Histological studies, however, show that there is no actual loss of thickness: after an initial period of hypertrophy, the epidermis tends to regain its normal thickness over time. The dermis, in turn, undergoes persistent remodeling, with the expansion of the papillary layer and formation of new collagen and elastic matrix, which remains thickened even years after the procedure. The clinical appearance of "thin" skin should therefore be understood as an optical result of skin lightening and melanocyte reduction, contrasting with the histological reality of dermal thickening and sustained neocollagenesis.

The greater tendency towards an atrophic appearance after dermabrasion, compared to phenol–croton oil peeling, can be explained by the distinct nature of the tissue trauma. Dermabrasion mechanically removes a large proportion of cutaneous appendages, such as hair follicles and sebaceous glands, which are fundamental structures for epidermal regeneration, thus favoring irregular healing. Phenol–croton oil, on the other hand, through its diffuse and relatively homogeneous chemical action, preserves a greater number of these units, promoting more uniform epidermal regeneration. The concentration of croton oil used is also a determining factor: higher doses in areas of thin skin may induce disproportionate damage, increasing the likelihood of clinical changes interpreted as atrophy.

Textural changes are another common finding after deep chemical peels (Fig. 10.10). Apparently enlarged pores may appear in the first weeks as a result of stratum corneum removal, and are generally transient. Persistent surface irregularities, often described as "coarse texture" or "mottling," are mainly the result of technical errors, such as insufficient depth or uneven agent penetration, leading to a heterogeneous scarring response. This phenomenon is more common in deep rhytids or in areas of severe actinic damage, when the injury does not reach the depth required for uniform remodeling.

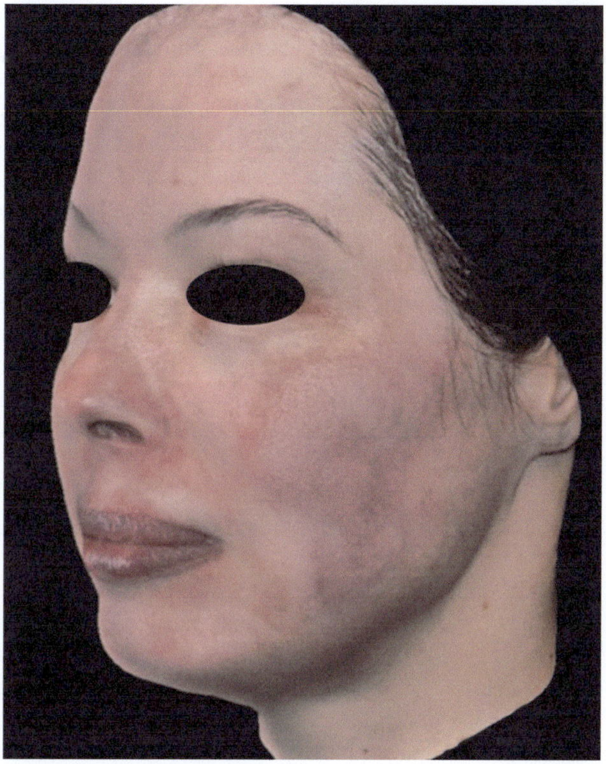

Fig. 10.10 Textural changes after deep phenol–croton oil peel. Heterogeneity of the skin surface is observed in the malar region, with areas of enlarged pores and slight irregularity, findings that may occur in the first weeks as a result of stratum corneum removal. While follicular dilation is usually transient, persistent irregularities—described as coarse texture or *mottling*—generally result from uneven penetration or insufficient depth of the agent, leading to heterogeneous dermal remodeling, especially in areas of marked actinic damage. *Source: Personal archive of Dr. Carolina Marçon and Dr. Carlos Wambier*

Several risk factors are associated with the development of atrophy and textural changes: excessive peel depth; type and concentration of the chemical agent, especially when more concentrated croton oil formulations are used; anatomical areas of thin or previously manipulated skin; inadequate technique, with multiple passes or uneven application; previously photodamaged, scarred or vascular altered skin; advanced age, due to lower collagen and elastic fiber density; recent use of isotretinoin; higher phototypes, which are predisposed to scarring complications and dyschromias; and situations of local vascular compromise, such as in areas of previous surgical undermining.

Prevention of these complications depends on careful patient and formula selection, adaptation of the technique to the regional skin thickness, and the adoption of appropriate postoperative measures. In more delicate areas, it is recommended to use lower concentrations of croton oil and to apply with a smooth transition to avoid demarcation lines. The choice of occlusion is equally important: older methods of rigid occlusion with adhesive tapes increase complications, whereas moist occlusion with petrolatum or semipermeable dressings provides a controlled and safe environment for healing. During the repair phase, measures such as strict photoprotection, gradual reintroduction of topical retinoids after complete re-epithelialization, intensive hydration, and the use of film-forming gels promote physiological recovery.

In mild cases, textural changes tend to resolve spontaneously with supportive care, while persistent or clinically significant cases may require further intervention. Repetition of the peel with deeper agents should only be considered after complete scar maturation, generally after six months. In specific situations, complementary technologies such as ablative fractional lasers (CO_2 and Er:YAG), microneedling, and even dermal grafts may be used to improve skin texture and elasticity.

In summary, both apparent atrophy and textural changes after deep peels are possible complications and should be understood within the pathophysiology of the procedure. The former most often corresponds to an optical phenomenon resulting from skin lightening, rather than histological loss of thickness, while the latter is more frequently related to technical inadequacies. Prevention is always the most effective approach, through appropriate agent selection, formula adjustment according to the treated area, and careful postoperative management, as treatment of established cases is often challenging and yields variable results (Table 10.5).

10.2.7 Ocular Complications

Ocular complications, although less frequent than other adverse events, are possible outcomes of phenol-croton oil peel, particularly when the procedure involves the periocular region. Cicatricial ectropion is the most feared complication, resulting from retraction of the lower eyelid during the healing process, which may lead to scleral exposure, ocular dryness, and risk of exposure keratitis, especially in patients with pre-existing eyelid laxity identified by a positive snap test (Fig. 10.11). Another

Table 10.5 Atrophy and textural changes after phenol–croton oil peel

Complication	Risk factors	Prevention	Management
Apparent cutaneous atrophy	Repeated use of deep peels; high-concentration croton oil in thin areas (periorbital); aggressive technique; advanced age; pre-existing atrophic skin	Adjust concentration according to area; uniform technique; avoid multiple passes in delicate regions	Explain the optical nature to the patient; supportive care (hydration, retinoids after re-epithelialization); in persistent cases, consider fractional laser or microneedling
Texture changes (irregularities, *mottling*, visible pores)	Uneven agent penetration; inadequate technique; insufficient number of passes in deep rhytids; photodamaged skin; prior use of isotretinoin	Homogeneous technique; pre-peel skin preparation; use of calibrated formulation (Hetter); smooth transitions at anatomical borders	Mild cases → spontaneous resolution with supportive care; persistent cases → repeat deep peel after ≥6 months; alternatives: fractional laser (CO_2/Er:YAG), microneedling, dermal grafts in selected cases

Apparent cutaneous atrophy and texture changes after phenol-croton oil peel, with risk factors, preventive measures, and suggested therapeutic approaches. *Notes: CO_2 = carbon dioxide; Er:YAG = erbium:yttrium-aluminium-garnet. Source: Table prepared by the author (Dr Carolina Marçon)*

common finding is marked eyelid edema, which is usually self-limiting within a few days, but in more severe cases may temporarily interfere with eyelid function and cause significant discomfort (Fig. 10.11). Severe globe displacement due to edema may also predispose susceptible patients, such as those with high myopia or keratoconus, to retinal detachment, which is why prior ophthalmological assessment should be considered in such cases. Other changes, such as epiphora, may also occur, generally related to transient edema compromising lacrimal drainage. More rarely, there are reports of accidental burns to the conjunctiva or cornea resulting from direct contact of the solution with the globe, constituting emergencies that require immediate irrigation and specialist assessment to prevent sequelae. In addition to the risk of direct chemical contact, it should be noted that phenol vapors during the procedure, as well as intense post-peel secretion, may cause conjunctival irritation and ocular discomfort even in the absence of direct injury. In such cases, preservative-free lubricating eye drops, such as hyaluronic acid, carboxymethylcellulose, or polyethylene glycol in unit dose formulations (Optive® UD, Systane® UD, Refresh Tears® UD), may be prescribed for greater comfort and protection of the ocular surface, avoiding the cumulative toxicity associated with preservatives.

Several factors increase the risk of ocular complications, including eyelid laxity associated with aging, history of blepharoplasty, inadequate application technique, and lack of appropriate ocular protection. Lower eyelid ectropion may occur when the peel is performed in conjunction with blepharoplasty, which is why a minimum interval of six months between procedures is recommended. There are reports of cases even in patients who have not undergone blepharoplasty, treated only with phenol-croton oil (Fig. 10.12), highlighting the need for caution when treating individuals with signs of partial or subclinical ectropion. Mild scarring may regress over time, with compression using a silicone sheet or massage, although more aggressive treatments are often employed, such as intralesional corticosteroids, fluocinonide-impregnated tapes, or a combination of laser excision and steroids.

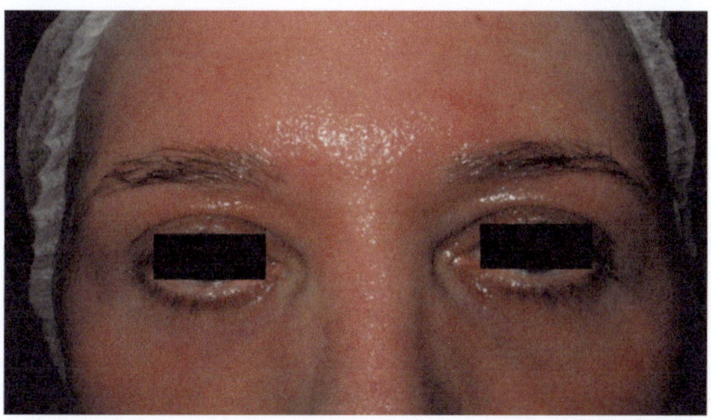

Fig. 10.11 Temporary lower eyelid ectropion after deep phenol-croton oil peel. This is a relatively common and generally self-limiting complication, which gradually resolves over time with local massage and supportive measures. It differs from permanent cicatricial ectropion, the most feared complication, which may occur in cases of severe lower eyelid retraction or when the procedure is combined with blepharoplasty. *Source: Author's personal archive (Dr Carolina Marçon)*

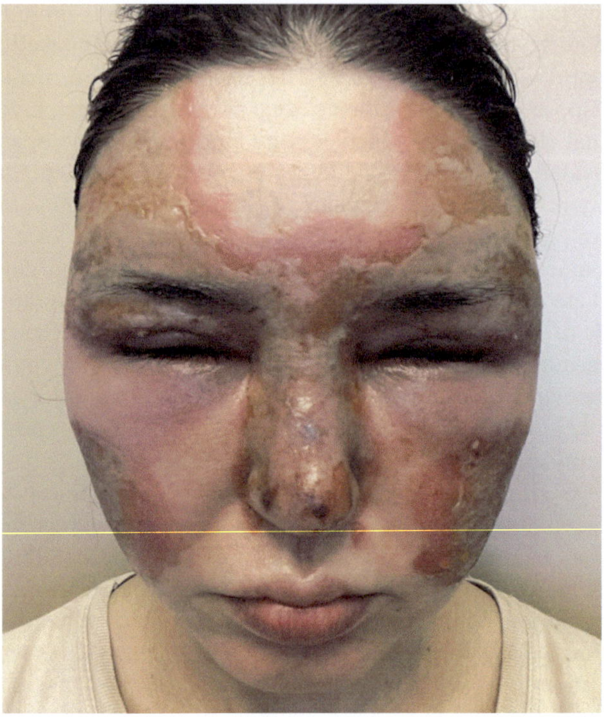

Fig. 10.12 Intense eyelid edema 36 h after deep phenol-croton oil (0.8%) peel performed in the periorbital and lateral forehead regions. Marked eyelid edema is a common finding and is generally self-limiting within a few days, but in more severe cases, it may temporarily interfere with eyelid function and cause significant discomfort. In susceptible patients, such as those with high myopia or keratoconus, pronounced displacement of the globe due to edema may predispose to more serious complications, such as retinal detachment, underscoring the importance of prior ophthalmological assessment in selected cases. *Source: Author's personal archive (Dr Carolina Marçon)*

Prevention of ocular complications depends on proper technique and effective protection of the corneal surface. The eyes should remain closed during the procedure, with an assistant responsible for drying any tears that may accumulate. Applicators soaked in peeling solution should never be passed near the eyelashes or directly over the eyes to avoid accidental dripping. The use of opiates during sedation may reduce tearing due to their anticholinergic effect, which is an additional benefit. The most effective and practical strategy for ocular protection is the application of a thick layer of sterile ophthalmic ointment over the cornea, forming an oily film that acts as a physical and chemical barrier. Unlike metallic or acrylic shields, which, although providing good protection, may become difficult to remove due to intense eyelid edema, ointments ensure adequate protection without this risk. The most commonly used formulations include sterile lubricating ointments based on petrolatum or mineral oil, such as *Lacri-Lube®, Lacrilan®, Refresh PM® and Duratears®*, and sterile antibiotic ointments, such as erythromycin or tobramycin in an oil base, may be added in cases of higher risk of abrasion. Application should be performed immediately before the peel, with reapplication as needed in lengthy procedures. To reduce the risk of solution leakage onto the globe, it is recommended to keep the head elevated, avoid excess product on the applicator, and dry tears throughout the procedure. Ointments with regenerative properties, such as *Regencel®* (hyaluronic acid and dexpanthenol) and *Epitezan®* (vitamin A), are more suitable for the treatment of established abrasions or chemical keratitis, promoting healing, but should not be used as intraoperative prophylaxis, as they do not provide the same mechanical protection as classic oily ointments.

Early recognition of complications is essential. In the acute phase, signs include conjunctival hyperemia, severe pain, tearing, photophobia, foreign body sensation, eyelid edema, corneal opacification, and epithelial defects. In more severe cases, corneal ulceration, limbal ischemia, corneal neovascularization, and, in more serious situations, structural changes detectable by ancillary tests, such as thinning of the retinal nerve fiber layer, may occur. Increased intraocular pressure may also result from severe chemical injury, leading to the development of secondary glaucoma, which presents with pain, blurred vision, halos, and, in advanced stages, irreversible visual loss.

Management should be guided by the severity of the condition. Immediate and copious irrigation of the eye exposed to the caustic agent is the priority measure, using balanced saline solution (BSS) for at least 15 min, ideally in large volume. This solution, formulated to mimic the ionic composition of aqueous humor, has osmolarity and pH similar to those of the ocular surface and is preferable to simple saline, although the latter may also be used if BSS is unavailable. After irrigation, treatment includes preservative-free ocular lubricants, cycloplegic eye drops for pain relief, prophylactic topical antibiotics in cases of extensive epithelial defect, anti-inflammatories, and topical corticosteroids, carefully monitored for inflammation control. Cruz et al. demonstrated that ophthalmic meloxicam is more effective than diclofenac in reducing croton oil-induced inflammation in rabbits, favorably modulating inflammatory cytokines without causing histological damage. Severe lesions may require amniotic membrane, autologous serum, or therapeutic lenses as adjunctive measures. Palpebral complications, such as persistent cicatricial ectropion, may require surgical correction.

Clinical reports reinforce the relevance of this topic. Ozturk et al. described a complication with 30% TCA in a patient undergoing facelift, who developed chemosis, chemical uveitis, and grade 3 corneal erosion, confirming that even with a protective gel, severe injury may occur if the substance leaks. Villena et al. in an experimental model, demonstrated that croton oil applied at 3% induces anterior uveitis with intense corneal edema, marked increase in PGE2, and leucocyte infiltration, evidencing the agent's capacity to provoke significant intraocular inflammation. Choi et al. in a retrospective study, showed that 37.5% of eyes with chemical burns progressed to glaucoma, usually within a few months, with elevated intraocular pressure at initial examination and pupillary involvement being the main risk factors for poor visual prognosis. These data corroborate the need for close monitoring, rigorous prevention, and immediate, individualized treatment.

In summary, although rare, ocular complications of phenol-croton oil peeling can significantly compromise visual function and periocular aesthetics. The risk can be reduced through careful patient selection, appropriate use of sterile protective ointments during the procedure, refined technique and careful monitoring in the post-operative period. Immediate irrigation in the event of an accident, early pharmacological management, and referral for ophthalmological assessment are essential to ensure safety and preserve the outcomes of aesthetic treatment (Table 10.6).

The following is a summary of the main local complications of phenol-croton oil peel, organized into six practical axes: warning signs, risk factors, preventive measures, initial management, and situations in which escalation to advanced treatment or specialist referral is recommended (Table 10.7).

Table 10.6 Ocular changes after phenol-croton oil peel

Complication	Risk factors	Prevention	Management
Cicatricial ectropion	Eyelid laxity; positive snap-test; previous blepharoplasty; aggressive application to lower eyelid	Careful patient selection; avoid deep peels on lax eyelids; observe interval $\geq$ 6 months after blepharoplasty	Massage; silicone; intralesional corticosteroids; surgical correction in persistent cases
Marked eyelid edema	Aggressive peels; individual predisposition; excessive product	Precise technique; avoid excess phenol/croton; head elevation	Usually self-limiting; cold compresses; NSAIDs; ocular lubricants if discomfort
Epiphora	Eyelid edema compromising lacrimal drainage	Edema control; appropriate technique	Self-limiting; ocular lubricants; rarely requires intervention
Ocular chemical burn	Direct contact of solution with conjunctiva/cornea; inadequate technique; lack of ocular protection	Protection with sterile ophthalmic ointment (Lacri-Lube®, Duratears®); avoid shields that are difficult to remove under edema; assistant to dry tears	Immediate irrigation with BSS or 0.9% saline; preservative-free lubricants; cycloplegics; topical antibiotics if epithelial defect; monitored topical corticosteroids; in severe cases → amniotic membrane/autologous serum
Conjunctival irritation from vapor's/phenol/secretion	Exposure to vapors during application; intense secretion post-peel	Adequate ventilation; ocular protection; head elevation	Preservative-free single-dose ocular lubricants (hyaluronic acid, CMC, PEG)
Severe complications (keratitis, uveitis, secondary glaucoma, retinal detachment)	Severe chemical contact; high myopia; keratoconus; lack of early treatment	Prior ophthalmological assessment in at-risk patients; prevention of agent leakage	Immediate referral to an ophthalmologist; individualized pharmacological management; risk of irreversible visual loss if not treated early

Ocular changes after phenol-croton oil peel, with risk factors, preventive measures, and therapeutic management organized in a practical format for dermatology clinics. *Notes: BSS = balanced salt solution; SF = saline solution; CMC = carboxymethylcellulose; PEG = polyethylene glycol. Source: Table prepared by the author (Dr Carolina Marçon)*

Table 10.7 Local complications of phenol-croton oil peel

Complication	Warning signs	Main risk factors	Targeted prevention	First-line management	Escalate/refer
Infections (bacterial, viral, fungal, mycobacterial)	Progressive erythema, disproportionate pain, purulent discharge/foul odor; fever, grouped vesicles (HSV); greenish exudate (Pseudomonas)	Immunosuppression, advanced age, diabetes, prolonged occlusive dressing, poor hygiene	Strict hygiene, avoid thick crusts, plain petrolatum (not topical antibiotics), universal antiviral prophylaxis	Cultures + oral antibiotics (cephalexin; clindamycin if allergic); acyclovir/valaciclovir if HSV; ciprofloxacin if Pseudomonas; oral/topical antifungals; mycobacteria = clarithromycin ± combination	Severe/systemic cases → IV antibiotics; SJS → hospitalization + intensive support; mycobacteria = infectious diseases specialist
Hypertrophic scars/keloids	Persistent erythema > 6–8 weeks, induration, nodules, intense pruritus	Previous history of pathological scars, darker skin phototypes, young age, associated infection, dynamic tension, previous surgery	Appropriate selection, avoid high-risk areas, reduce mechanical tension, avoid prior cosmetics/dyes, early Botox in critical areas	Potent topical corticosteroids; silicone sheets/gels; PDL or IPL; fractional CO_2 + corticosteroid/5-FU drug delivery; intralesional triamcinolone ± 5-FU	Refractory keloid → multimodal (bleomycin, cryotherapy, CO_2 + infiltration)
Pigmentary changes	Hyperpigmentation >6 months, focal hypopigmentation (islands), diffuse depigmentation, pseudo melanoma	Darker skin phototypes (IV–VI), prolonged inflammation, sun exposure, hormones, use of high doses of croton/phenol under occlusion	Preparation with lightening agents (HQ, retinoids, ATX), strict photoprotection, tinted sunscreen for ≥ 6 months	HQ 4–5%, vitamin C, oral/topical ATX, niacinamide; tacrolimus/pimecrolimus for hypopigmentation; 308 nm excimer; microneedling + drug delivery; excision of suspicious lesions	Refractory dyschromia → Q-switched lasers; persistent hypopigmentation → excimer + immunomodulators

(continued)

Complication	Warning signs	Main risk factors	Targeted prevention	First-line management	Escalate/refer
Delayed re-epithelialization/ necrosis	Incomplete epithelialization >14 days, persistent ulcerations, focal necrosis, prolonged erythema >6 months	Excessive dose/volume of phenol/croton, intense friction, smoking, diabetes, malnutrition, AFF, associated surgery	Avoid phenol-croton oil in AFF; precise technique; do not apply to undermined flaps; intensive monitoring	Local support, antibiotics if infection; early debridement in necrosis; mild corticosteroids for prolonged erythema	Severe cases → hospitalization; chronic EPD → topical corticosteroids, tacrolimus, dapsone, isotretinoin, fractional CO_2 laser
Milia	Whitish/firm papules, 1–2 mm, asymptomatic.	Excessive use of oily ointments, overly occlusive dressings, thick skin	Prepare/reintroduce tretinoin; avoid excessive occlusion	Simple mechanical extraction; mild electrodessication	Multiple/recurring cases → low-intensity CO_2/ Er:YAG
Atrophy/texture changes	Thin/translucent skin appearance; enlarged pores, persistent irregularity.	Areas of thin skin, concentrated croton, multiple passes, irregular technique, prior isotretinoin	Adjust concentration by region; avoid multiple passes; prefer petrolatum to rigid occlusion	Supportive measures, photoprotection; reintroduce retinoids; intensive hydration; fractional laser in persistent cases	Severe cases → repeat deep peel after 6 months; consider dermal grafts
Ocular complications	Ectropion, marked edema, epiphora, severe ocular pain, conjunctival/ corneal burn.	Eyelid laxity, previous blepharoplasty, inadequate technique, absence of ocular protection.	Protect the cornea with sterile oily ointment; meticulous technique; avoid excess near the eyelashes.	Immediate irrigation (BSS or saline); preservative-free lubricating eye drops; topical antibiotics if epithelial defect is present; topical corticosteroids with monitoring.	Severe lesions → amniotic membrane, autologous serum, therapeutic lenses; persistent ectropion → surgery

Local complications of phenol-croton oil peeling, summarized with their clinical warning signs, most relevant risk factors, prevention strategies, recommended initial management, and situations in which therapeutic escalation or specialist referral is indicated. *Notes. TSS = toxic shock syndrome; MRSA* = Methicillin-resistant Staphylococcus aureus*; TXA = tranexamic acid; FFA = frontal fibrosing alopecia; HQ = hydroquinone; PDL* = pulsed dye laser*; IPL* = intense pulsed light*; CO_2 = carbon dioxide; RGM = rapidly growing mycobacteria. Source: Table prepared by the author (Dr Carolina Marçon)*

10.3 Systemic Complications

10.3.1 Introduction

Despite advances in the standardization of formulations and the scientific consolidation of phenol-croton oil peeling, systemic complications remain a highly relevant clinical concern. This chapter differs from the one dedicated to toxicity, which focused on the pharmacological and pathophysiological aspects of phenol and croton oil. Here, the emphasis is practical: understanding how these complications present in the patient, assessing their potential severity, and, above all, defining safe and immediate management in the event of adverse events.

Although the procedure is topical, phenol has a high capacity for cutaneous absorption and can reach systemic concentrations capable of triggering acute effects on the heart, respiratory system, and central nervous system. *Croton tiglium* oil, even when used in minimal doses, contains biologically active phorbol esters that can induce intense and unpredictable inflammatory responses. This interplay between therapeutic efficacy and potential risk underscores the need for in-depth clinical knowledge to ensure the safe performance of the peel.

Since the nineteenth century, the medical literature has documented fatal cases of phenol poisoning via various routes of exposure. In the context of peeling, it is known that the severity of systemic complications is strongly related to the extent of the treated area, the speed of application, and the body's ability to eliminate the substance. Reports describe manifestations ranging from non-specific symptoms such as nausea, dizziness, and lethargy to severe events such as cardiac arrhythmias, seizures, pulmonary edema, renal failure, and, in extreme cases, death.

On the one hand, such data reinforce the importance of caution in clinical practice; on the other, it is essential to recognize that complications are largely preventable when the procedure is performed by qualified physicians, in an appropriate setting, and with strict protocols. The widespread use of these substances by non-medical professionals, combined with the sale of unregulated and uncontrolled formulations, further increases the risks and highlights the need for ongoing education and systematic knowledge.

The purpose of this section, therefore, is to objectively organize the most relevant systemic complications, correlating their clinical presentation with appropriate management. More than emphasizing the aesthetic potential of phenol-croton oil peeling, this chapter highlights that patient safety is directly linked to the physician's technical preparation and ability to respond promptly to high-severity situations.

10.3.2 Cardiovascular Complications

Reviewed by Dr André Luís Wambier

Cardiovascular complications represent the most feared systemic effect of phenol-croton oil peeling. Phenol exerts direct toxicity on the myocardium, reducing its contractility, altering electrical conduction, and promoting autonomic imbalance—effects already demonstrated in animal models, where decreased contractile force and slowed electrical activity were observed after systemic exposure. Clinically, these changes manifest as a spectrum ranging from sinus tachycardia, bradycardia, and ventricular extrasystoles to more severe arrhythmias such as ventricular tachycardia, atrial fibrillation, and ventricular fibrillation, which may culminate in cardiorespiratory arrest and death (Fig. 10.13).

Individual susceptibility to these complications does not show a consistent relationship with age, sex, cardiac history, or even serum phenol levels. Classic studies, such as those by Truppman and Ellenberg, demonstrated that the most relevant risk factor is the extent of the skin area treated within a short period of time. When 50% or more of the face was treated in less than 30 min, 23% of patients developed arrhythmias, whereas the risk disappeared when the same procedure was performed over 60 min. Gross reported a similar incidence, with arrhythmias in 30% of patients undergoing rapid peels, including cases of atrial fibrillation that resolved spontaneously after serum phenol clearance. Beeson, in a series of 43 patients, observed 10 cases of arrhythmias, including premature ventricular contractions, bigeminy, paroxysmal atrial tachycardia, and ventricular tachycardia. In a retrospective study of 181 patients, the incidence was 6.6%, more frequent in individuals with hypertension, diabetes, and depression, highlighting the role of comorbidities as a vulnerability factor. Kadunc and Vanti, in their evaluation of 60 women with rigorous Holter monitoring and urinary gas chromatography, identified four cases of sustained ventricular tachycardia. More recently, Rullan et al. reinforced the importance of intraoperative monitoring by demonstrating that, among 196 patients undergoing peeling with multiparametric monitoring, only 5% developed benign and transient arrhythmias.

Although rare, there are reports of death associated with phenol-croton oil peels in the literature, including recent publications such as the case documented by our group in 2024. Most of these events occurred in situations of excessive systemic

Fig. 10.13 Examples of electrocardiographic tracings observed during phenol-croton oil peeling, including sinus rhythm (P waves preceding each QRS complex, with regular interval), sinus tachycardia (regular rhythm with heart rate above 100 bpm), sinus bradycardia (regular rhythm with heart rate below 60 bpm), ventricular extra systole (premature and widened QRS complex, followed by a compensatory pause), ventricular bigeminy (alternation between sinus beat and ventricular extra systole), atrial fibrillation (irregularly irregular rhythm, without discernible P waves), ventricular fibrillation (disorganized electrical activity, with complexes of variable amplitude and morphology), and asystole (isoelectric line indicating absence of ventricular electrical activity). *Source: Figure created by the author (Dr Carolina Marçon)*

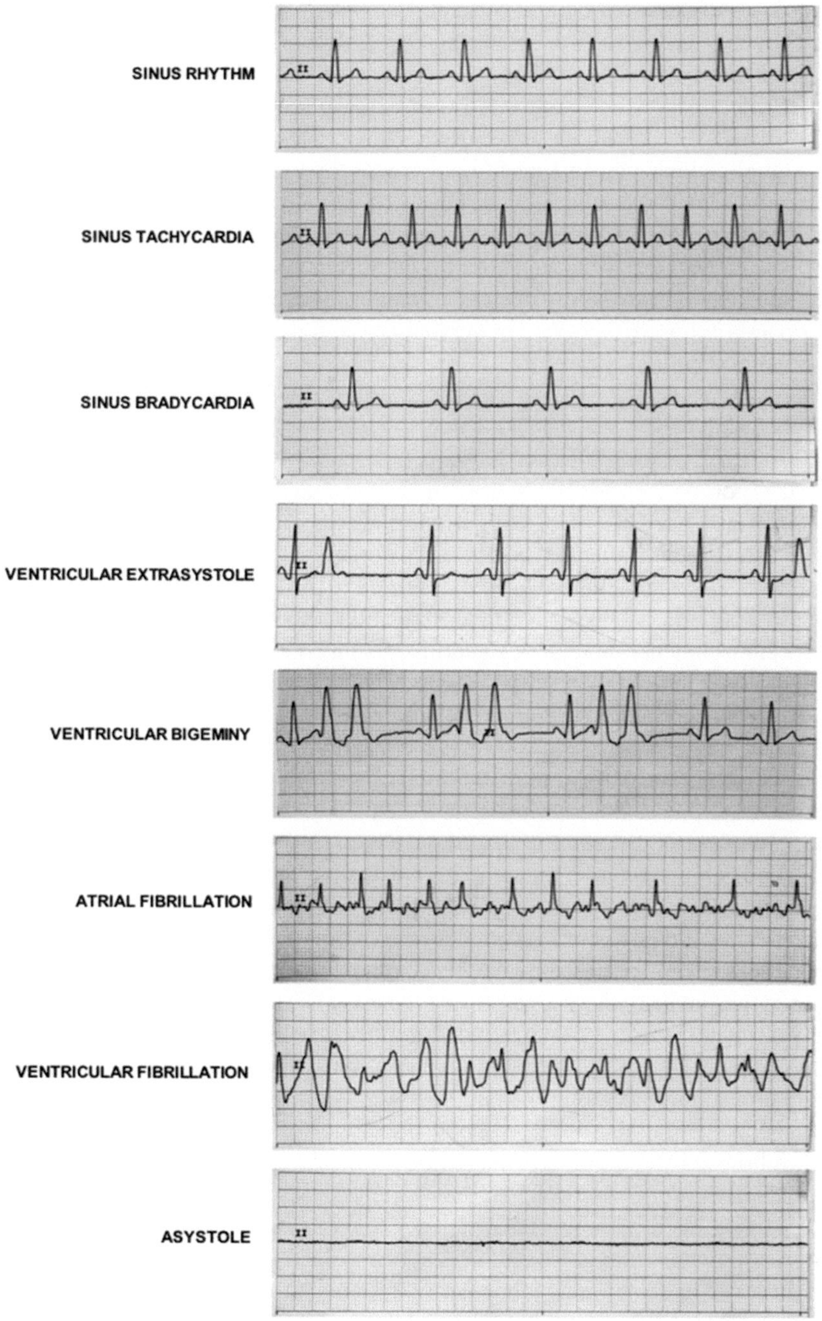
SINUS RHYTHM
SINUS TACHYCARDIA
SINUS BRADYCARDIA
VENTRICULAR EXTRASYSTOLE
VENTRICULAR BIGEMINY
ATRIAL FIBRILLATION
VENTRICULAR FIBRILLATION
ASYSTOLE

absorption, either due to the use of high doses, application to large areas in a short period, or inadequate techniques, often performed outside the medical setting. In addition to formally published cases, there are also anecdotal reports among experienced specialists, which reinforce the possibility of fatal outcomes when the procedure is performed without appropriate safety criteria. There are also records of fatal complications via unconventional routes of exposure, such as the episode reported by Li and colleagues, in which a 21-year-old man died after subcutaneous injection of phenol in an attempt to remove a tattoo, illustrating the extreme risks of improper use of the substance. These findings demonstrate that the fatal toxicity of phenol-croton oil is not solely dependent on the concentration used, but above all on the skin area exposed, the speed of application, and the safety of the environment in which the procedure is performed.

Prevention is an essential part of procedural safety. The peel should be performed in segments, dividing the face into five to eight aesthetic units, with intervals of 10–20 min between each area, allowing for metabolism and partial excretion of phenol. Vigorous intravenous hydration is also mandatory: it is recommended to administer at least 500 ml of Ringer's lactate prior to the procedure and around 1000 ml during and after its execution, in order to promote diuresis and phenol elimination. Animal studies have confirmed that forced diuresis substantially reduces the occurrence of arrhythmias and cardiotoxicity. In addition, it is essential that the environment is adequately ventilated, that continuous multiparametric monitoring with ECG, blood pressure, and oximetry is in place, and that the team is trained in advanced life support, with immediate access to a defibrillator and all emergency drugs.

The clinical management of arrhythmias should follow the updated protocols of Advanced Cardiac Life Support (ACLS), adapted to the context of peeling. The first step in the event of any rhythm disturbance is to immediately suspend the application, ensure supplemental oxygen, maintain a patent intravenous line with vigorous hydration, and proceed with intensive monitoring. Sinus tachycardia, generally related to pain, anxiety, or initial phenol absorption, may be reversed by temporarily suspending the peel, optimizing analgesia, oxygenation, and fluid therapy; if persistent or symptomatic, short-acting beta-blockers such as esmolol (0.5 mg/kg bolus followed by infusion of 50–200 mcg/kg/min) may be used. Isolated ventricular extrasystoles or bigeminy, although common, may signal a risk of progression and require interruption of the procedure, oxygen administration, and hydration; when recurrent or symptomatic, intravenous lidocaine is recommended (1–1.5 mg/kg bolus, followed by continuous infusion of 1–4 mg/min). Supraventricular tachycardias and paroxysmal atrial tachycardia, often associated with rapid applications, should be managed with immediate suspension of the procedure and oxygenation; in cases of hemodynamic instability, synchronized cardioversion is mandatory, while in stable patients, vagal maneuvers or adenosine (6 mg IV rapid bolus, repeatable with a second dose of 12 mg) may be attempted. Atrial fibrillation, although less common, requires immediate electrical cardioversion (120–200 J biphasic) in cases of instability; in stable patients, ventricular rate control may be achieved with beta-blockers (metoprolol 5 mg IV every 5 min up to 15 mg) or calcium channel blockers such as diltiazem (15–20 mg IV over 2 min, repeatable after 15 min) or verapamil (5–10 mg IV over 2 min), reserving amiodarone (150 mg IV over 10 min followed of continuous infusion) for refractory cases (Table 10.8).

Sustained ventricular tachycardia is a serious and potentially fatal complication. In cases of instability, immediate electrical cardioversion (100 J biphasic) is the recommended approach. When the patient remains stable, intravenous antiarrhythmics such as amiodarone (150 mg over 10 min, followed by continuous infusion), procainamide (20–50 mg/min until arrhythmia suppression, hypotension, or a maximum dose of

Table 10.8 Management of arrhythmias during phenol-croton oil peeling

Arrhythmia	Management
General initial steps	Immediately discontinue application; provide supplemental O_2; maintain intravenous access with vigorous hydration; continue intensive monitoring
Sinus tachycardia	**If persistent/symptomatic:** esmolol 0.5 mg/kg IV bolus followed by infusion at 50–200 mcg/kg/min
Ventricular extrasystoles/bigeminy	**If recurrent/symptomatic:** lidocaine 1–1.5 mg/kg IV bolus, followed by infusion at 1–4 mg/min
Supraventricular tachycardia/ paroxysmal atrial tachycardia	**Unstable:** synchronized cardioversion **Stable:** vagal maneuvers or adenosine 6 mg IV (may repeat with a second dose of 12 mg)
Atrial fibrillation	**Unstable:** electrical cardioversion 120–200 J biphasic **Stable:** ventricular rate control (metoprolol 5 mg IV up to 15 mg; diltiazem 15–20 mg IV; verapamil 5–10 mg IV). Amiodarone 150 mg IV over 10 min if refractory
Sustained ventricular tachycardia	**Unstable:** immediate electrical cardioversion 100 J biphasic **Stable:** amiodarone 150 mg IV over 10 min; procainamide 20–50 mg/min up to a maximum dose of 17 mg/kg; sotalol 1.5 mg/kg over 5 min (contraindicated if prolonged QT)
Ventricular fibrillation/ pulseless VT	Immediate CPR + early defibrillation 120–200 J biphasic. Epinephrine 1 mg IV every 3–5 min. Amiodarone 300 mg IV bolus (may repeat 150 mg) or lidocaine 1–1.5 mg/kg IV
Torsades de Pointes	Suspend procedure, provide O_2 and IV hydration. Magnesium sulfate 2 g IV over 10–15 min, followed by infusion (1–2 g/h) if recurrent. If bradycardic, consider isoproterenol 2–10 mcg/min or temporary pacing at 90–110 bpm. Unstable: immediate electrical cardioversion. Avoid QT-prolonging drugs (amiodarone, sotalol). Lidocaine may be considered only in refractory cases.
Symptomatic sinus bradycardia	Discontinue the procedure, provide O_2 and volume replacement. Atropine 1 mg IV every 3–5 min (max 3 mg). If refractory: dopamine 5–20 mcg/kg/min or epinephrine 2–10 mcg/min; consider transcutaneous pacing
Asystole/PEA	Immediate CPR, epinephrine 1 mg IV every 3–5 min, correction of reversible causes (5H and 5T). Defibrillation is not indicated in asystole

Management adapted from the ACLS protocol to the context of phenol-croton oil peeling. *Notes: ACLS = Advanced Cardiac Life Support; CPR = cardiopulmonary resuscitation; PEA = pulseless electrical activity;* O_2 *= supplemental oxygen; IV = intravenous; bpm = beats per minute; mcg = micrograms; mg = milligrams; g = grams; min = minute(s); J = joules. Source: Table prepared by the author (Dr Carolina Marçon)*

17 mg/kg), or sotalol (100 mg IV, 1.5 mg/kg over 5 min) may be used, the latter being contraindicated in patients with prolonged QT. Ventricular fibrillation and pulseless ventricular tachycardia are medical emergencies requiring immediate cardiopulmonary resuscitation combined with early defibrillation at 120–200 J biphasic, in addition to administration of epinephrine (1 mg IV every 3–5 min) and antiarrhythmics such as amiodarone (300 mg IV bolus, followed by 150 mg if necessary) or, alternatively, lidocaine (1–1.5 mg/kg IV bolus, repeating 0.5–0.75 mg/kg every 5–10 min up to a maximum dose of 3 mg/kg). In cases of symptomatic sinus bradycardia, management includes discontinuation of the application, supplemental oxygen, fluid resuscitation, and atropine (1 mg IV every 3–5 min up to a maximum of 3 mg); if refractory, dopamine infusion (5–20 mcg/kg/min) or epinephrine (2–10 mcg/min) may be used, and transcutaneous pacing should be considered. Asystole and pulseless electrical activity, in turn, should be managed with immediate resuscitation, epinephrine every 3–5 min, and correction of reversible causes (5 Hs and 5 Ts), with no indication for defibrillation in the case of asystole (Fig. 10.14).

Another critical aspect is the transient prolongation of the heart rate-corrected QT interval, described during phenol-croton oil peels. For this reason, it is recommended to perform a baseline electrocardiogram before a full-face procedure, as well as to discontinue any drugs that may prolong the QT interval. The interval is considered pathological when it exceeds 440 ms in men and 470 ms in women, a condition that increases the risk of severe arrhythmias by promoting early afterdepolarizations, which may progress to torsades de pointes, ventricular fibrillation, and sudden death (Fig. 10.15). Acquired QT prolongation is more prevalent than the congenital form, and in the context of peeling, it generally resolves within 15 min after completion of the procedure. The presence of atrial or ventricular ectopic beats should be interpreted as a warning sign, justifying longer pauses, reduction of the treated area in each application, optimization of analgesia, and intensification of fluid therapy. It is important to emphasize that a full-face peel should not be performed in less than one hour.

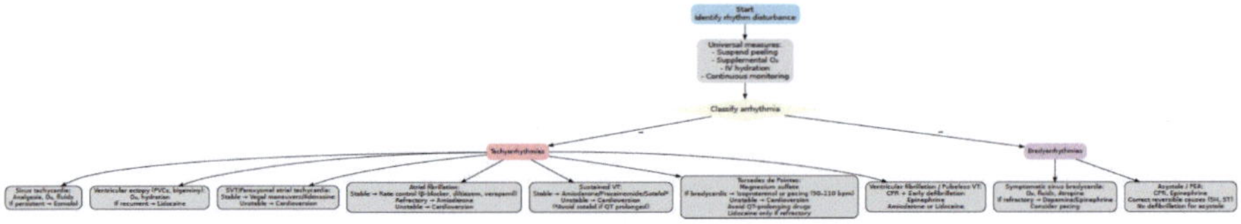

Fig. 10.14 Flowchart for the management of arrhythmias during phenol-croton oil peeling, adapted from *Advanced Cardiac Life Support (ACLS)* recommendations. The algorithm begins with rhythm identification and universal support measures (immediate discontinuation of the procedure, supplemental oxygen, intravenous hydration, and continuous monitoring). It then specifies management according to arrhythmia type: tachyarrhythmias (sinus tachycardia, ventricular ectopy, supraventricular tachycardia, atrial fibrillation, sustained ventricular tachycardia, *torsades de pointes*, ventricular fibrillation/pulseless tachycardia) and bradyarrhythmias (symptomatic sinus bradycardia and asystole/pulseless electrical activity). The flowchart emphasizes the need for immediate and systematic intervention following advanced life support protocols. Source: Figure prepared by the author (Dr. Carolina Marçon). *Source: Figure prepared by the author (Dr Carolina Marçon)*

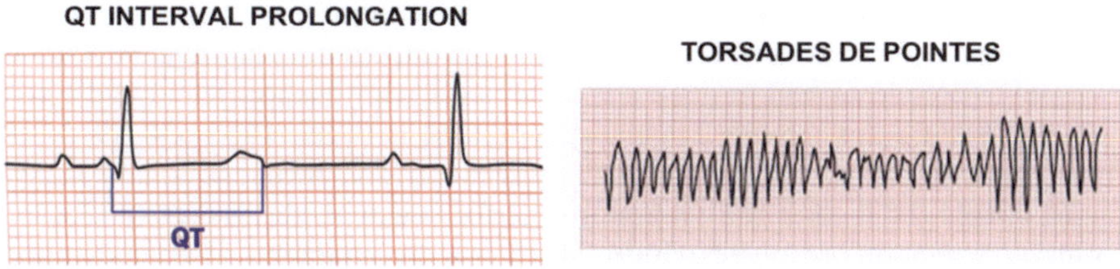

Fig. 10.15 Schematic electrocardiographic tracings illustrating, on the left, QT interval prolongation (interval between the start of the QRS complex and the end of the T wave visibly increased) and, on the right, the typical polymorphic ventricular tachycardia known as Torsades de Pointes, characterized by QRS complexes of varying morphology that appear to twist around the baseline. *Source: Figure prepared by the author (Dr Carolina Marçon)*

The management of torsades de pointes (TdP), a polymorphic ventricular tachycardia associated with QT interval prolongation, requires immediate and specific measures. The first-line therapy is intravenous magnesium sulfate (2 g IV over 10–15 min), regardless of baseline serum magnesium levels, followed by continuous infusion (1–2 g/h) if recurrences occur. In hemodynamically unstable patients, immediate electrical cardioversion is mandatory. A key aspect of TdP is its frequent association with bradycardia, which favors early afterdepolarizations and increases arrhythmogenic risk; in such cases, increasing the heart rate by temporary transcutaneous pacing (90–110 bpm) or intravenous isoproterenol infusion (2–10 mcg/min) is recommended, provided there are no contraindications such as acute coronary syndromes. Antiarrhythmics that further prolong the QT interval, such as amiodarone and sotalol, should be strictly avoided. Lidocaine, as a class IB antiarrhythmic that does not prolong QT, is not a first-line option but may be considered in refractory situations when magnesium and pacing are ineffective or unavailable.

Thus, cardiac arrhythmias, although rare when peeling is performed under appropriate conditions, represent a critical and potentially fatal systemic complication. Early recognition and immediate management are crucial for patient safety, and simple discontinuation of the application may be sufficient in benign cases. However, unstable arrhythmias require immediate advanced response, according to ACLS protocols, always in a prepared environment, with multiparametric monitoring, a trained team, and access to all necessary drugs and equipment. This set of measures reaffirms that phenol-croton oil peeling, although highly effective for rejuvenation, should remain exclusively under the domain of qualified physicians and in conditions of complete safety for the patient.

10.3.3 Respiratory Complications

Inhalation of phenol vapors can cause upper and lower airway compromise, with the potential to induce anything from local irritation to severe cases of glottic edema and acute pulmonary edema. These effects result from the corrosive nature of the substance, which can damage the respiratory epithelium and trigger an intense inflammatory response. Although uncommon, laryngeal edema is a complication described in deep chemical peels with phenol. Klein and Little reported three cases among 245 patients treated between 1965 and 1975, all female and smokers, who developed laryngeal stridor, hoarseness, and tachypnoea within 24 h after the procedure, performed with the Baker & Gordon formula. Symptoms resolved within 24–48 h with inhalation of heated vapor, without the need for orotracheal intubation, tracheostomy, or permanent sequelae. The authors attributed the phenomenon to a hypersensitivity reaction in larynges chronically irritated by tobacco, and after these episodes, instituted an empirical prophylactic protocol consisting of hydrochlorothiazide (50 mg orally (PO) twice daily), chlorpheniramine combined with phenylpropanolamine (Ornade® - 1 tablet PO 2x/day) and chymotrypsin (Chymoral®—100 mg PO 4x/day). The regimen was initiated 24 h prior to the peel and maintained in the immediate postoperative period, with discontinuation of hydrochlorothiazide and chlorpheniramine on the second day, and continuation of chymotrypsin for one week. The authors themselves emphasized the empirical and unvalidated nature of this protocol, which appeared to reduce the incidence of laryngeal edema in their case series.

Laryngeal edema requires prompt diagnosis and immediate intervention. Initial measures include oxygen supplementation and inhalation of heated vapor, as described in classical reports. Currently, immediate oxygen supplementation, inhalation of heated vapor, administration of antihistamines via intramuscular (IM) or intravenous (IV) routes (for example, diphenhydramine 25–50 mg IM or slow IV), combined with systemic corticosteroids (such as dexamethasone 4–8 mg IV or methylprednisolone 1 mg/kg), may help reduce inflammatory edema. In cases of severe stridor or imminent risk of airway obstruction, nebulized adrenaline (1 mg diluted in 5 mL of 0.9% saline) or intramuscular adrenaline (0.3–0.5 mg of 1:1000 solution) may be used. When there is significant ventilatory compromise, early orotracheal intubation in a hospital setting with advanced life support is mandatory (Table 10.9).

Pulmonary toxicity from phenol is not limited to inhalation. Systemic cutaneous absorption or exposure via other routes may also cause severe respiratory failure. Gupta et al. described a case of accidental intramuscular exposure to phenol, which resulted in acute pulmonary edema and respiratory failure, highlighting the severity of alveolar involvement regardless of the route of absorption. The pathophysiology is related to the direct action of phenol on pneumocytes and endothelial cells, increasing the permeability of the alveolocapillary membrane. The cytotoxic effect induces cellular necrosis and triggers an intense inflammatory response, with neutrophilic infiltration and release of inflammatory mediators, resulting in alveolar microhemorrhages, fibrin deposition, and accumulation of protein-rich fluid in the alveolar space. The clinical picture, similar to acute respiratory distress syndrome (ARDS), leads to progressive and refractory hypoxemia, characteristic of noncardiogenic pulmonary edema.

Table 10.9 Management of respiratory complications of phenol

Complication	Management	Medications and dosages
Laryngeal edema	Immediate oxygen therapy Inhalation of heated vapour IM/IV antihistamine IV corticosteroid Adrenaline (nebulized or IM) if severe stridor Early orotracheal intubation in refractory cases	Diphenhydramine 25–50 mg intramuscularly or by slow intravenous injection Chlorpheniramine 10 mg intramuscularly or intravenously Dexamethasone 4–8 mg intravenously or Methylprednisolone 1 mg/kg IV Nebulized adrenaline: 1 mg in 5 mL 0.9% saline Intramuscular adrenaline: 0.3–0.5 mg (1:1000 solution), in cases of imminent obstruction
Acute pulmonary edema	High-flow oxygen therapy Non-invasive or invasive ventilation with PEEP in severe cases IV diuretic to reduce congestion Hemodynamic support as required Multiparametric monitoring in an intensive care setting	Furosemide 20–40 mg intravenous bolus (repeat as needed) Oxygen therapy/mechanical ventilation with adjusted PEEP Vasodilators (IV nitroglycerin) if hypertensive congestion Vasoactive drugs (noradrenaline, dopamine) if associated shock Continuous hemodynamic support

Recommended management of respiratory complications associated with the use of phenol in deep chemical peels. Laryngeal edema requires rapid intervention with ventilatory support and specific pharmacological measures, while acute pulmonary edema demands intensive management with oxygen therapy, protective mechanical ventilation, and hemodynamic support. The dosages and routes of administration of the medications follow recommendations based on emergency and intensive care protocols, supplemented by classical literature reports. The empirical preventive protocol proposed by Klein and Little has not been validated in clinical trials and is of historical interest only. *Source: Table prepared by the author (Dr Carolina Marçon)*

Management of acute pulmonary edema must be instituted immediately. Measures include supplemental oxygen therapy, non-invasive or mechanical ventilation with positive end-expiratory pressure (PEEP) to recruit alveoli and improve oxygenation, as well as intensive monitoring. Administration of diuretics, such as furosemide 20–40 mg IV bolus, helps reduce pulmonary congestion, especially in cases with an associated cardiogenic component. In situations of hemodynamic instability, support with vasodilators or vasoactive drugs may be required.

More recently, a fatal case in Brazil, published by Marçon et al. in the *Journal of the American Academy of Dermatology*, highlighted the risks of severe pulmonary complications resulting from systemic absorption of phenol. The patient developed acute pulmonary edema associated with diffuse alveolar hemorrhage (Fig. 10.16), as well as inflammatory erosions in the larynx (Fig. 10.17) and trachea, confirming a pattern of fulminant respiratory toxicity. This case had regulatory repercussions and led to the temporary suspension of phenol by ANVISA in 2024, underscoring

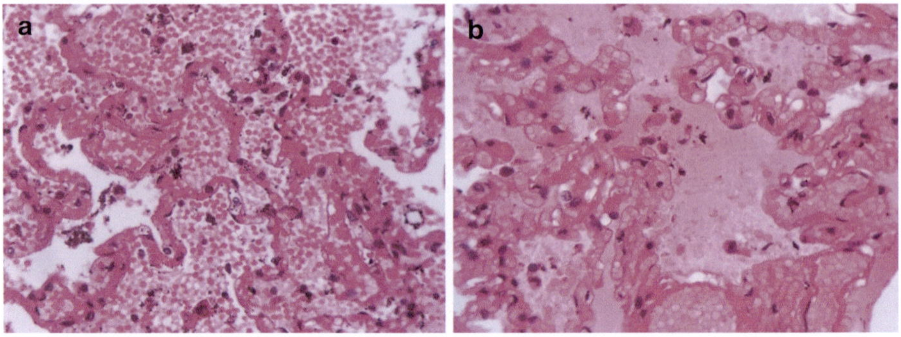

Fig. 10.16 Lung tissue sections showing pathological changes. Hematoxylin-eosin stain, original magnification: ×400. (**a**) Alveolar hemorrhage. (**b**) Alveolar edema. *Source: Adapted from Marçon CR et al. Fatal Phenol Peel by an Unlicensed Social Media Practitioner: A Forensic Medical Analysis. J Am Acad Dermatol. 2025 Aug 5:S0190-9622(25)02555-1. doi:10.1016/j.jaad.2025.05.1461. Epub ahead of print. PMID: 40774430. Reproduced with permission from the publisher*

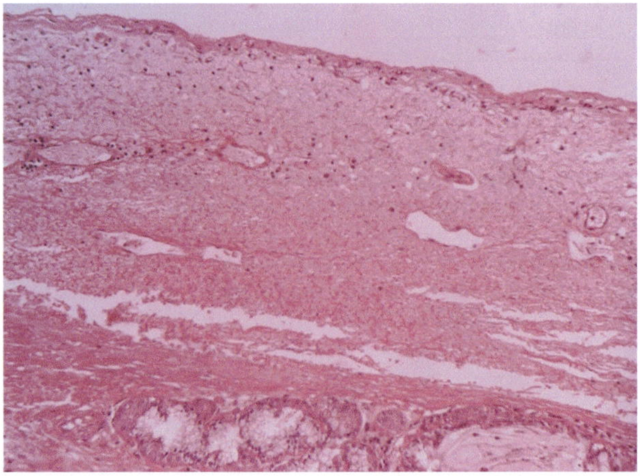

Fig. 10.17 Section of infraglottic laryngeal mucosa showing erosion associated with hemorrhage in the chorion. Hematoxylin-eosin stain, original magnification: ×400. *Source: Adapted from Marçon CR et al. J Am Acad Dermatol. 2025 Aug 5:S0190-9622(25)02555-1. doi:10.1016/j.jaad.2025.05.1461. Epub ahead of print. PMID: 40774430. Reproduced with permission from the publisher*

the magnitude of the risks involved when the substance is used outside an appropriate medical setting.

Respiratory compromise following phenol exposure may manifest as either central depression or acute pulmonary edema, the latter frequently implicated in fatal outcomes. Although some post-mortem reports attribute this to direct inhalation of vapors, most experts consider the edema, in the majority of cases, to be secondary to cardiac toxicity, particularly severe arrhythmias. Regardless of the exact mechanism, immediate availability of resources for intubation and assisted ventilation is mandatory in any setting where phenol peeling is performed.

10.3.4 Neurological Complications

The central nervous system may also be affected by systemic phenol toxicity. At toxic doses, the substance can induce dizziness, headache, confusion, agitation, tremors, seizures, and even coma, potentially progressing to multiorgan failure and death. The mechanism is related to direct depressant action on the CNS, with a narcotic effect that impairs both higher and spinal centers, accounting for the rapid loss of consciousness and profound collapse in massive exposures.

During phenol-croton oil peeling, it is relatively common for the patient to experience psychomotor slowing, mild drowsiness, and slight confusion in the first hours after the procedure, symptoms that are generally transient. However, changes such as altered speech patterns, progressive reduction in consciousness level, psychomotor agitation, tremors, central-origin vomiting, or seizures should be considered signs of systemic toxicity. In such cases, the procedure must be stopped immediately and vigorous intravenous hydration instituted to accelerate renal clearance of phenol. Intensive clinical and neurological monitoring is recommended throughout the procedure and for 12–24 h afterward, the critical period during which systemic absorption may reach high concentrations. In sedated patients, there is a risk of masking early signs of neurotoxicity, making it essential to monitor objective parameters such as respiratory pattern, oxygen saturation, and motor response.

Treatment of neurological complications associated with systemic phenol exposure is fundamentally supportive and symptomatic, as there is no specific antidote. Seizure episodes require immediate intervention with intravenous benzodiazepines—diazepam 5–10 mg slow IV or midazolam 0.1–0.2 mg/kg IV—together with ventilatory support and multiparametric monitoring. In addition to benzodiazepines, experimental studies have shown that phenobarbital can reverse phenol-induced motor symptoms and restore altered cerebral enzymatic activity, constituting an alternative in the management of refractory seizures. Central-origin vomiting should be managed with airway protection and administration of metoclopramide 10 mg slow IV, with dexamethasone 4–8 mg IV as an adjunctive measure. Anti-emetics such as ondansetron should be avoided due to the risk of QT interval prolongation and the potential to precipitate arrhythmias, especially in patients already vulnerable to phenol-induced cardiotoxicity.

In cases of coma or multiorgan failure, advanced life support measures become mandatory, including mechanical ventilation, serial neurological monitoring, and hemodynamic support. Severity assessment can be performed through clinical signs of cortical, subcortical, and brainstem dysfunction. Indicators of poor prognosis include: decreased level of consciousness progressing to stupor or coma; absence of brainstem reflexes such as pupillary and corneal, especially after 24 h; mid-position or dilated pupils with slow or absent reactivity; abnormal motor postures such as decerebration; absence of motor response to painful stimuli; contralateral Babinski reflex to hemiparesis; involuntary movements such as multifocal myoclonus or myoclonic status; severe respiratory disturbances, such as irregular rhythm or loss of chemical control of breathing; acute decline of ≥2 points on the Glasgow Coma Scale (GCS); and signs of dysautonomia, such as urinary retention, autonomic instability, and sphincter disturbances. The absence of motor and pupillary responses after 24 h of acute insult is highly predictive of an unfavorable prognosis.

Cases of peripheral nerve injury associated with phenol have also been documented. Inadvertent application to cranial nerves can cause focal deficits, such as facial paralysis, as reported in a case of facial nerve injury following tympanostomy in which 89% phenol was inadvertently instilled into the auditory canal. The patient developed tympanic necrosis, ossicular injury, and complete peripheral facial paralysis, with partial recovery after corticosteroid therapy, but required surgical reconstruction and had persistent conductive hearing loss. In such cases, management is conservative, including physiotherapy and motor rehabilitation, with reconstructive surgery indicated for persistent anatomical sequelae.

Classic reports underscore the severity of phenol neurotoxicity. Griffiths described an industrial accident in which a 23-year-old man died within minutes after extensive skin contact with liquid phenol. The worker was dismantling a filter without protective equipment when he was struck by a jet of the substance, affecting about 25% of his body surface area. Within minutes, he developed seizures, cardiorespiratory collapse, and died. Autopsy revealed extensive caustic lesions, cerebral congestion, laryngeal edema, hemorrhagic pulmonary congestion, renal edema, and a phenol concentration of 7 mg%. This case illustrates the lethal potential of massive cutaneous absorption of phenol. Abrahams reported the death of a newborn after indirect contact with phenol present on a nanny's hands. Even in small amounts, absorption was sufficient to trigger seizures, coma, and death within about 10 h, highlighting the vulnerability of neonatal skin.

Recent cases also illustrate the devastating potential of phenol neurotoxicity. Kissoon et al. reported a 53-year-old woman who underwent intercostal blocks with 3% phenol, resulting in extensive myelopathy from T1 to L1 due to epidural diffusion, leading to permanent paraparesis and neurogenic bladder. Kowalewski et al. described a 55-year-old man who received 7.5% aqueous phenol for intercostal neurolysis and developed irreversible paraplegia below T11, with cerebrospinal fluid confirming high phenol concentrations. Both cases highlight that even small volumes of phenol can cause extensive and disabling spinal cord injury when inadvertently in contact with the neuroaxis.

The literature further emphasizes that early skin decontamination with isopropyl alcohol or polyethylene glycol can reduce systemic absorption of phenol in cases of cutaneous exposure, minimizing the risk of neurological complications. The use of water for decontamination may increase systemic absorption and is therefore not recommended as the first choice.

Several patient groups are at increased risk of neurological complications associated with systemic phenol exposure. These include: children and infants, due to a higher body surface area-to-weight ratio, thin skin, and immature detoxification systems; the elderly, due to reduced hepatic and renal function and a higher prevalence of comorbidities; patients with pre-existing liver or kidney disease, who have reduced capacity for metabolism and excretion; individuals with pre-existing neurological disorders, who are at risk of clinical decompensation; immunocompromised patients; and those with pre-existing disabilities, especially neurological, who have reduced capacity for functional recovery.

In summary, neurological complications of phenol encompass a broad spectrum, from mild symptoms to irreversible manifestations. Management is based on intensive supportive measures, anticonvulsants such as benzodiazepines and, in some scenarios, phenobarbital, as well as motor rehabilitation for peripheral sequelae. Early decontamination in cases of cutaneous accident and intensive monitoring are essential to reduce the risk of severe progression. In the context of phenol-croton oil peeling, strict monitoring of consciousness level and readiness for immediate intervention are mandatory to ensure that the therapeutic benefits of the procedure are achieved safely (Table 10.10).

10.3.5 Renal and Hepatic Complications

The mechanism by which phenol induces renal injury is not fully understood, but includes direct damage to tubular epithelial cells by phenol-derived free radicals, impaired regeneration of reduced glutathione, excretion of unconjugated phenol with glomerular injury, renal ischemia, formation of intratubular casts due to hemoglobin precipitation, as well as pigment nephropathy secondary to rhabdomyolysis or intravascular hemolysis. These processes culminate in acute tubular necrosis (ATN), cortical and papillary necrosis, and may progress to severe acute kidney injury (AKI) requiring dialysis.

Several reports have documented renal complications following systemic exposure to phenol. Gupta et al. described the case of a 50-year-old man who was inadvertently injected with 10 mL of 89% phenol, corresponding to approximately 105 mg/kg. Within a few hours, he developed severe pain, dyspnea, profound hypoxemia (pO_2 38 mmHg), massive proteinuria, myoglobinuria, lactic acidosis, and a rise in creatinine to 8 mg/dL, consistent with ATN. He developed persistent oliguria and required daily hemodialysis for 12 days, followed by a polyuric phase exceeding 5 L/day. Renal function normalized after six months, although polyuria persisted for several weeks. The authors attributed the renal toxicity to the accumulation of reactive phenol metabolites, oxidative stress, and glutathione depletion in tubular cells.

Similarly, Parikh reported the case of a 35-year-old man who suffered an occupational burn with 94% phenol over 37% of his body surface area. He was admitted 90 min after exposure, already presenting with myoclonus, severe metabolic acidosis, and early signs of renal failure. Despite immediate decontamination with pressurized water and application of glycerol, he developed oliguria, hyperkalemia, and a creatinine of 7.9 mg/dL within the first 24 h, requiring multiple dialysis sessions. The clinical course was complicated by severe hypoalbuminemia, large pleural effusion, and ARDS, necessitating ventilatory support and intensive protein

Table 10.10 Monitoring and management of neurological complications associated with phenol

Clinical situation	Signs/manifestations	Recommended management
Post-peel observation	Mild psychomotor slowing Subtle mental confusion Mild (transient) drowsiness	Common and expected symptoms Continuous observation during the procedure and for 12–24 h afterward Record level of consciousness, speech, and motor response
Early warning signs	Altered speech Progressive decrease in the level of consciousness Psychomotor agitation Tremors or myoclonus Vomiting of central origin	Discontinue the peel immediately Initiate vigorous IV hydration Multiparametric monitoring Protect airway if vomiting occurs Consider intensive care support
Seizures	Generalized tonic-clonic or focal seizures	Diazepam 5–10 mg slow IV or Midazolam 0.1–0.2 mg/kg IV Ventilatory support and intensive monitoring Repeat dose if necessary Consider transfer to ICU
Vomiting of central origin	Persistent nausea and emesis, risk of aspiration	Ensure airway patency Metoclopramide 10 mg slow IV (first choice) Dexamethasone 4–8 mg IV (adjuvant/late prophylaxis) Avoid ondansetron (risk of QT prolongation)
Coma/multiorgan failure	Deep loss of consciousness Respiratory/circulatory depression	Advanced life support Mechanical ventilation, vasoactive drugs Immediate transfer to ICU Monitor renal function and consider hemodialysis
Patient under sedation	Risk of masking early warning signs	Observe objective parameters (ventilation, O_2 saturation, motor response) Heightened vigilance during the first 12–24 h Document subtle changes in consciousness

Monitoring and management of neurological complications associated with phenol. Mild symptoms, such as psychomotor slowing and transient confusion, may be expected after phenol-croton oil peeling, but warning signs such as altered speech, decreased level of consciousness, tremors, seizures, or vomiting of central origin indicate systemic toxicity and require immediate intervention. Treatment is essentially supportive, as there is no specific antidote, and should include intravenous anticonvulsants, airway protection, vigorous intravenous hydration, and intensive care support when necessary. Continuous monitoring is recommended during the procedure and for 12–24 h afterward, which is the critical period for systemic absorption. In sedated patients, vigilance should be increased, with attention to objective parameters that may indicate early neurological deterioration. Source: *Table prepared by the author (Dr Carolina Marçon)*

replacement. After 24 days of hospitalization, there was complete recovery of renal and pulmonary function. This case highlights that even non-fatal exposures (<40% of body surface area) can trigger multiorgan failure.

Another classic report was published by Foxall et al., who documented a 41-year-old worker exposed to a 40% phenol solution in dichloromethane, with skin contact over approximately 50% of his body surface area. The patient rapidly developed anuria, metabolic acidosis, and progressive creatinine elevation, requiring hemodialysis for three weeks. After clinical and laboratory recovery, he continued to experience persistent polyuria (up to 3 L/day) for over a year, suggesting residual renal injury. A distinguishing feature of this study was the pioneering use of urinary Proton Nuclear Magnetic Resonance—^{1}H-NMR, which enabled monitoring of lesion progression: initial aminoaciduria and glycosuria consistent with cortical necrosis, followed by markers of papillary necrosis (succinate, dimethylamine, and N,N-dimethylglycine). These findings demonstrated that, even after conventional laboratory normalization, metabolic alterations could persist, indicating incomplete renal recovery.

Regarding hepatic involvement, phenol can induce acute hepatotoxicity due to the formation of toxic metabolites during hepatic biotransformation, leading to oxidative stress, mitochondrial dysfunction, and hepatocellular necrosis. Clinical manifestations include elevated transaminases, jaundice, and, in severe cases, acute liver failure. Although hepatic complications are less frequently described in modern medical protocols, they may theoretically occur in extensive or poorly monitored procedures.

Hepatorenal toxicity from phenol is related to its metabolism and excretion, with the kidneys and liver being the main organs responsible for clearance. In severe cases, dysfunction of these systems may lead to multiple organ failure, which is a determinant of fatal outcome.

From a clinical perspective, the main early signs of renal involvement include oliguria (<0.5 mL/kg/h for more than 6 h), anuria, peripheral edema, nausea, vomiting, hypertension, and laboratory abnormalities (creatinine increase ≥ 0.3 mg/dL above baseline, proteinuria, or hematuria). In severe cases, fluid overload, dyspnea, and acute pulmonary edema may occur. Early recognition of these signs, together with strict monitoring of urine output and serial laboratory tests, is essential to prevent progression to dialysis-dependent AKI.

The management of renal and hepatic complications associated with phenol is based on supportive and preventive measures. Early intravenous hydration should be initiated in the initial phases, while there is a risk of systemic absorption, with the aim of diluting the toxin, increasing urinary flow, and promoting renal clearance. However, once oliguric or anuric acute kidney injury is established, excessive fluid administration should be avoided, as it does not restore diuresis and may precipitate fluid overload and acute pulmonary edema; in such cases, support should be shifted to early hemodialysis. Strict monitoring of electrolytes and hepatorenal function, adequate protein replacement, and, in selected situations, the use of antioxidants such as N-acetylcysteine are important complementary measures (Table 10.11). Phenol-croton oil peeling should be avoided in patients with pre-existing renal or hepatic disease, as phenol clearance is reduced, increasing the risk of systemic toxicity.

Therefore, acute renal failure and hepatotoxicity, although rare in safe medical protocols, represent potentially fatal complications when there is excessive systemic absorption. Careful patient selection, limitation of the treated area, and

Table 10.11 Management of renal complications associated with phenol toxicity

Clinical phase	Recommended management
Prevention (initial phase, risk of systemic absorption)	Early and vigorous intravenous hydration with crystalloids (e.g., 0.9% saline at 250–500 mL/h, adjusted according to body weight and hemodynamic status) Monitoring of urine output and electrolytes Early correction of fluid and electrolyte imbalances Use of antioxidants, such as N-acetylcysteine, in selected situations
Established acute renal failure (oliguria/anuria)	Avoid excessive hydration (risk of fluid overload and acute pulmonary edema) Maintenance fluids only for basal support Early initiation of hemodialysis Continuous monitoring of hepatorenal function and fluid balance Nutritional support with adequate protein replacement

Summary of management recommendations for renal complications associated with systemic phenol toxicity. In the initial phase, when there is a risk of systemic absorption, early intravenous hydration aims to increase renal clearance and reduce the risk of acute tubular necrosis. Once oliguric or anuric acute renal failure is established, excessive hydration should be avoided due to the risk of fluid overload, and early hemodialysis is indicated, together with intensive monitoring of renal and hepatic function. *Source: Table prepared by the author (Dr Carolina Marçon)*

intra- and post-procedure monitoring for at least 24 h are essential measures to ensure safety in the therapeutic use of phenol-croton oil peel.

10.3.6 Hematological and Metabolic Complications

Acute and intense systemic exposure to phenol can trigger a range of hematological and metabolic disturbances, resulting from its caustic and oxidative action and interference with cellular biochemical processes. Although less frequent than neurological, respiratory, and renal complications, these events can significantly worsen the clinical picture and contribute to multiorgan failure in severe intoxications.

Among the hematological complications, the most significant is acute intravascular hemolysis, resulting from the direct action of phenol on the erythrocyte membrane and oxidative stress generated by its metabolites. Massive red cell lysis can lead to acute anemia, hemoglobinuria, and pigment nephropathy, favoring the development of acute renal failure. Another reported event is methemoglobinemia, characterized by oxidation of the haem iron in hemoglobin ($Fe^{2+} \rightarrow Fe^{3+}$), which reduces oxygen-carrying capacity and may result in severe tissue hypoxia. Isolated cases have also reported disseminated intravascular coagulation (DIC), attributed to diffuse endothelial injury and release of tissue thromboplastin, as well as platelet abnormalities such as transient thrombocytopenia and functional impairment, which contribute to hemorrhagic risk in critical scenarios.

In metabolic terms, high anion gap metabolic acidosis is one of the most consistent findings in cases of systemic phenol intoxication. This disorder results from the accumulation of acidic metabolites, such as catechol, hydroquinone, p-benzoquinone, and lactate, associated with mitochondrial dysfunction and inhibition of energy metabolism enzymes. Fluid and electrolyte disturbances are also common: hyperkalemia may occur due to cell lysis and renal failure; hypokalemia and hypophosphatemia are more common during the recovery phase. Hypocalcemia, as described by Foxall et al., reflects both calcium deposition in damaged tissues and systemic metabolic imbalance. Rhabdomyolysis, secondary to seizures or direct toxic action on muscle fibers, contributes to myoglobin release and an additional risk of renal injury. There are also reports of hypoglycemia, probably related to increased glucose consumption during phenol metabolism and hepatic enzymatic inhibition of gluconeogenesis.

Management of these complications should be immediate and targeted. Hemolysis requires serial laboratory monitoring (full blood count, LDH, indirect bilirubin, haptoglobin) and transfusional support as needed. Symptomatic methemoglobinemia should be treated with intravenous methylene blue (1–2 mg/kg by slow infusion, repeated if necessary), which acts as an electron donor, restoring hemoglobin to its functional form. Severe metabolic acidosis (pH < 7.2) should be corrected with intravenous sodium bicarbonate, together with removal of the underlying cause and dialytic support when indicated. Electrolyte disturbances should be corrected individually, with particular attention to hyperkalemia, which may precipitate fatal arrhythmias. In cases of rhabdomyolysis, in addition to fluid and electrolyte replacement, early hemodialysis should be considered to prevent pigment nephropathy (Table 10.12).

In summary, the hematological and metabolic complications of phenol range from transient laboratory abnormalities to severe cases of hemolysis, methemoglobinemia, DIC, profound metabolic acidosis, and rhabdomyolysis. It is important to emphasize, however, that these complications are described in cases of massive systemic exposure and accidents involving high concentrations of the substance, and are extremely unlikely in the context of phenol-croton oil peeling performed under controlled medical conditions. Nevertheless, understanding these events and their pathophysiology is essential, both for the adoption of preventive measures and for the early recognition of signs of toxicity in exceptional situations.

10.3.7 Complications Related to Croton Oil

Although the systemic toxicity of phenol is better documented, the risks associated with croton oil (*Croton tiglium*), which is rich in bioactive phorbol esters, should not be overlooked. Experimentally, these compounds are potent activators of protein kinase C (PKC), triggering inflammatory cascades and significant cytotoxic effects. There are historical records and clinical reports of poisoning following ingestion, presenting with nausea, vomiting, abdominal pain, profuse diarrhea, severe dehydration and, in some cases, hemorrhagic gastroenteritis and death after the ingestion of only a few drops of the oil—an indication of its narrow safety margin for systemic use. In animal models, studies with isolated proteins from *Croton tiglium* demonstrate induction of gastrointestinal inflammation and renal injury associated with activation of pro-inflammatory pathways (e.g., p38-MAPK),

Table 10.12 Hematological and metabolic complications associated with phenol toxicity

Complication	Clinical manifestations	Recommended management
Intravascular hemolysis	Acute anemia Hemoglobinuria Jaundice Risk of pigment nephropathy	Serial monitoring (full blood count, LDH, bilirubin, haptoglobin) Transfusion support when necessary Prevention of renal failure with hydration/dialysis
Methemoglobinemia	Cyanosis Hypoxia refractory to oxygen therapy Altered level of consciousness	Methylene blue 1–2 mg/kg slow IV (may repeat) Oxygen therapy Ventilatory support if severe
High anion gap metabolic acidosis	Lactic acidosis Depressed level of consciousness Hemodynamic instability	Correction with intravenous sodium bicarbonate if pH < 7.2 Hemodialysis if refractory Intensive support
Fluid and electrolyte disturbances	Hyperkalemia (arrhythmias, muscle weakness) Hypokalemia/ hypophosphatemia during recovery Hypocalcemia (tetany, arrhythmias)	Individualized correction of electrolytes Continuous cardiac monitoring Immediate treatment of severe hyperkalemia
Rhabdomyolysis	Myalgia Weakness Myoglobinuria Acute renal failure	Early intravenous hydration (initial phase) Fluid and electrolyte correction Early hemodialysis if necessary
Hypoglycemia	Sweating Confusion Seizures Coma in severe cases	Immediate intravenous glucose administration Serial blood glucose monitoring

Summary of the main hematological and metabolic complications associated with systemic phenol toxicity. It should be emphasized that such complications are described in cases of massive systemic exposure and are unlikely to occur in the context of phenol-croton oil peel performed in a controlled medical environment. However, knowledge of these complications is essential for the adoption of safe protocols and early recognition of signs of toxicity. *Source: Table prepared by the author (Dr Carolina Marçon)*

reinforcing the toxic potential when systemic exposure occurs. Conversely, recent cutaneous evidence points to a predominantly local action profile. Justo et al. showed that isolated *Croton tiglium* oil, when applied topically in animal models, induces epidermal thickening, acanthosis and persistent inflammation, suggesting that part of the histological effects of phenol-croton oil peeling is directly attributable to the croton component; however, this study was limited to cutaneous assessment and did not investigate possible systemic repercussions in internal organs. Justo et al. observed that topical application induces a marked dermal inflammatory response, with increased fibroblast density and, at higher concentrations, focal necrosis of the deep reticular dermis; in addition, they examined the lungs, liver, kidneys and heart of treated animals, without finding histological changes in these organs, suggesting an absence of measurable systemic toxicity under the experimental conditions tested.

From a historical and ethnopharmacological perspective, *Croton tiglium* is native to tropical Asia and, for millennia, has been part of traditional Chinese medicine (as ba dou, 巴豆) and Ayurveda (as jamal gota/kuchila taila), mainly as a drastic purgative. These traditions have always recommended prior purification of the seeds (shodhana) to mitigate toxicity, foreshadowing the risks associated with the raw material. In the West, between the seventeenth and nineteenth centuries, oil was described as a violent purgative—being referred to as "hell oil"—and, although incorporated in a limited way into allopathic prescriptions for severe constipation, it was historically accompanied by strict warnings regarding dose and route of administration. This trajectory consolidated the duality of *Croton tiglium*: pharmacological potency with a high toxicological risk when used outside strict controls.

In the modern dermatological context, croton oil has assumed a central role in deep peeling formulations in combination with phenol. In carefully calibrated concentrations (as in Hetter's standardized formulations), its phorbol esters produce a controlled inflammatory stimulus, dermal remodeling, increased collagen synthesis and matrix restructuring, findings reproduced in histological analyses. However, such benefits are realized within narrow safety margins: excessive concentrations, non-standardized formulations, extensive applications or compromised skin barrier (e.g., due to dermabrasion or microneedling) may theoretically increase absorption and heighten the risk of adverse reactions. In humans, the toxic spectrum via the oral route includes severe (sometimes hemorrhagic) gastroenteritis and dehydration with potential progression to collapse; via the cutaneous route, consistently documented complications mainly concern chemical dermatitis, burns and local necrosis in cases of misuse. Systemic symptoms via the cutaneous route are not robustly characterized in the modern clinical literature and, when mentioned, are extrapolated from occupational or experimental exposures, not from controlled studies in aesthetic dermatology.

Crucially, to date there are no studies specifically evaluating the systemic toxicity of croton oil when used in combination with phenol in the context of chemical peels. This gap precludes the precise definition of systemic risks and safe doses of the croton component in this combined application. In light of current knowledge—that is, a potent, local and dose-dependent cutaneous effect in animal models and a history of systemic toxicity by ingestion—clinical practice should remain anchored in qualified raw materials, standardized formulations, exclusive medical execution, monitoring and a controlled environment, with rejection of crude extracts, products of dubious origin or uncontrolled compounding. In parallel, future studies are needed to elucidate cutaneous pharmacokinetics, safety thresholds and the potential systemic contribution of croton when combined with phenol, providing a more robust basis for practice recommendations and regulatory policies.

In summary, croton oil remains a biologically potent agent whose safe use depends on rigorous standardization and medical expertise. In trained hands and under established protocols, it can be used with good efficacy rates; outside this context, compositional variability, the potency of phorbol esters and lack of monitoring constitute a significant public health risk.

10.3.8 Considerations Regarding the Risk of Death

Although rare, death is a possible complication in the context of phenol-croton oil peeling, generally associated with refractory arrhythmias, cardiorespiratory arrest, or acute pulmonary edema secondary to the systemic and myocardial toxicity of phenol. Since the empirical era of *lay peelers*, there have been anecdotal reports of sudden deaths linked to extensive and rapid applications over large body surfaces, without prior assessment, monitoring, or life support—a pattern which, although historically described in a non-systematic manner, already indicated the potentially lethal nature of the procedure when performed outside safe medical standards.

In the scientific literature and official documents, there are few formal but consistent reports that reinforce this risk. In 1998, in New Zealand, the case of a patient who underwent facial peeling with Exoderm (a phenol-based formulation) was described; the procedure was performed by a doctor practicing "appearance medicine" in a marketing-driven context and without the minimum safety infrastructure. There was no continuous monitoring (no functional oximeter), and oxygen, airway equipment, and resuscitation devices were lacking. Sedation was administered without another physician responsible for monitoring, in breach of the then-current guidelines (ANZCA). Approximately 30 min after the procedure began, the patient developed gasping, had cardiorespiratory collapse, and, despite late rhythm reversal during transport, suffered irreversible neurological damage, dying three weeks later in the hospital. The decision of the Medical Disciplinary Tribunal highlighted multiple failures in pre-procedure assessment, inadequate sedation management, and the absence of monitoring and support, characterizing a serious deviation from professional standards.

In 1999, the regulatory agency Medsafe published a warning in the Prescriber Update reporting a death associated with Exoderm Lift and emphasizing the potential toxicity of phenol, including via topical application, with significant systemic absorption. The agency noted that such formulations had not undergone safety or efficacy evaluation in the country and had no ministerial authorization, advising against their use and stressing the duty to fully inform patients and to report serious adverse events.

In addition to fatalities, there are cases of severe systemic intoxication with imminent risk of death. In 2004, intoxication was reported in an 11-year-old boy with xeroderma pigmentosum, who underwent dermabrasion followed by phenol peeling on multiple areas ($\approx$15% of body surface area), developing multifocal ventricular arrhythmias with a rate of up to 220 bpm at the end of the procedure. There was an increase in urinary phenol (58.9 mg/dl; reference $\leq$20.7 mg/dl) and a need for intravenous lidocaine, forced diuresis (furosemide and mannitol), vigorous fluid therapy, and intensive monitoring for 5 days until resolution. The report discusses the extremely rapid absorption of phenol through the skin (with up to 70% absorbed in about 30 min) and the typical occurrence of arrhythmias within the first 20 min when large areas are treated in a short interval. It is emphasized that prior dermabrasion likely facilitated accelerated systemic penetration of phenol, acting as an additional risk factor. These findings support recommendations for fractionated application, adherence to safety intervals between areas, and performing the procedure only with continuous cardiac monitoring and immediate availability of cardiopulmonary resuscitation (CPR).

More recently, in 2025, the *Journal of the American Academy of Dermatology* published the case of a 27-year-old man who died following facial phenol peeling performed by a non-medical individual promoting themselves on social media. The procedure included prior microneedling, followed by application of an unidentified phenol-containing formula. Minutes later, the patient developed tremors, profuse sweating, loss of consciousness, and cardiorespiratory arrest, with no trained team or basic support equipment on site. Post-mortem examination revealed deep chemical burns on the face and acute pulmonary edema with diffuse alveolar hemorrhage as the direct cause of death; toxicology (Headspace Gas Chromatography–Mass Spectrometry HS-GC/MS) identified phenol as the sole agent. Prior microneedling was identified as a factor that enhanced systemic absorption. The article further endorses safety protocols advocated by the International Peeling Society (IPS): physician-dependence, standardized formulas (Hetter/Baker-Gordon), adequate room ventilation, safety pauses ($\geq$10 min per cosmetic unit), and, when the treated area exceeds ~1.5% of body surface area (half the face), mandatory multiparametric monitoring and intravenous crystalloid infusion.

In summary, the available official documents and clinical reports—from anecdotal records of the lay peelers' era to formal cases in both medical and non-medical settings—converge on the same conclusion: lethality does not arise from the procedure per se, but from incompetence, recklessness, and negligence in its execution. The common pattern includes rapid and/or extensive application, inadequate technique, lack of prior assessment, absence of monitoring, and lack of advanced life support—as well as non-standardized formulations and interventions that increase permeation (e.g., dermabrasion/microneedling), which accelerate absorption and raise the risk of cardiac and pulmonary toxicity.

In light of this, emphasizing the risk of death is essential to contextualize the seriousness of phenol-croton oil peeling and to reinforce that it should be performed exclusively by trained physicians, in appropriate settings, with strict protocols, continuous monitoring, and advanced life support readily available.

10.3.9 Risk Factors and Preventive Measures

The occurrence of systemic complications is strongly related to risk factors that, to a large extent, can be prevented. Among these, the most significant are the application over large areas in a single session, performing the peel without adequate intervals between treated regions, the use of non-standardized formulations or excessive concentrations, as well as procedures carried out by professionals without specific training. Patients with cardiovascular, renal, or hepatic comorbidities are at increased risk, as are those with reduced functional reserve due to advanced age or poor nutritional status.

Prevention requires strict patient selection, with thorough clinical assessment and laboratory tests, including renal, hepatic, and cardiac profiles. The use of recognized formulations, such as those proposed by Hetter, combined with fractionated application in cosmetic units with intervals of 15–20 min, significantly reduces the systemic absorption of phenol. Continuous monitoring throughout the procedure, including electrocardiogram, pulse oximetry, and blood pressure control, is essential, as is the immediate availability of advanced life support resources, including a defibrillator, oxygen, emergency medications, and a trained team.

Additional precautions must be taken regarding the storage, handling, and disposal of phenol. The substance should be kept in restricted areas, in secure and clearly labeled containers, away from routinely used medications to prevent administration errors. Preparation should be carried out under controlled conditions, ensuring the quality and provenance of the ingredients used. It is also essential that the application environment is adequately ventilated, reducing occupational exposure to potentially toxic vapors, and that all staff are trained and equipped with appropriate protective measures to prevent accidents.

Furthermore, errors inherent to the handling of the formulation can exacerbate complications. Partial evaporation of the aqueous base, for example, may inadvertently concentrate the solution, increasing its toxicity. Ideally, solutions should be freshly prepared for each procedure, as they are not miscible and present a risk of instability.

10.4 Ethical and Legal Considerations

The management of complications arising from phenol-croton oil peel requires technical expertise, a safe environment, and the availability of advanced life support. In light of all that has been discussed in this book, it is clear that both the procedure itself and the handling of formulations must be performed exclusively by qualified medical professionals. The application of phenol by non-medical personnel constitutes the illegal practice of medicine and should be regarded as a serious offense, subject to penalties commensurate with the risk posed to the public.

The path to safety is not the prohibition of the procedure—which would deprive doctors and patients of a technique capable of delivering transformative results in appearance, health, self-esteem, and quality of life—but rather strict regulation and oversight. It is urgent that the marketing, distribution, and application of these formulations be controlled by the competent authorities in each country, ensuring the quality, provenance, and traceability of the products, as well as protecting society from unqualified and dangerous practices. The need for safety protocols, team training, and absolute respect for the toxic potential of the substance is therefore emphasized.

Thus, ensuring that phenol-croton oil peel remains a medical act, governed by clear regulations and effective oversight, is the only way for it to continue as a procedure of significant aesthetic and human impact, performed with safety, responsibility, and ethics.

Another essential aspect is the doctor–patient relationship. In deep peeling procedures, this relationship must be strong and based on mutual trust, supporting even the most delicate phases of the postoperative period. Pre-procedure counseling should align expectations, clarify risks, and prepare the patient for the recovery period, which may cause anxiety due to the temporary appearance. Often, family members, friends, or professionals unfamiliar with the technique may misinterpret post-peel clinical findings and induce insecurity in the patient. It is the doctor's responsibility to reinforce their availability for close and continuous follow-up, providing reassurance and confidence at every stage of the process.

10.5 Future Perspectives and Conclusion

The future of phenol-croton oil peel is closely linked to the consolidation of safety protocols, advances in research, and the standardization of its use.

Current challenges include the trivialization of the technique by non-medical professionals, the lack of clear regulation in some countries, and the spread of formulations of dubious origin, which expose patients to unnecessary risks.

Future research directions should focus on elucidating the cutaneous pharmacokinetics of phenol and croton oil, studying early toxicity biomarkers, characterizing safe dosages, and, above all, assessing the systemic risk of croton oil in combination with phenol—a field not yet explored in the scientific literature and representing a fundamental knowledge gap.

From a regulatory perspective, it is imperative to establish official standards restricting the use of phenol and croton oil to qualified medical settings, setting minimum requirements for monitoring, infrastructure, and substance preparation. Only with clear regulation and universal protocols will it be possible to ensure safety and efficacy, reducing the current variability in practice.

Ethical considerations remain central. Phenol-croton oil peel must be conducted with full awareness of its therapeutic potency and associated risks. The physician's responsibility involves not only technical execution but also the duty to inform, transparency with the patient, and a commitment to prioritizing safety.

10.6 Final Considerations

The success of phenol-croton oil peeling is not limited to the aesthetic outcome, but above all depends on its safe execution, technical preparation, and the ability to manage complications. A thorough understanding of the risks, the adoption of preventive measures, and prompt intervention in the face of complications are the pillars that ensure not only therapeutic efficacy but also the patient's safety and trust.

Given the potential for systemic toxicity of phenol and croton oil, it is essential that their use remains restricted to controlled environments, with continuous monitoring and by trained physicians. The literature shows that serious complications are rare when appropriate protocols are followed, but the margin between benefit and toxicity is narrow. For this reason, utmost caution, rigorous preparation, and adherence to medical standards are recommended.

Systemic complications of phenol-croton oil peeling, although rare, are severe and have been historically documented. Recognizing this risk does not mean abandoning the practice, but rather assuming the responsibility to perform it with excellence, in accordance with the highest technical and ethical standards. The safety of the procedure lies not in denying its risks, but in the commitment to prevent and manage them appropriately.

Final Message

We hope that this book will help dermatologists to enhance their practice, delivering excellent results with ethics, responsibility, and care. May it serve as a guide for practice grounded in science, caution, and respect for patient integrity, reinforcing the importance of safe protocols and qualified medical training.

Our wish is that this work not only complements existing knowledge but also represents a milestone in the history of phenol in medicine, helping to consolidate its use in a modern, regulated, and responsible manner. May it inspire new generations of specialists to practice dermatology with technical excellence, ethical commitment, and profound respect for the human being.

The authors

Sources

1. Yoon ES, Ahn DS. Report of phenol peel for Asians. Plast Reconstr Surg. 1999;103(1):207–14. discussion 215-217
2. Garman ME, Orengo I. Unusual infectious complications of dermatologic procedures. Dermatol Clin. 2003;21(2):321–35.
3. Deichmann WB. Local and systemic effects following skin contact with phenol; a review of the literature. J Ind Hyg Toxicol. 1949;31:146–54.
4. Rullan P, Lin EM, Schaut E, Wambier CG. Cardiac safety in full-face phenol-croton oil peels: A 22-year retrospective study. J Am Acad Dermatol. 2024;91(4):762–3.
5. Deichmann WB, Miller T, Roberts JB. Local and systemic effects following application of dilute solutions of phenol in water and in camphor-liquid petrolatum on the skin of animals. AMA Arch Ind Hyg Occup Med. 1950;2:454–61.
6. Perkins SW, Sklarew EC. Prevention of facial herpetic infections after chemical peel and dermabrasion: new treatment strategies in the prophylaxis of patients undergoing procedures of the perioral area. Plast Reconstr Surg. 1996;98(3):427–33. discussion 434-435
7. Vemula S, Maymone MBC, Secemsky EA, Widjajahakim R, Patzelt NM, Saade D, Vashi NA. Assessing the safety of superficial chemical peels in darker skin: a retrospective study. J Am Acad Dermatol. 2018;79(3):508–513.e2.
8. McDermott J, Kao LS, Keeley JA, Grigorian A, Neville A, de Virgilio C. Necrotizing soft tissue infections: a review. JAMA Surg. 2024;159(11):1308–15.

9. Evans L, Rhodes A, Alhazzani W, Antonelli M, Coopersmith CM, French C, Machado FR, Mcintyre L, Ostermann M, Prescott HC, Schorr C, Simpson S, Wiersinga WJ, Alshamsi F, Angus DC, Arabi Y, Azevedo L, Beale R, Beilman G, Belley-Cote E, Burry L, Cecconi M, Centofanti J, Coz Yataco A, De Waele J, Dellinger RP, Doi K, Du B, Estenssoro E, Ferrer R, Gomersall C, Hodgson C, Møller MH, Iwashyna T, Jacob S, Kleinpell R, Klompas M, Koh Y, Kumar A, Kwizera A, Lobo S, Masur H, McGloughlin S, Mehta S, Mehta Y, Mer M, Nunnally M, Oczkowski S, Osborn T, Papathanassoglou E, Perner A, Puskarich M, Roberts J, Schweickert W, Seckel M, Sevransky J, Sprung CL, Welte T, Zimmerman J, Levy M. Surviving sepsis campaign: international guidelines for management of sepsis and septic shock 2021. Intensive Care Med. 2021;47(11):1181–247.
10. Lynch TJ. Choosing optimal antimicrobial therapies. Med Clin North Am. 2012;96(6):1079–94.
11. Nanni CA, Alster TS. Complications of carbon dioxide laser resurfacing. An evaluation of 500 patients. Dermatol Surg. 1998;24(3):315–20.
12. Smack DP, Harrington AC, Dunn C, Howard RS, Szkutnik AJ, Krivda SJ, Caldwell JB, James WD. Infection and allergy incidence in ambulatory surgery patients using white petrolatum vs bacitracin ointment. A randomized controlled trial. JAMA. 1996;276(12):972–7.
13. Christian MM, Behroozan DS, Moy RL. Delayed infections following full-face CO2 laser resurfacing and occlusive dressing use. Dermatol Surg. 2000;26(1):32–6.
14. Gilbert S, McBurney E. Use of valaciclovir for herpes simplex virus-1 (HSV-1) prophylaxis after facial resurfacing: A randomized clinical trial of dosing regimens. Dermatol Surg. 2000;26(1):50–4.
15. Draelos ZD, Rizer RL, Trookman NS. A comparison of postprocedural wound care treatments: do antibiotic-based ointments improve outcomes? J Am Acad Dermatol. 2011;64(3 Suppl):S23–9.
16. Stevens DL, Bisno AL, Chambers HF, Dellinger EP, Goldstein EJ, Gorbach SL, Hirschmann JV, Kaplan SL, Montoya JG, Wade JC, Infectious Diseases Society of America. Practice guidelines for the diagnosis and management of skin and soft tissue infections: 2014 update by the Infectious Diseases Society of America. Clin Infect Dis. 2014;59(2):e10-52. Erratum in: Clin Infect Dis. 2015;60(9):1448
17. Daum RS, Miller LG, Immergluck L, Fritz S, Creech CB, Young D, Kumar N, Downing M, Pettibone S, Hoagland R, Eells SJ, Boyle MG, Parker TC, Chambers HF, DMID 07-0051 Team. A placebo-controlled trial of antibiotics for smaller skin abscesses. N Engl J Med. 2017;376(26):2545–55.
18. Bassetti M, Magnasco L, Del Puente F, Giacobbe DR. Role of new antibiotics in the treatment of acute bacterial skin and skin-structure infections. Curr Opin Infect Dis. 2020;33(2):110–20.
19. Wang W, Chen W, Liu Y, Siemieniuk RAC, Li L, Martínez JPD, Guyatt GH, Sun X. Antibiotics for uncomplicated skin abscesses: systematic review and network meta-analysis. BMJ Open. 2018;8(2):e020991.
20. Brody HJ. Complications of chemical resurfacing. Dermatol Clin. 2001;19(3):427–38.
21. Brody HJ. Complications of chemical peeling. J Dermatol Surg Oncol. 1989;15(9):1010–9.
22. LoVerme WE, Drapkin MS, Courtiss EH, Wilson RM. Toxic shock syndrome after chemical face peel. Plast Reconstr Surg. 1987;80(1):115–8.
23. Dmytryshyn JR, Gribble MJ, Kassen BO. Chemical face peel complicated by toxic shock syndrome. A case report. Arch Otolaryngol. 1983;109(3):170–1.
24. Katz TM, Glaich AS, Goldberg LH, Friedman PM. 595-nm long pulsed dye laser and 1450-nm diode laser in combination with intralesional triamcinolone/5-fluorouracil for hypertrophic scarring following a phenol peel. J Am Acad Dermatol. 2010;62(6):1045–9.
25. Basson R, Bayat A. Skin scarring: latest update on objective assessment and optimal management. Front Med (Lausanne). 2022;9:942756.
26. Carrière ME, Mokkink LB, Tyack Z, Westerman MJ, Pijpe A, Pleat J, van de Kar AL, Brown J, de Vet HCW, van Zuijlen PPM. Development of the Patient Scale of the Patient and Observer Scar Assessment Scale (POSAS) 3.0: a qualitative study. Qual Life Res. 2023;32(2):583–92.

27. Stratis C, Haider SA, Oleru O, Seyidova N, Sbitany H, Henderson PW. Paper tape may improve scar aesthetics and prevent wound closure complications. Plast Aesthet Nurs (Phila). 2024;44(1):59–69.
28. Salameh F, Shumaker PR, Goodman GJ, Spring LK, Seago M, Alam M, Al-Niaimi F, Cassuto D, Chan HH, Dierickx C, Donelan M, Gauglitz GG, Haedersdal M, Krakowski AC, Manuskiatti W, Norbury WB, Ogawa R, Ozog DM, Paasch U, Victor Ross E, Clementoni MT, Waibel J, Bayat A, Goo BL, Artzi O. Energy-based devices for the treatment of Acne Scars: 2022 International consensus recommendations. Lasers Surg Med. 2022;54(1):10–26.
29. Walsh LA, Wu E, Pontes D, Kwan KR, Poondru S, Miller CH, Kundu RV. Keloid treatments: an evidence-based systematic review of recent advances. Syst Rev. 2023;12(1):42.
30. Ogawa R. The most current algorithms for the treatment and prevention of hypertrophic scars and keloids: a 2020 update of the algorithms published 10 years ago. Plast Reconstr Surg. 2022;149(1):79e–94e.
31. Bronte J, Zhou C, Vempati A, Tam C, Khong J, Hazany S, Hazany S. A comprehensive review of non-surgical treatments for hypertrophic and keloid scars in skin of colour. Clin Cosmet Investig Dermatol. 2024;17:1459–69.
32. Yang S, Luo YJ, Luo C. Network meta-analysis of different clinical commonly used drugs for the treatment of hypertrophic scar and keloid. Front Med (Lausanne). 2021;8:691628.
33. Grigoryan KV, Fusco I, Ronconi L, Zingoni T. Fractional CO_2 laser therapy for effective treatment of facial traumatic hypertrophic scar: a case report. Am J Case Rep. 2024;25:e942706.
34. Clementi A, Cannarozzo G, Guarino L, Zappia E, Cassalia F, Alma A, Sannino M, Longo C, Nisticò SP. Sequential fractional CO_2 and 1540/1570 nm lasers: a narrative review of preclinical and clinical evidence. J Clin Med. 2025;14(11):3867.
35. Haji Mohammadi A, Seirafianpour F, Khosravi M, Jafarzadeh A, Neshastesaz Kashi H, Baradaran H, Goodarzi A. A systematic review of comparative clinical trials on the efficacy, safety, and patient satisfaction of ablative and non-ablative laser therapies for atrophic, hypertrophic, and keloid scars. Lasers Med Sci. 2025;40(1):280.
36. Hetter GP. An examination of the phenol-croton oil peel: part IV. Face peel results with different concentrations of phenol and croton oil. Plast Reconstr Surg. 2000;105(3):1061–83. discussion 1084-1087
37. Lotter AM. Human pigment factors relative to chemical face peeling. Ann Plast Surg. 1979;3(3):231–40.
38. Langsdon PR, Milburn M, Yarber R. Comparison of laser and phenol chemical peel in facial skin resurfacing. Arch Otolaryngol Head Neck Surg. 2000;126(10):1195–9.
39. Park JH, Choi YD, Kim SW, Kim YC, Park SW. Effectiveness of modified phenol peel (Exoderm) on facial wrinkles, acne scars and other skin problems in Asian patients. J Dermatol. 2007;34(1):17–24.
40. Lee JH, Kwon HS, Jung HM, Lee H, Kim GM, Yim HW, Bae JM. Treatment outcomes of topical calcineurin inhibitor therapy for patients with vitiligo: a systematic review and meta-analysis. JAMA Dermatol. 2019;155(8):929–38.
41. Jha AK, Prasad S, Sinha R. Bimatoprost ophthalmic solution in facial vitiligo. J Cosmet Dermatol. 2018;17(3):437–40.
42. Marçon CR. Phenol in dermatology: updated evidence on efficacy and safety. An Bras Dermatol. 2025;100(5):501200.
43. Mina M, Elgarhy L, Al-Saeid H, Ibrahim Z. Comparison between the efficacy of microneedling combined with 5-fluorouracil vs microneedling with tacrolimus in the treatment of vitiligo. J Cosmet Dermatol. 2018;17(5):744–51.
44. Hofer A, Hassan AS, Legat FJ, Kerl H, Wolf P. Optimal weekly frequency of 308-nm excimer laser treatment in vitiligo patients. Br J Dermatol. 2005;152(5):981–5.
45. Bae JM, Choo JY, Chang HS, Kim H, Lee JH, Kim GM. Effectiveness of the 308-nm excimer laser on hypopigmentation after lichen striatus: a retrospective study of 12 patients. J Am Acad Dermatol. 2016;75(3):637–9.

46. Passeron T, Ostovari N, Zakaria W, Fontas E, Larrouy JC, Lacour JP, Ortonne JP. Topical tacrolimus and the 308-nm excimer laser: a synergistic combination for the treatment of vitiligo. Arch Dermatol. 2004;140(9):1065–9.
47. Nikalji N, Godse K, Sakhiya J, Patil S, Nadkarni N. Complications of medium depth and deep chemical peels. J Cutan Aesthet Surg. 2012;5(4):254–60.
48. Castagna RD, Stramari JM, Chemello RML. The recurrent nevus phenomenon. An Bras Dermatol. 2017;92(4):531–3.
49. Grunwald MH, Gat A, Amichai B. Pseudomelanoma after Solcoderm treatment. Melanoma Res. 2006;16(5):459–60.
50. Mervak JE, Gan SD, Smith EH, Wang F. Facial erosive pustular dermatosis after cosmetic resurfacing. JAMA Dermatol. 2017;153(10):1021–5.
51. Ibrahim O, Arndt KA, Dover JS. Pathophysiology and treatment considerations for erosive pustular dermatosis. JAMA Dermatol. 2017;153(10):971–2.
52. Van Exel CE, English JC 3rd. Erosive pustular dermatosis of the scalp and nonscalp. J Am Acad Dermatol. 2007;57(2 Suppl):S11–4.
53. Landau M, Tosti A, Kroumpouzos G, Eims E, Goldust M. Frontal fibrosing alopecia-A new absolute contraindication for deep chemical peels. Clin Dermatol. 2024;42(6):696–700.
54. Gonser P, Kaestner S, Jaminet P, Kaye K. Histological case-control study of peeling-induced skin changes by different peeling agents in surgically subcutaneous undermined skin flaps in facelift patients. J Plast Reconstr Aesthet Surg. 2017;70(11):1660–5.
55. Hopley G, Shaharan S, Bailey C, Markeson D, Jones I. Erosive Pustular Dermatosis: an important differential diagnosis for the non-healing burn wound. J Plast Reconstr Aesthet Surg. 2025;104:14–7.
56. Stone PA, Lefer LG. Modified phenol chemical face peels: recognizing the role of application technique. Clin Plast Surg. 2001;28(1):13–36. Erratum in: Clin Plast Surg 2001;28(3):preceding xi
57. Justo AS, Lemes BM, Nunes B, Antunes KA, Capote ACMO, Lipinski LC, Campagnoli EB, Emiliano J, Meurer EC, Ezemma O, Miot HA, Beltrame FL, Wambier CG. Characterization of the activity of *Croton tiglium* Oil in Hetter's very heavy phenol-croton oil chemical peels. Dermatol Surg. 2021;47(7):944–6.
58. de Oliveira CN, Bisson GB, Ferreira JO. Adverse effects associated with the irresponsible use of phenol peeling: literature review. Oral Surg Oral Med Oral Pathol Oral Radiol. 2025;139(2):161–5.
59. Sun C, Lim D, Bekhor P. Extensive facial scarring after ablative laser resurfacing in a patient with frontal fibrosing alopecia. JAAD Case Rep. 2022;23:123–7.
60. Pozo J, Castiñeiras I, Fernández-Jorge B. Variants of milia successfully treated with CO(2) laser vaporization. J Cosmet Laser Ther. 2010;12(4):191–4.
61. Stegman SJ. A comparative histological study of the effects of three peeling agents and dermabrasion on normal and sun-damaged skin. Aesthetic Plast Surg. 1982;6(3):123–35.
62. Kligman AM, Baker TJ, Gordon HL. Long-term histological follow-up of phenol face peels. Plast Reconstr Surg. 1985;75(5):652–9.
63. Giese SY, McKinney P, Roth SI, Zukowski M. The effect of chemosurgical peels and dermabrasion on dermal elastic tissue. Plast Reconstr Surg. 1997;100(2):489-98; discussion 499-500.
64. Spring LK, Krakowski AC, Alam M, et al. Isotretinoin and timing of procedural interventions: a systematic review with consensus recommendations. JAMA Dermatol. 2017;153(8):802–9.
65. Singh S, Chauhan A. Comparative analysis of efficacy of lactic acid 30% with ferulic peel 12% (Combination Peel) versus TCA 10% with ferulic peel 12% (Combination Peel) for photoaged skin. Aesthetic Plast Surg. 2024;48(19):4007–13.
66. Roberts WE, Miller N. Optimised patient outcomes with the novel modality of corrective chemical peel and neurotoxin on same-day treatment. J Drugs Dermatol. 2024;23(1):1349–54.
67. Ocampo-Candiani J, Saint Aroman M, Carballido F, Darde MS, Vázquez Martínez O, Garza-Rodríguez V, Chavez-Alvarez S, Aardewijn T. Efficacy of a repair cream based on Rhealba

Oat plantlet extract and active healing compounds in peelings: benefit to patient's downtime and pain. J Eur Acad Dermatol Venereol. 2019;33(Suppl 5):3–12.
68. Bruce S, Roberts W, Teller C, Colvan L. The effects of a daily skincare regimen on maintaining the benefits obtained from previous chemical resurfacing treatments. J Drugs Dermatol. 2016;15(9):1145–50.
69. Weinstein C, Ramirez OM, Pozner JN. Postoperative care following CO2 laser resurfacing: avoiding pitfalls. Plast Reconstr Surg. 1997;100(7):1855–66.
70. Gatti JE. Eyelid phenol peel: an important adjunct to blepharoplasty. Ann Plast Surg. 2008;60(1):14–8. discussion 19-20
71. Soon SL, Wambier CG, Rullan PR, Sterling JB, Brody HJ, Lee KC, Kreyden OP, Landau M, International Peeling Society. Phenol-croton oil chemical peeling induces durable improvement of constitutional periorbital dark circles. Dermatol Surg. 2023;49(4):368–73.
72. Poon SHL, Wong WHL, Bu Y, Lo ACY, Jhanji V, Chan YK, Shih KC. A systematic review of emerging therapeutic strategies in the management of chemical injuries of the ocular surface. Eye Contact Lens. 2020;46(6):329–40.
73. Dang DH, Riaz KM, Karamichos D. Treatment of non-infectious corneal injury: review of diagnostic agents, therapeutic medications, and future targets. Drugs. 2022;82(2):145–67.
74. Hewett Brumberg EK, Douma MJ, Alibertis K, Charlton NP, Goldman MP, Harper-Kirksey K, Hawkins SC, Hoover AV, Kule A, Leichtle S, McClure SF, Wang GS, Whelchel M, White L, Lavonas EJ, American Heart Association and American Red Cross. 2024 American Heart Association and American Red Cross Guidelines for First Aid. Circulation. 2024;150(24):e519–79.
75. Ozturk MB, Ozkaya O, Karahangil M, Cekic O, Oreroğlu AR, Akan IM. Ocular complication after trichloroacetic acid peeling: a case report. Aesthetic Plast Surg. 2013;37(1):56–9.
76. Skruodyte J, Olechnovic J, Serpytis P. Changes in retinal nerve fibre and ganglion cell layers after chemical injury: a prospective study. J Clin Med. 2025;14(15):5601.
77. Choi SH, Kim MK, Oh JY. Glaucoma after ocular chemical burns: incidence, risk factors, and outcome. Sci Rep. 2020;10(1):4763.
78. Villena C, Vivas JM, Villar AM. Ocular inflammation models by topical application: croton-oil induced uveitis. Curr Eye Res. 1999;18(1):3–9.
79. Lucas RC, Lane WA. Two cases of carbolic acid coma induced by the application of carbolic compresses to the skin. Lancet. 1895;145:1362–4.
80. Turtle WRM, Dolan T. A case of rapid and fatal absorption of carbolic acid through the skin. Lancet. 1922;200:1273–4.
81. Miller FG. Poisoning by Phenol. Can Med Assoc J. 1942;46:615–6.
82. Giri PP, Sinha R, Sikka S, Meur S. Acute carbolic acid poisoning: a report of four cases. Indian J Crit Care Med. 2016;20:668–70.
83. Cohen N, Modai D, Khahil A, Golik A. Acute resin phenol-formaldehyde intoxication. A life threatening occupational hazard. Hum Toxicol. 1989;8:247–50.
84. Hassan AB, Seligmann H, Bassan HM. Intravascular hemolysis induced by pentachlorophenol. Br Med J (Clin Res Ed). 1985;291:21–2.
85. Todorović V [Acute phenol poisoning]. Med Pregl. 2003;56:37–41. Serbian.
86. Lewin JF, Cleary WT. An accidental death caused by the absorption of phenol through skin. A case report. Forensic Sci Int. 1982;19:177–9.
87. Griffiths GJ. Fatal acute poisoning by intradermal absorption of phenol. Med Sci Law. 1973;13:46–8.
88. Abrahams R. A fatal case of carbolic acid poisoning in an infant, due to absorption by the skin. Pediatrics. 1900;9:241–2.
89. Litton C. Observations after chemosurgery of the face. Plast Reconstr Surg. 1963;32:554–6.
90. Stagnone GJ, Orgel MG, Stagnone JJ. Cardiovascular effects of topical 50% trichloroacetic acid and Baker's phenol solution. J Dermatol Surg Oncol. 1987;13:999–1002.
91. Truppman ES, Ellenby JD. Major electrocardiographic changes during chemical face peeling. Plast Reconstr Surg. 1979;63:44–8.

92. Gross BG. Cardiac arrhythmias during phenol face peeling. Plast Reconstr Surg. 1984;73:590–4.
93. Matarasso SL. Phenol chemical peels. In: Wheeland RG, editor. Cutaneous surgery. 1st ed. Philadelphia: Saunders; 1994. p. 491–508.
94. Wexler MR, Halon DA, Teitelbaum A, Tadjer G, Peled IJ. Prevention of cardiac arrhythmias induced in an animal model by the topical application of a commonly used phenol preparation for facial peeling. Plast Reconstr Surg. 1984;73:595–8.
95. Beeson WH. The importance of cardiac monitoring in superficial and deep chemical peels. J Dermatol Surg Oncol. 1987;13:949–50.
96. Li Z, Zhang H, Li SH, Byard RW. Fatal phenol toxicity following attempted tattoo removal. J Forensic Sci. 2016;61:1143–5.
97. Seak CK, Lin CC, Seak CJ, Hsu TY, Chang CC. A case of black urine and dark skin - cresol poisoning. Clin Toxicol (Phila). 2010;48:959–60.
98. Foxall PJ, Bending MR, Gartland KP, Nicholson JK. Acute renal failure following accidental cutaneous absorption of phenol: application of NMR urinalysis to monitor the disease process. Hum Toxicol. 1989;8:491–6.
99. Rodgers GC. Ellenhorn's medical toxicology: diagnosis and treatment of human poisoning. JAMA. 1997;278:1201.
100. Soares ER, Tift JP. Phenol poisoning: three fatal cases. J Forensic Sci. 1982;27:729–31.
101. Fu HS, Chu YK, Liao SQ, Liu RS. Scintigraphic appearance in Lysol-induced pulmonary toxicity. Clin Nucl Med. 2001;26:655–6.
102. Gupta S, Ashrith G, Chandra D, Gupta AK, Finkel KW, Guntupalli JS. Acute phenol poisoning: a life-threatening hazard of chronic pain management. Clin Toxicol (Phila). 2008;46:250–3.
103. Ghosh S. Self-injection of intravenous carbolic acid and multiorgan failure. Indian J Crit Care Med. 2014;18:43–5.
104. Rendon MI, Berson DS, Cohen JL, Roberts WE, Starker I, Wang B. Evidence and considerations in the use of chemical peels for skin disorders and aesthetic resurfacing. J Clin Aesthet Dermatol. 2010;3:32–43.
105. Wambier C. Brown Dermatology Phenol-croton oil peeling: standard operating procedure v1.1 [Internet]. 2023 [cited 2024 Oct 15].Available from: https://www.peelingsociety.com/fileadmin/user_upload/pdf/press/2024/Brown_SOP_Phenol-croton_oil_2023.pdf
106. Bruce RM, Santodonato J, Neal MW. Summary review of the health effects associated with phenol. Toxicol Ind Health. 1987;3:535–68.
107. Botta SA, Straith RE, Goodwin HH. Cardiac arrhythmias in phenol facial peeling: a suggested protocol for prevention. Aesthetic Plast Surg. 1988;12(2):115–7.
108. Kadunc BV, Vanti AA. Evaluation of the systemic toxicity of phenol in facial peels. Surg Cosmet Dermatol. 2009;1:10–4.
109. Agency for Toxic Substances and Disease Registry (US). Relevance to public health. In: Toxicological profile for phenol [Internet]. Atlanta, GA: ATSDR; 2008. [cited data]. Available from: https://www.ncbi.nlm.nih.gov/books/NBK599443/.
110. Piotrowski JK. Evaluation of exposure to phenol: absorption of phenol vapour in the lungs and through the skin and excretion of phenol in urine. Br J Ind Med. 1971;28(2):172–8.
111. Landau M. Cardiac complications in deep chemical peels. Dermatol Surg. 2007;33:190–3.
112. Yun JW, Kwon E, Kim YS, Kim SH, You JR, Kim HC, Park JS, Che JH, Lee SK, Jang JJ, Kim HH, Kang BC. Assessment of acute, 14-day, and 13-week repeated oral dose toxicity of Tiglium seed extract in rats. BMC Complement Altern Med. 2018;18(1):251.
113. Zhang XL, Wang L, Li F, Yu K, Wang MK. Cytotoxic phorbol esters from *Croton tiglium*. J Nat Prod. 2013;76(5):858–64.
114. Saputera MD, Raharja S, Kardono LB, Iswantini D. Characteristics, efficacy and safety assessment of standardized extract of *Croton tiglium* seed from Indonesia as a laxative agent. Pak J Biol Sci. 2008;11(4):618–22.

115. Shahid M, Tayyab M, Naz F, Jamil A, Ashraf M, Gilani AH. Activity-guided isolation of a novel protein from *Croton tiglium* with antifungal and antibacterial properties. Phytother Res. 2008;22(12):1646–9.
116. Pal PK, Nandi MK, Singh NK. Detoxification of *Croton tiglium* L. seeds by the Ayurvedic Śodhana process. Anc Sci. Life. 2014;33(3):157–61.
117. Klein DR, Little JH. Laryngeal edema as a complication of chemical peel. Plast Reconstr Surg. 1983;71(3):419–20.
118. Marçon CR, Coppinger AJ, Salomão C, Alves Dos Reis V, Alves Dos Reis VN, de Menezes Gomes JL, Gianvecchio VAP, Medeiros de Aquino E, de Seixas Alves MT, Canzian M, Coelho Frenkelis Brandão SA, Fusel de Ue RR, Ribeiro F, Bageorgou F, Wambier CG. International Peeling Society (IPS) and São Paulo's Legal Medical Institute (IML-SP). Fatal phenol peel by an unlicensed social media practitioner: a forensic medical analysis. J Am Acad Dermatol. 2025;93(6):e211–3.
119. American Heart Association. ACLS Algorithms. [Internet]. Dallas, TX: American Heart Association; 2020. [cited 25 Aug 2025]. Available from: https://cpr.heart.org/en/resuscitation-science/cpr-and-ecc-guidelines/algorithms
120. Fulton MR 2nd, Nordquist E. Advanced Cardiac Life Support (ACLS). In: StatPearls [Internet]. Treasure Island, FL: StatPearls Publishing; 2025. [updated 2025 Feb 11; cited data]. Available from: https://www.ncbi.nlm.nih.gov/books/NBK613285/.
121. Panchal AR, Bartos JA, Cabañas JG, Donnino MW, Drennan IR, Hirsch KG, et al. 2020 American Heart Association guidelines for cardiopulmonary resuscitation and emergency cardiovascular care. Circulation. 2020;142(16 Suppl 2):S366–468.
122. Fan E, Del Sorbo L, Goligher EC, Hodgson CL, Munshi L, Walkey AJ, et al. An Official American Thoracic Society/European Society of Intensive Care Medicine/Society of Critical Care Medicine Clinical Practice Guideline: mechanical ventilation in adult patients with acute respiratory distress syndrome. Am J Respir Crit Care Med. 2017;195(9):1253–63.
123. Menzikov SA, Morozov SG. Involvement of brain GABAAR-coupled Cl-/HCO3--ATPase in phenol-induced head-twitching and tremor responses in rats. Neurotoxicology. 2019; 71: 122-131.
124. Kowalewski R, Schurch B, Hodler J, Borgeat A. Persistent paraplegia after an aqueous 7.5% phenol solution to the anterior motor root for intercostal neurolysis: a case report. Arch Phys Med Rehabil. 2002;83(2):283–5.
125. Kissoon NR, Graff-Radford J, Watson JC, Laughin RS. Spinal cord injury from fluoroscopically guided intercostal blocks with phenol. Pain Physician. 2014;17(2):E219–24.
126. Cerda J. Oliguria: an earlier and accurate biomarker of acute kidney injury? Kidney Int. 2011;80(7):699–701.
127. Parikh TJ. Acute concentrated phenol dermal burns: complications and management. Indian J Crit Care Med. 2015;19(5):280–2.
128. Unlü RE, Alagöz MS, Uysal AC, Orbay H, Kilinç H, Tekin F, Sensöz O, Erk G. Phenol intoxication in a child. J Craniofac Surg. 2004;15(6):1010–3.
129. Liu L, Yu H, Wu H, Yang X, Pan Y, Chen Y, Wang K, Wang W, Zhang W, Jin Y, Zhang C, Jiang A, Xia C. Toxic proteins from *Croton tiglium* L. exert a proinflammatory effect by inducing the release of proinflammatory cytokines and activating the p38-MAPK signaling pathway. Mol Med Rep. 2017;16(1):631–8.
130. Matsuura NC, Toledo C, Santana VLM, Steiner D, Pessotti NS. Intense pulsed light therapy for treatment of facial erythema and hypertrophic scar after phenol peeling. Surg Cosmet Dermatol. 2024;16:e20240292.
131. Cruz R, Quintana-Hau JD, González JR, Tornero-Montaño R, Baiza-Durán LM, Vega L. Effects of an ophthalmic formulation of meloxicam on COX-2 expression, PGE2 release, and cytokine expression in a model of acute ocular inflammation. Br J Ophthalmol. 2008;92(1):120–5.

Index

C. Marçon, C. Wambier, *Phenol-Croton Oil Peel*,
https://doi.org/10.1007/978-3-032-25993-6

Q

R

S

T

MIX
Papier aus verantwortungsvollen Quellen
Paper from responsible sources
FSC® C105338

If you have any concerns about our products,
you can contact us on
ProductSafety@springernature.com

In case Publisher is established outside the EU,
the EU authorized representative is:
Springer Nature Customer Service Center GmbH
Europaplatz 3, 69115 Heidelberg, Germany

Printed by Libri Plureos GmbH
in Hamburg, Germany